T0401252

NEW DEVELOPMENTS IN MEDICAL RESEARCH

RECENT DEVELOPMENTS IN PHYTOMEDICINE TECHNOLOGY

NEW DEVELOPMENTS IN MEDICAL RESEARCH

Additional books in this series can be found on Nova's website under the Series tab.

Additional e-books in this series can be found on Nova's website under the eBooks tab.

NEW DEVELOPMENTS IN MEDICAL RESEARCH

RECENT DEVELOPMENTS IN PHYTOMEDICINE TECHNOLOGY

LUIS ALEXANDRE PEDRO DE FREITAS,
CRISTIANE CARDOSO CORREIA TEIXEIRA
AND
CRISTINA MARA ZAMARIOLI
EDITORS

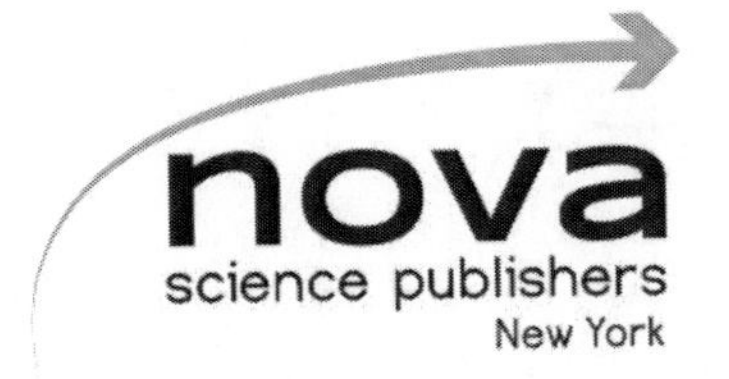

NOTICE TO THE READER

Additional color graphics may be available in the e-book version of this book.

Library of Congress Cataloging-in-Publication Data

ISBN: 978-1-53611-977-0
Library of Congress Control Number: 2017941341

Published by Nova Science Publishers, Inc. † New York

CONTENTS

PREFACE

Phytomedicines have been playing an important role since the beginning of civilization, curing many diseases and alleviating different symptoms for the wellbeing of humans and animals. The millenary history of medicinal plant use and its derivatives give credibility to the development of new and advanced pharmaceutical forms of phytomedicines, which may play an important role in social medicine for developing countries. A renewed interest for herbal medicines and phytomedicine has been observed in recent years. However, adulteration and misidentification of crude drugs still exist. Thus, the development of standardization and quality control of herbal medicines needs to be prioritized at the earliest stage.

Furthermore, the increasing demand for natural food antioxidants has fostered worldwide research for extracting biologically active substances from a variety of raw vegetal materials. However, the modern use of plant-derived medicines must be based on reliable and reproductive processes as well as manufacturing techniques to preserve chemical composition and therapeutic effectiveness of the plant extract.

This can be achieved only through the knowledge and scientific approach to all steps involved in phytomedicine production, such as the pharmacognostic evaluation, extraction process, drying of the extracts and pharmacotechnical preparation of the final pharmaceutical form.

This book will compile the recent advances in the pharmaceutical industrial process and phytomedicine carries development. It is suitable for different levels of undergraduate study and/or the facilitation of pharmaceutical industrial processes.

Luis Alexandre Pedro de Freitas
Cristiane Cardoso Correia Teixeira
Cristina Mara Zamarioli

INTRODUCTION

In this book the recent advances in the phytopharmaceutical process and in the field of new carriers for phytomedicines will be presented. It is recommended in different levels of undergraduate and/or pharmaceutical industrial processes.

Figure 1 shows the themes discussed in each chapter.

The first chapter showed the main variations found among the plant organs most commonly used as drugs and the use of the variation of plant morphological attributes in order to detect adulteration and misindentification of crude drugs. The second included the recent development in pharmacognostic evaluation to assure the quality regarding the chemical composition and concentrations of active compounds in plant products, in all phases of its production chain. The chapter three gives a overall view of the Quality by Design, QbD, approach in the development of industrial operations in the manufacture of phytomedicines, based on optimization in all phases of its production chain. Chapter four aims to show the importance of experimental design in standardization of development of analytical methodologies. In the fifth chapter the recent developments in extraction process were discussed. In the sixth chapter, the recent developments in drying of the extracts were described. In chapters seven and eight the recent development in preparation methods of polymeric micro/ nanoparticle and solid lipid carries to phytomedicine and liposomal production were presented. And finally in ninth chapter standardization and quality control of herbal medicines were discussed.

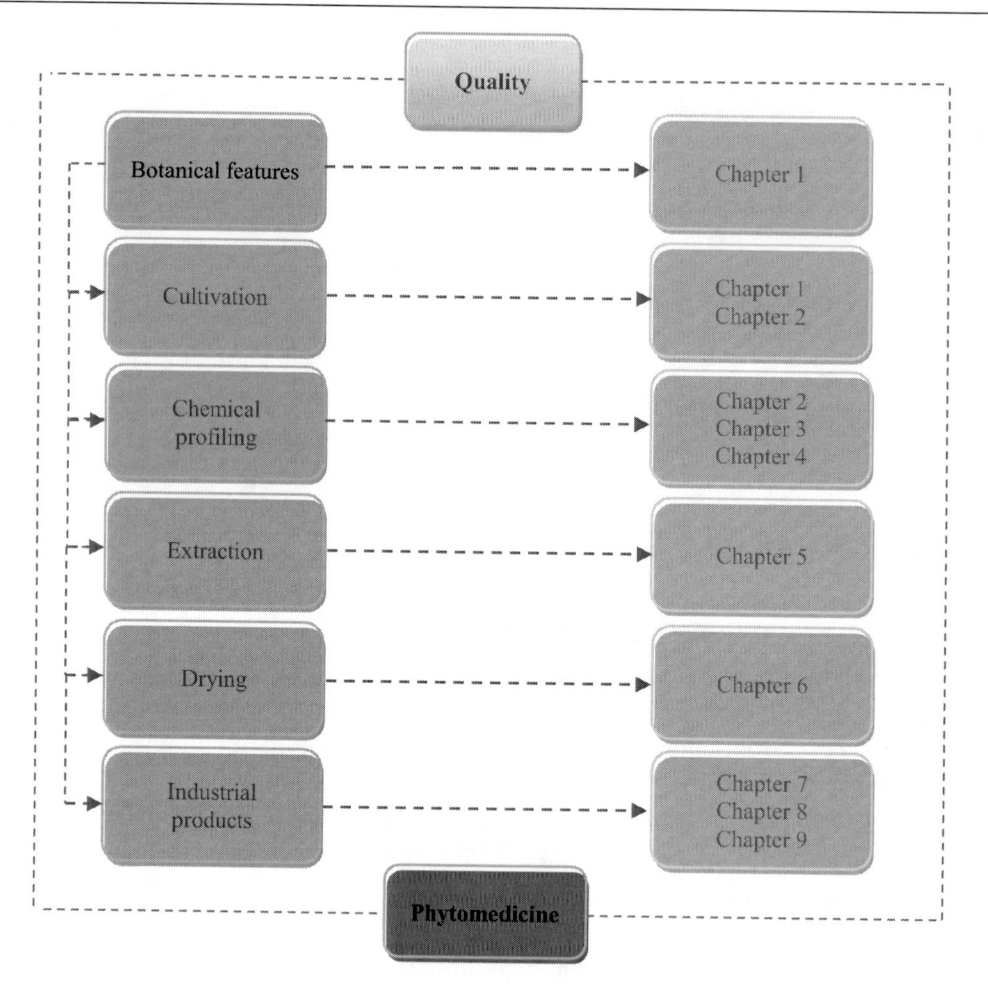

Figure 1. The book organization diagram.

It is noteworthy that this book will show the importance of the process control in all stages of the production in phytomedicine.

Luis Alexandre Pedro de Freitas
Cristiane Cardoso Correa Teixeira
Cristina Mara Zamarioli

In: Recent Developments in Phytomedicine Technology ISBN: 978-1-53611-977-0
Editors: L. A. Pedro de Freitas et al.

Chapter 1

ADULTERATION AND MISIDENTIFICATION OF CRUDE DRUGS

***Simone P. Teixeira*[1,*] *and Juliana V. Paulino*[2]**

[1]Universidade de São Paulo (USP), Faculdade de Ciências Farmacêuticas de Ribeirão Preto, Departamento de Ciências Farmacêuticas, Ribeirão Preto, SP, Brasil

[2]Universidade Federal do Rio de Janeiro, Faculdade de Farmácia, Centro de Ciências da Saúde, Departamento de Produtos Naturais e Alimentos, Ilha do Fundão, Rio de Janeiro, RJ, Brasil

ABSTRACT

All parts of the plant body can be used as drugs: root, stem (rhizome, bark, wood), leaf, flower, fruit, seed. The chemical class and amount of the bioactive compounds present in these plant parts depend on the family, genus or even species to which the plant belongs. If the material is not fragmented, each plant part used as a drug can be easily recognized by gross morphology. However, the plant drug is generally marketed in fragments, splinters or even powdered. In such cases, there must be an additional anatomical study based on cyto-histological techniques, i.e., considering the distribution and types of cells and tissues that compose the organ under examination. This is because the plant species, despite having a general organization of tissues along the body, can exhibit histological variations that permit a safe identification of plant drugs from certain species, thus preventing adulteration and misidentification. These variations involve the presence, size, number of layers and types of cells that form the tissues, as well as the tissue location and distribution in the different plant organs. Indeed, organs of closely related plant species, but with different bioactive compounds, used as adulterants, can be recognized by such an analysis. Quantitative traits must be carefully evaluated because

* Corresponding Author Email: spadua@fcfrp.usp.br.

plants of the same species exposed to different environmental conditions can vary, for example, in number and thickness of cells and tissues. Thus, this chapter aims (1) to show the main variations found among the plant organs most commonly used as drugs, adopting as examples tropical plant species, well known for their biological activities and their main adulterants, and (2) to use the variation of plant morphological attributes in order to detect adulteration and misidentification of crude drugs. Conventional and advanced light and electron microscopy techniques and their applications to drug identification studies based on gross morphology and anatomy will be discussed. We will highlight that the recognition of the part of the plant used as a drug and its taxonomic identity depend on the comparison of the sampled data to those of the literature such as pharmacopoeia monographs, dissertations and scientific articles or reference materials properly identified by a specialist.

Keywords: anatomy, bioactive substance, diagnostic character, microscopy, plant drug, plant structure

INTRODUCTION

All parts of the plant body may be used as crude drugs for the pharmaceutical industry: root, stem (rhizome, bark, wood) and leaf are vegetative organs; flower, fruit and seed are involved in plant reproduction. Among the most used parts, stems (aerial and underground, bark), leaves and flowers are among the most cited in pharmacopoeia compendia since roots and seeds are less used. The type and amount of bioactive substances present in these organs depend on the species and the family to which the plant belongs.

The identification and correct name of the plant part used and the plant species are essential steps of quality control recommended by the World Health Organization (WHO). These steps, when properly taken, including the use of the scientific names according to the International Code of Botanical Nomenclature [1], give credibility to the pharmaceutical product, ensure the reproducibility of phytomedicines and avoid adulterations that are the result of confusion and misidentification, particularly by the attribution of several regionally defined popular names to the plant species.

To avoid misidentification of plant drugs, three types of analyses are important: organoleptic, macroscopic and microscopic. Organoleptic analysis involves features that impress the senses, such as color, odor, flavor and texture. Macroscopic analysis refers to the external appearance such as shape and size and is usually performed with the naked eye or with a magnifying aid (stereomicroscopy). Macroscopic analysis by scanning electron microscopy (SEM) has permitted the detection of a wider range of detailed external features, e.g., surface ornamentation of epidermal cells, detailed information about seed coat and trichome morphology [2]. Although this technique has a higher cost, it permits a very rapid analysis.

If the drug is whole, i.e., not fragmented, its identity (organ, species) can be determined by using simple macroscopic analysis. Some features are important in this recognition, such as the presence of buds on stems and their general absence in roots, for example.

However, the plant drug is generally marketed in fragments, splinters and even powdered. In these cases it is difficult to check whether the drug is a root, stem, leaf, flower, fruit or seed by only characterizing its external morphology. This characterization should be also based on internal morphology (= anatomy), studied by histology, i.e., considering the distribution and types of tissues that compose the sampled organ. Although the tissues are continuously distributed in the plant body, histological variations always occur, permitting the identification of organ type and the taxon from which the drug originates. Variations in the composition of plant organs occur regarding the presence, size, number of layers and types of cells that make up the tissues, as well as the location and distribution of different tissues in a certain organ. Quantitative traits must be carefully evaluated because plants of the same species, for example, may differ in the number and thickness of cells and tissues under different environmental conditions. Anyway, to assess quantitative and qualitative characteristics it is essential to analyze a large number of samples, ensuring the credibility of the results. Such macroscopic and microscopic analyses have been recommended by the WHO since 1998.

The data obtained for the sample to be identified should be compared to those already published in pharmacopoeia monographs, dissertations, scientific papers and herbarium specimens, a procedure that we believe is the basis for success in the aforementioned steps. Pharmacopoeias regulate the quality specifications of pharmaceutical products from raw materials to packaging, as well as relations with foreign trade, besides providing parameters for the actions of the local Health Surveillance. Scientific papers should be selected among those published in periodicals with international circulation and with a reliable editorial board. Herbarium specimens (= exsiccates) should be consulted in renowned herbaria included in the Index Herbariorum and identified by expert taxonomists. With due acquiescence of the curators, it is possible to extract morphological, chemical, geographical, and phenological information from herbarium specimens. It is noteworthy that similar organs of closely related species may contain different bioactive substances, and can be employed as adulterants.

Thus, this chapter aims (1) to show the main variations found among the plant organs most commonly used as drugs, adopting as examples tropical plant species, well known for their biological activities and their main adulterants; (2) to use the variation of plant morphological attributes to avoid and detect adulteration and misidentification of crude drugs.

AVOIDING MISIDENTIFICATION AND ADULTERATION OF CRUDE DRUGS CONSISTING OF RHIZOME AND ROOT

Species for which the rhizome is the raw material for the pharmaceutical industry are highly represented among Zingiberaceae (turmeric, galangal, ginger, and zedoary). Species whose roots are raw materials for the pharmaceutical industry are spread among eudicotyledons, and the most representative families are Convolvulaceae (jalapa), Menispermaceae (abutua and calumba), Polygalaceae (poligala and rhubarb) and Ranunculaceae (aconite and goldenseal) [3-4]. Families with species well known for the use of root and rhizome are Valerianaceae (valerian), Fabaceae (licorice), Apocynaceae (rauvolfia), and Solanaceae ("jurubeba"). Among the monocotyledons, the best known are Smilacaceae (sarsaparilla) and Araceae (aromatic calamus) [3-4].

Many ethnopharmacological articles and even books and some pharmacopoeia monographs mention incorrectly drugs obtained from rhizomes (= underground stems) as roots, such as ginger, turmeric, and burdock. This probably occurs because stem and root are generally cylindrical organs, and also because there are aerial roots and underground stems. Thus, the combination of macroscopic and microscopic analyses becomes essential to the search for diagnostic features that allow the correct identification of these plant crude drugs.

Rapid observations can be performed with the naked eye at low cost by distinguishing the rhizome from the root. The rhizome is an underground stem and hence is characterized by the presence of nodes and internodes. The nodes are the regions from where the lateral buds emerge. The root is in general a cylindrical underground organ, devoid of chlorophyll, nodes or buds, generally with positive geotropism combined with negative phototropism. When a root has buds, such as shoot bud-forming roots found in some tropical species ("quebra-mironga"), the buds are endogenous. Exceptions are the reparative buds of exogenous origin [5-6]. The roots usually exhibit longitudinal grooves and striations, as well as lateral roots with scars. The stems can have spines, thorns, trichomes, scars, exudate, and variable texture (smooth, lacy, flaky, grooved, striate, fissured, and corky) [7].

In eudicotyledons, magnoliids and gymnosperms the root emerges during the embryonic stage of the plant, develops and becomes the principal (= axial) root, penetrates the soil and emits branches that will form lateral roots. In contrast, in monocotyledons and a few eudicotyledons such as fig trees, clusias and red mangrove, the embryonic root degenerates, and all the roots emerge from the stem base. In this case, roots are termed adventitious. The adventitious roots are radially positioned on the stem, and one is not considerably larger than the other, forming the fascicular root system that has lower penetration into the soil than the axial roots of eudicotyledons [7].

Anatomically, stem and root in primary structure such as that of herbs, vines and small shrubs can be recognized by the position of the xylem cells. In the root, the protoxylem (the first xylem cells to differentiate) is external to the metaxylem (xylem cells that differentiate after protoxylem cells) and phloem cells occur intercalated with those of the xylem (Figure 1A). In the stem, the protoxylem is internal to the metaxylem and phloem cells are grouped to the xylem cells in individual vascular bundles (Figure 1B) or in a continuous vascular cylinder [6, 8].

In some species, the distinction between root and stem is not an easy task, especially if the ontogenetic stages of the organ are not analyzed. For example, carrot and radish are considered to be tuberous roots in the literature; however, the ontogeny shows that the stem and the transition region (between root and stem) also participate in the tuberization process. Thus, they are considered mixed structures [6].

After verifying that the drug consists of root or stem, it is necessary to identify which taxonomic group it belongs to, if possible up to the species level. The identification can be initiated by the distinction into two major taxonomic groups of angiosperms: monocotyledons and eudicotyledons. The root of eudicotyledons is a protostele (= central region occupied by primary xylem) forming arcs with up to five xylematic poles (Figure 1A), and the root of monocotyledons is a siphonostele (= central region occupied by pith – Figure 1C) [8]. In addition, in eudicotyledons the stem is usually a eustele (= vascular bundles delimiting cortex and pith - Figure 1B) and in monocotyledons it is usually an atactostele (= vascular bundles distributed throughout the organ, without the delimitation of cortex and pith - Figure 1D).

Drugs consisting of root and stem, in general, are in an early secondary structure (= thickness growth). Roots and stems in secondary structure are less easily distinguished because the thickness growth promotes a radiate appearance in both types of organs and the remnants of the primary structure can be ephemeral or imperceptible.

For the identification of drugs at the familial, generic and specific levels, it is necessary to consider a combination of characters in order to obtain a good diagnosis: (a) number of epidermal layers; (b) the presence and type of crystal idioblasts; (c) cellular composition of the cortex and medulla; (d) collenchyma arrangement (whether continuous as in medicinal lavender - Figure 2A, or discontinuous forming strands as in ornamental lavender - Figure 2B); (e) type (e.g., bicollateral in Cucurbitaceae, Solanaceae) and distribution of vascular bundles (cortical and medullary in Cactaceae and Rutaceae vs. only medullary in Apocynaceae, Asteraceae, Crassulaceae, Didieriaceae, Euphorbiaceae, Geraniaceae, and Vitaceae); (f) type of reserve substance present in the parenchyma of cortex and medulla.

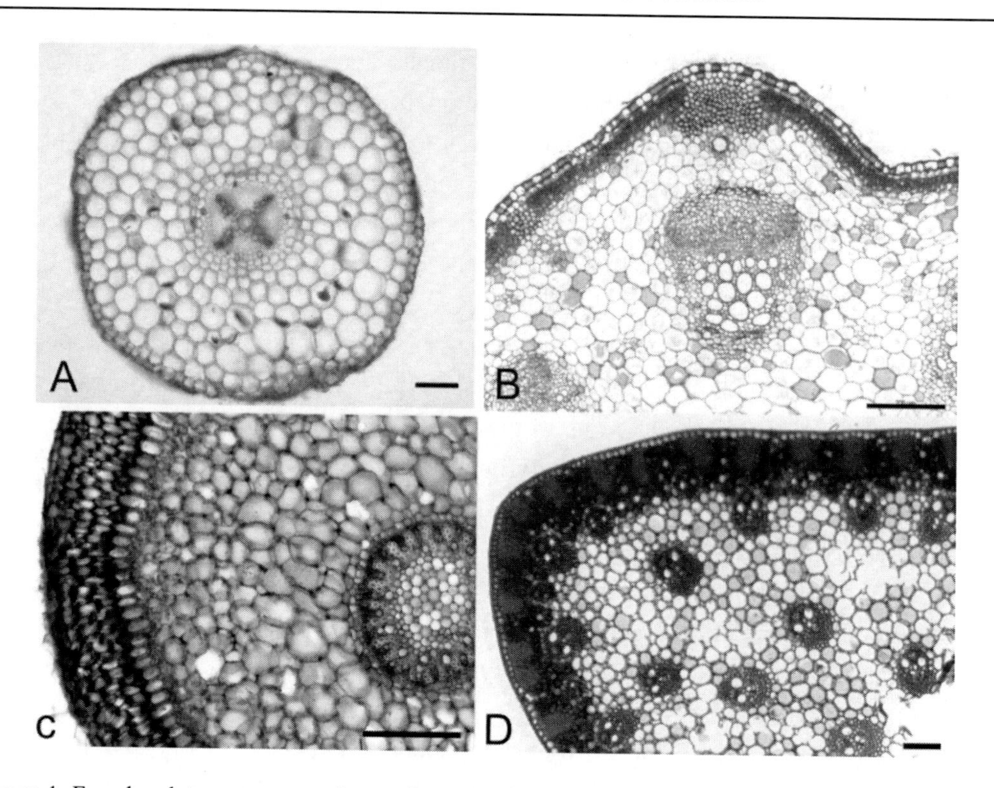

Figure 1. Free hand transverse sections of root and stem (fresh material - light microscopy). A. Barbatimao (*Stryphnodendron adstringens* (Mart.) Coville, eudicot) root stained with ferric chloride. B. Fennel (*Foeniculum vulgare* Mill., eudicot) stem stained with safranin and astra blue. C. Orchid (*Cattleya* sp., monocot) adventitious root stained with toluidine blue. D. Nutsedge (*Cyperus rotundus* L., monocot) stem stained with toluidine blue. Compare the root and stem structure in A and B. Compare the root of eudicots and monocots in A and C. Compare the stem of eudicots and monocots in B and D. Scale bars: A, C, D = 100 μm; B = 200 μm.

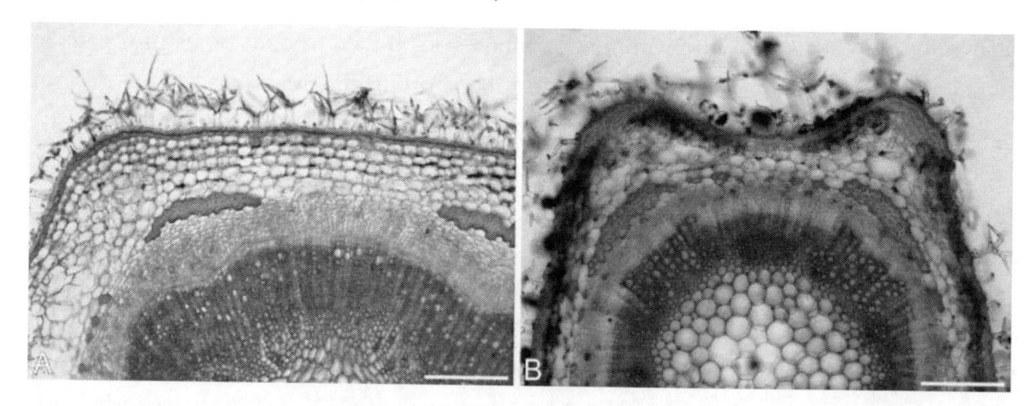

Figure 2. Free hand transverse sections of lavender stems (fresh material) stained with toluidine blue (light microscopy). A. Medicinal lavender (*Lavandula officinalis* Chaix). B. Ornamental lavender (*Lavandula angustifolia* Mill.). Observe a continuous arrangement of subepidermal collenchyma in A (medicinal lavender) and a discontinuous arrangement, forming strands, in B (ornamental lavender). Scale bars: 200 μm.

How to Identify Bark and Wood Drugs of Renowned Value

Bark and wood are defined regions of the stem and root and are the result of secondary growth that promotes thickening of the plant body. Secondary growth is common in gymnosperms, eudicotyledons and woody magnoliids, and rare in monocotyledons. It also occurs in some herbs that are not woody (e.g., tomato, potato, carrot, sweet potato) [8]. Some species also exhibit secondary growth in the leaf, but have been seldom reported in the literature [9].

Bark is a term defining the set of periderm tissues (suber, phellogen and phelloderm) and secondary phloem in stems and roots. It also includes remnants of primary tissues such as cortical parenchyma and primary phloem. Wood is a term attributed exclusively to the secondary xylem. The wood is internal to the bark [7-8].

Barks formed on the stems of plant species of pharmaceutical interest are found among Anacardiaceae (cashew, marula and mastic), Fabaceae (true barbatimao, coral tree, purple-sandalwood, balsam of Peru, “mulungu”), Lauraceae (sassafras and cinnamon). Examples of well known species from whose bark economically important substances are extracted are the rubber tree (rubber), the yew (taxol) and the weeping willow (salicylic acid) [3-4].

Drugs made from wood are not mentioned in the pharmacopoeias, but the guaico, quassia, citrin sandalwood, cassau, clove vine, bittersweet, “jurubeba”, and pine are used in folk medicine. The most representative family is Simarubaceae (quassia) [3-4].

The anatomy of the bark and wood provides secure identification of the sample in question since their characteristics are surveyed in close taxonomic groups for comparative purposes without simply taking into account the adulterants. Anyway, it is difficult to check whether the bark/wood is from the stem or the root, because remnants of the primary structure, that provide diagnostics traits for stem and root, are temporary or imperceptible in the secondary structure.

The plants subjected to secondary growth have a cambium, i.e., an annular band of meristematic cells that produce xylem inside and phloem outside in the plant body. Since xylem tissues are mainly formed by lignified dead cells, subsequent xylematic rings can be added to those previously formed, forming a rigid and resistant structure that provides support for the plants while at the same time improving the transport of water and assimilates. With the increment of the conduction system, the epidermis ruptures and a periderm emerges, performing the same functions (protection, reduction of water loss). The periderm consists of tissues produced by another lateral meristem called phellogen. The cambium and phellogen are established after the primary structure of the plant body is finalized [7-8].

The cambium is the first lateral meristem to be installed and become active. In the stem, it results from the resumption of activity of procambium remnants found between the xylem and phloem in the vascular bundles (fascicular cambium) and of pericycle cells located between the vascular bundles (interfascicular cambium). In the root, it results from the resumption of activity of procambium remnants between the xylem and phloem and of pericycle divisions located in front of the protoxylem poles. This difference between root and stem is no longer observed in the drugs (bark and wood), and therefore cannot be used as a diagnostic character. The cambium formed from the procambium produces all conductive elements of the axial and radial systems and the cambium formed from pericycle cells only produces radial parenchyma. Thus, secondary xylem and phloem exhibit axial and radial systems [7-8].

The frontal anatomical analysis of the organ permits to observe a radiated structure, an important characteristic of organs in the secondary structure. Some sets of traits can be used to diagnose drugs made from the bark such as: (a) presence of crystal cells forming a sheath in the secondary phloem (cascara, ipe-purple, buckthorn, true barbatimao), or sparse in the phelloderm (condurango); (b) cork arranged in layers containing thin-walled cells alternating with layers of thick-walled cells (mastic); (c) presence of stone cells in the cortex and libriform fibers in the secondary phloem (cinnamon-of-China) and idioblasts with prismatic crystals and raphids (cinnamon-of-India); (d) phenolic cells spread throughout all tissues of periderm and phloem (true barbatimao – Figure 3A) and phenolic cells only in the phelloderm and cortical cells (false barbatimao – Figure 3B).

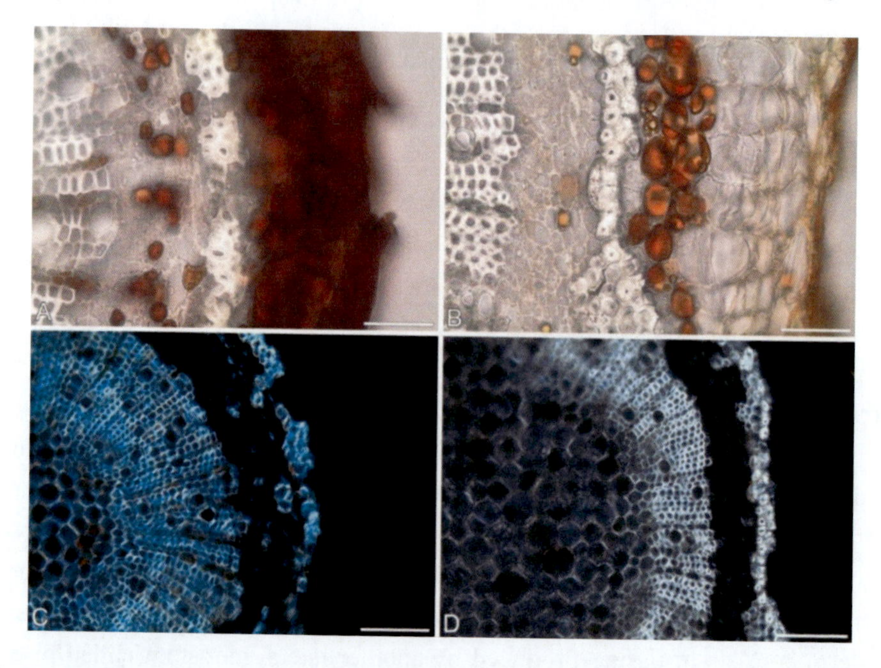

Figure 3. Free hand transverse sections of barbatimao bark (fresh material). Compare the sections stained with ferric chloride to detect phenolic cells (in brown) (light microscopy) and observe the presence of phenolics in the periderm and phloem cells in true barbatimao (*Stryphnodendron adstringens* (Mart.) Coville) (A) and in the phelloderm and cortical cells in false barbatimao (*Dimorphandra mollis* Benth.) (B). Observe that the barks of true barbatimao (C) and false barbatimao (D) are very similar under polarized light. Scale bars: A, B = 50 μm; C, D = 100 μm.

To diagnose drugs made from wood, the same characters used in wood anatomy may be useful (see [10-12]): type of radial parenchyma, ray homogeneity, presence and type of fiber, presence of internal secretory structures (e.g., secretory ducts and cavities in pine, araucaria, guaco, copaiba).

Crude Drugs Made From Leaves and Flowers

Many drugs are made from leaves (guaco, mint, eucalyptus, tea tree, digitalis, belladonna, datura), flowers (dianthus, macela, papaya, kapok) or part of a flower (stigma of saffron and corn, petals of poppy and rose) or inflorescences (arnica, chamomile, lavender, and linden) [3-4].

The most representative families in pharmacopoeia monographs are Asteraceae and Lamiaceae, whose species are also well known by the population, e.g., chamomile, arnica, lavender, rosemary. Among the monocotyledons the best known are Iridaceae and Poaceae. Species whose leaves are the raw material for pharmaceutical purposes occur throughout eudicotyledons, and the most representative families are also Asteraceae, Lamiaceae in addition to Myrtaceae, Scrophulariaceae, Solanaceae and Verbenaceae [3-4].

The recognition of drugs made from leaves and floral organs is easy and safe, both by using macroscopic and microscopic analyses. The flower is a specialized stem branch containing shortened internodes and leaf appendages, modified to perform functions in angiosperm reproduction. Appendices are sepals, petals, stamens and carpels [13-14]. The flower is part of the asexual generation in the angiosperm cycle while the male gametophyte (pollen grain or pollen tube) and female gametophyte (embryo sac) are parts of the sexual generation and develop within the floral organs considered reproductive [15].

The leaf is a laminar stem appendix of limited growth, which contains chlorophyll. Unlike the flower, it widely occurs among the various groups of plants such as ferns and mosses. It is formed by a blade, a petiole and a sheath. The blade is generally greenish, thin and laminar; the petiole joins the blade to the stem and can exhibit various shapes (rounded, quadrangular, triangular, and winged). The sheath is the enlargement of the basal region of the blade [7].

The leaf and floral appendices, especially when fresh, can be recognized by external and internal morphology, which can help a lot for crude drug identification. The leaf is formed of typical tissues such as the palisade and spongy parenchyma (Figure 4A). The laminar floral appendices like sepals and petals also have a parenchyma protected by an epidermis which, however, is not differentiated into palisade and spongy types [8].

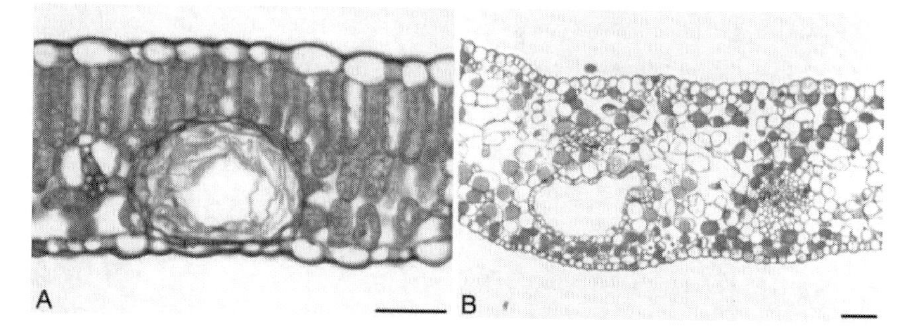

Figure 4. Microtome transverse sections of a leaf blade and a petal of two medicinal legume species. A. Rattle rattlesnake (*Poiretia punctata* (Willd.) Desv.). B. "Jatobá" (*Hymenaea courbaril* L.). Note that in A (leaf blade) the mesophyll is divided into palisade and spongy parenchyma, and in B (petal) the parenchyma cells are homogeneous and there are many intercellular spaces filled with air. Interestingly, a secretory cavity is seen in both species, although of different anatomic structure. Scale bars: A = 50 µm; B = 100 µm.

The floral organs exhibit wide variation among major taxonomic groups such as families, while they are less plastic within a particular taxon, such as genera. The Asteraceae family, for example, has an exclusive floral characteristic easily identified by macroscopic analysis that is the presence of a type of inflorescence named head or capitulum (= small sessile flowers arranged into a common discoid axis; the peripheral flowers can be different from those inside the disc; e.g., chamomile), which looks like a single flower to lay people [16]. Members of Apiaceae (e.g., hemlock, parsley and fennel) are characterized by inflorescences in the shape of an umbel (numerous pedicellate flowers arranged in an axis forming an angle of 180°), simple or compound, a feature that gave the name Umbelliferae for the family (currently not accepted, see APG IV [17]). The flowers of most species of Lamiaceae (e.g., lavender, mint, basil) have a corolla formed by five petals united so that the two upper petals form an upper lip opposite to the three lower petals that form the lower lip [18]. The presence of these corolla lips gave the name Labiatae to the family (currently not accepted, see APG IV [17]).

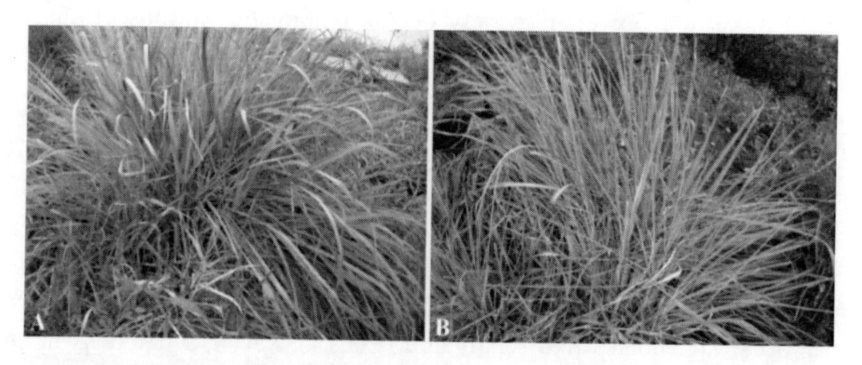

Figure 5. Aspect of the external leaf morphology of lemongrass (A) and citronella (B). Lemongrass (*Cymbopogon citratus* (DC) Stapf.) and citronella (*Cymbopogon winterianus* Jowitt) are both used as medicinal herbs. They belong to the same family (Poaceae) and genus (*Cymbopogon*) and, thus, they are closely similar in appearance and habit.

The leaf morphology is also highly variable, exhibiting features of both taxonomic and ecological interest. The external and internal morphology of the leaf can provide secure identification of the organ and of the species concerned when close taxonomic groups are compared for a diagnosis (see a comparative example of lemongrass and citronella in Figures 5 and 6).

Some sets of traits can be used to diagnose drugs made from the leaf, identifying both major taxonomic groups (monocotyledons versus eudicotyledons) at the familial, generic and specific levels: (a) presence and type of stomata; (b) presence and type of trichomes (e.g., *Malva sylvestris* can be distinguished from *Sida cordifolia* by trichome type and number); (c) presence and type of other specialized epidermal cells (siliceous, suberose, secretory); (d) type of mesophyll (e.g., indigo species can be distinguished by the type of mesophyll); (e) presence of mesophyll specializations (water storage parenchyma, air storage parenchyma); (f) presence and type of crystal cells; (g) distribution and arrangement of collenchyma or sclerenchyma (e.g., lemongrass and citronella - Figure 6); (h) type of vascular bundle; (i) cell type that forms the bundle sheath (endoderm); (j) venation pattern; (k) shape of the vascular system in the midrib and petiole.

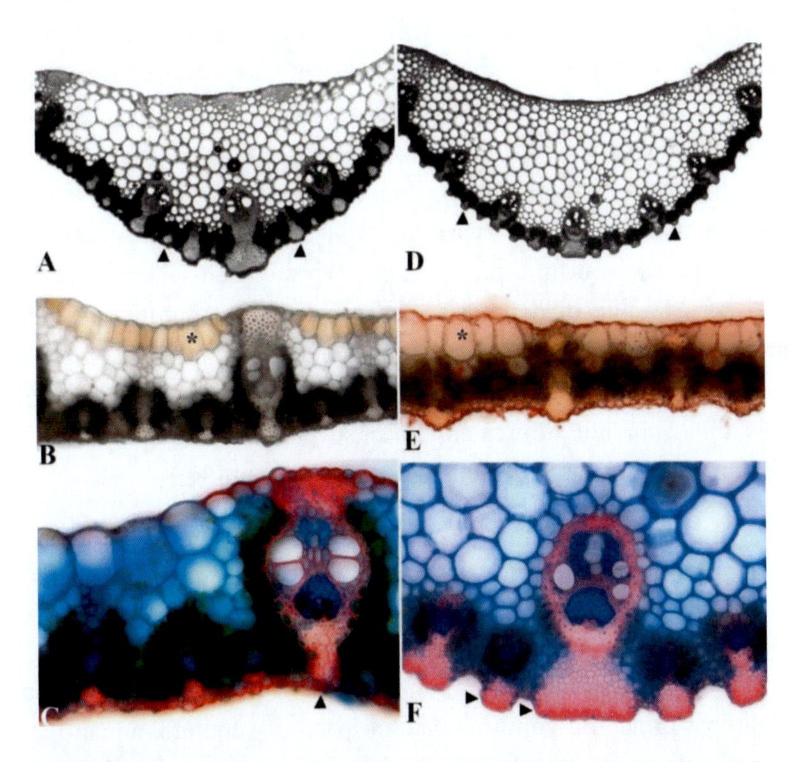

Figure 6. Free hand transverse sections of lemongrass (A-C) and citronella (D-F) fresh leaves (light microscopy). Compare the fiber quantity and arrangement of the two species (arrowheads). The fiber clusters in citronella are prominent in the abaxial leaf surface (D-F). In B and E, the symbol * shows bulliform (= motor) epidermal cells, that produce and store essential oil and likely play a role in the leaf roll. Stains: A, C, D, F – safranin plus astra blau; B, E – sudan III. Scale bars: A = 170 μm; B = 60 μm; C, E = 80 μm; D = 140 μm; F = 70 μm.

Crude Drugs Made from Fruit

Anise, fennel, hemlock, fava, "jatobá", and peppers are examples of drugs made from fruits. The most representative families are Apiaceae, Cucurbitaceae, Fabaceae and Solanaceae. Monocotyledons are poorly represented. Standing out among the basal lineages of angiosperms is star anise, of the Schisandraceae family [3-4].

As well as the flower, the fruit occurs only in angiosperms. It acts on seed protection and often on seed dispersal. It is a food resource for many animal species. The fruit develops in general after double fertilization, which occurs inside the flower and therefore is closely related to it. Exceptions are parthenocarpic species that produce fruit without fertilization. There are several concepts about fruit, most of them considering its origin. The latest concept says that the fruit represents the developed and ripened ovary or ovaries. Other parts of extracarpellar origin (flower or inflorescence) can be joined to the fruit during development when the fruit originates from the inferior ovary. Most authors consider the seed to be part of the fruit [19-20].

The fruit wall (= pericarp), both in fleshy and dry types, shows three distinct regions: exocarp, mesocarp and endocarp. In dried fruits the mesocarp (= median region) and endocarp (= internal) generally consist of sclerified tissues formed of fibers and/or sclereids. Some drugs can be made from the entire pericarp (vanilla, fennel), others from the exocarp plus mesocarp (e.g., bitter orange), or from the endocarp (e.g., tamarind) [19-20].

A range of diagnostic features can be found for drugs made from fruits, especially because there are many different types of fruits. These features are color, shape, consistency of the pericarp, origin, presence and types of dehiscence, presence and type of appendages. An example of diagnosis of drugs made from fruits is the distinction between fennel (*Foeniculum vulgare* Mill.) and anise (*Pimpinella anisum* L.), Apiaceae. The fennel fruit has a bifurcated stylopodium, whereas in anise the stylopodium is thick but not bifurcated; in anise the fruit shows several short tector trichomes, while in fennel fruit the trichomes are not present [3].

Crude Drugs Made from Seed

Pumpkin, cocoa, coffee, cardamom, brown guinea, strophanthus, guarana, flax, mustard, nhandiroba, projectile-vomiting walnut, pacova, sucupira, annatto, nutmeg aryl, and kola nut cotyledons are the drugs made from seeds most cited in the literature. Cucurbitaceae and Zingiberaceae are the families most extensively used [3-4].

The seed is the dispersion unit of gymnosperms and angiosperms. It is responsible for the survival of the species. Seeds are recognized by the presence of a coat, composed of testa and/or tegmen, usually consisting of fibers and/or sclereids, which protects the embryo and even prevents its germination. The ripe seed may or may not have endosperm cells. In the first case, the seed is considered albuminous; in the second, it is considered exalbuminous [21].

In general, the embryo results from fertilization of the egg cell (exceptions can be observed in apomictic species – see [22]). Double fertilization occurs in some gymnosperms and in almost all angiosperms, i.e., in addition to the egg cell, the middle cell is also gametic and is fertilized, leading to the formation of the endosperm, an organism whose tissues play a role in the storage of substances such as oil, starch or protein responsible for embryo nutrition. The retention of the female gametophyte inside the ovule and thus the embryo is called endospory and is a fundamental requirement for seed formation [23]. Some seeds may contain more than one embryo and are called polyembryonic (ex. mango tree, orange tree, and inga tree). Supernumerary embryos are clonal, derived from somatic cells (e.g., nucellus cells) that undergo mitotic divisions or from embryo sac cells that do not undergo or complete the meiotic process [24].

Important diagnostic features for drugs made from seeds are size, color, shape, surface ornamentation, structure and consistency of the coat, size, shape and presence of reserve tissue in the cotyledons, color and shape of scars, presence and type of appendages such as aryl, and location, quantity and nature of the reserve tissue. An example of successful diagnosis of a drug made from the medicinal indigo seed (Fabaceae) took into account size and seed shape, integument surface ornamentation, hilum shape, embryo size, and types of metabolites. These features permit distinguishing seeds of medicinal indigo (*Indigofera suffruticosa* Mill.) from those of toxic indigo (*I. truxillensis* Kunth.) [2, 25].

Drugs made from fruits and seeds or from parts of them are more easily identified by macroscopic analysis, whereas microscopic analysis is impaired by the rigidity and large amount of tissues composing the pericarp and the seed coat.

Glands Are Useful Structures in the Secretion of Bioactive Compounds and in Drug Identification

The plant body can contain cells or multicellular structures specialized in the secretion of various substances involved in biological interactions - the secretory structures or glands. They can be distributed on the surface of the organs (external) or immersed (internal). Such structures can occur in all plant organs and in different taxonomic groups, besides having great ecological and physiological importance. The type and organ distribution of secretory structures can be valuable taxonomic markers of families such as Lamiaceae (peltate and capitate glandular trichomes - Figure 7),

Rutaceae (secretory cavity), Lauraceae (oil-producing idioblast), and Moraceae (ramified laticifer) [8, 26-28]. Even at generic and specific levels [9] it is possible to use secretory structure morphology to provide a secure drug diagnosis.

Among the external secretory structures, glandular trichomes and osmophores are of special interest to the pharmaceutical area.

Glandular trichomes have variable morphology and distribution (e.g., boldo species - Figure 7) and their exudates have been associated with both plant attraction and defense. In general, the chemical compounds secreted by glandular trichomes have diverse biological activity, possibly as a result of co-adaptation of plant pathogens and herbivores, pollinators and other organisms [26, 29].

Osmophores are essential oil-secreting structures, mainly present in floral organs. When considering the *sensu stricto* concept, they are of protodermal origin and comprise localized areas of the epidermis, being composed of non-cuticularized papillae [13, 30].

Secretory idioblasts, secretory ducts and cavities, and laticifers are internal secretory structures that deserve attention.

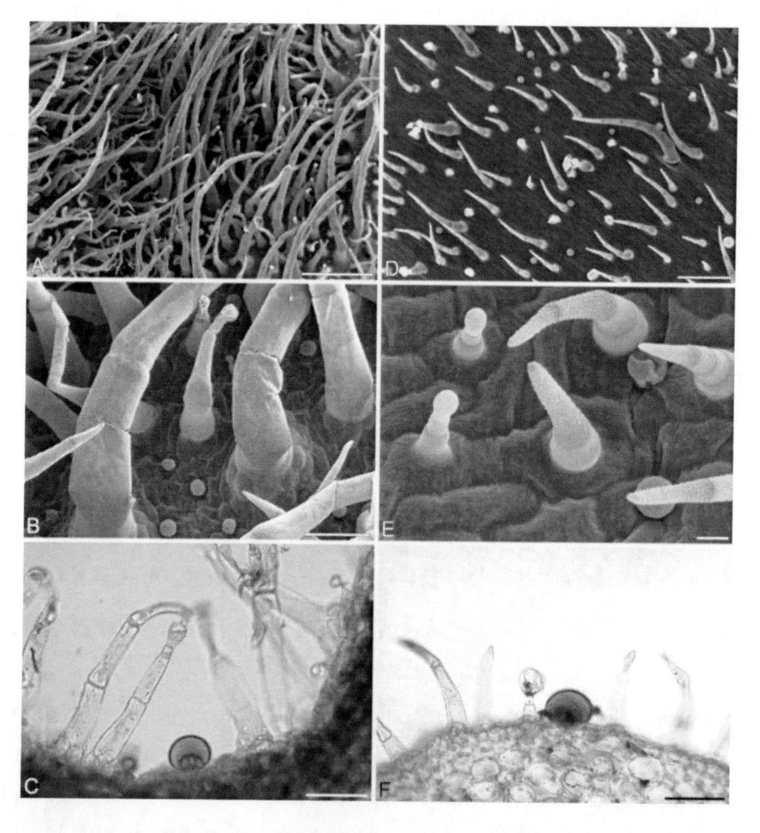

Figure 7. External and internal morphology of different types of trichomes (glandular and non-glandular) on the stem of two "boldo" species. A-C. Brazilian "boldo" (*Coleus barbatus* (Andrews) Benth.). D-F. Creeping "boldo" (*Plectranthus ornatus* Codd). A, B, D, E. Scanning electron microscopy. C, F. Light microscopy (free hand section). It is noteworthy that the true "boldo" (*Peumus boldus* Molina) belongs to the Monimiaceae rather than the Lamiaceae family, and has oily idioblasts and star-shaped trichomes. Scale bars: A = 500 µm; B, C, F = 100 µm; D = 200 µm; E = 50 µm.

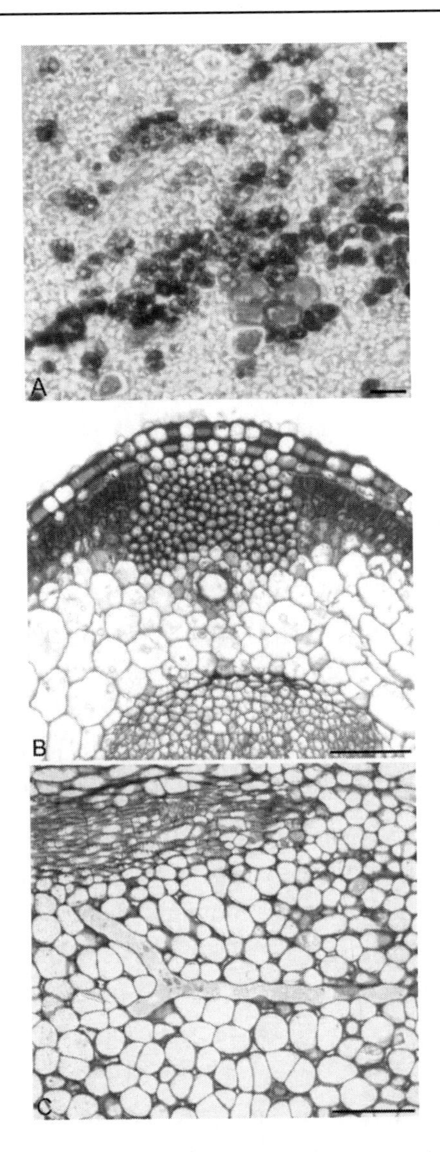

Figure 8. Microtome sections showing different types of secretory structures in different plant organs (light microscopy). A. Peridermic section of the Brazil wood pericarp (*Paubrasilia echinata* (Lam.) Gagnon, H.C.Lima & G.P.Lewis) stained with Comassie Brilliant Blue showing mixed-content idioblasts. B. Transverse section of the fennel stem (*Foeniculum vulgare* Mill.) stained with safranin and astra blue showing an oil duct. C. Longitudinal section of a fig tree developing fig (*Ficus obtusiuscula* (Miq.) Miq.) stained with PAS reagent showing a ramified laticifer. Scale bars: A = 6 µm; B, C = 100 µm.

A secretory idioblast is an individualized cell which differs from the others by its shape, size and mainly for its content. It can be immersed in any tissue of all organs of the plant, including the root [26]. The bark of barbatimao, for example, is rich in phenolic idioblasts (see Figure 2A). The fruits of Brazil wood and ironwood, Brazilian trees with medicinal properties, belong to the same family (Fabaceae) and are closely related species. They can be distinguished by the presence of secretory cells in the mesocarp of Brazil wood (Figure 8A) and the absence of these cells in ironwood [31].

Secretory ducts and cavities are structures found in subepidermal tissues or even in deeper regions. They have even been reported in roots, but most commonly occur in leaves, stems and fruits. They consist of a secreting epithelium that stores the produced substances in a lumen (isodiametric in a cavity or elongated in a duct) from where they are released outside the plant. They can originate from ground meristem, procambium or vascular cambium cells. In the last two cases, the ducts and cavities are formed in response to injuries suffered by the plant [26].

Mucilage ducts have been reported in mallow (Malvaceae); essential oil ducts in the pericarp of anise and fennel fruit (Apiaceae) (Figure 8B); resin ducts in pine (Pinaceae); and oil-resin ducts in copaiba (Fabaceae). Secretory cavities of essential oil and polyphenols have been recorded in eucalyptus (Myrtaceae) and secretory cavities of essential oil have been reported in clove (Myrtacaeae), in jaborandi leaf (Rutaceae) and in the pericarp of orange fruit (Rutaceae). In Myrtaceae leaves, secretory cavities are an important diagnostic marker because they appear as translucent points when viewed against the light with the naked eye. In addition to the chemical nature of the exudate, the presence of secretory cavities is also used as a diagnostic trait, as illustrated in two ichthyotoxic Brazilian legume trees of the genus *Dahlstedtia*, distinguished by the presence of secretory cavities in the leaf of one species (*D. pentaphylla* (Taub.) Burkart) and their absence in the other (*D. erythrina* (Vell.) M.J.Silva & A.M.G. Azevedo) [9].

Laticifers are complex secretory structures that occur within the plant and produce latex (= suspension of polyisoprene hydrocarbons, steroids, triterpenoids, fatty and aromatic acids, carotenes, phospholipids, proteins, alkaloids, inorganic compounds in a liquid with a differential refractive index). They consist of tubular cells connected or not by cell walls and usually positioned close to vascular bundles. Latex release occurs only when the plant suffers injury. They occur in about 20 families, more often among eudicotyledons and also in some gymnosperms. The types of laticifers (articulated, unarticulated, branched, unbranched) may or may not be exclusive to a family, as exemplified in Euphorbiaceae (articulated and non-articulated laticifers) and Moraceae (branched laticifers - Figure 8C). Contrary to popular belief, the latex color varies even from species to species and can be white and milky, yellow to brown, orange or colorless [8, 26], a trait that can be easily used for drug identification.

Conclusion

The advancement of knowledge of plant cell morphology and biology and, consequently, the identification of plant drugs depends on methodological and instrumental progress. Recent techniques in the field of electron microscopy (see illustrations in this chapter), immuno-fluorescence, confocal microscopy, freeze-fracture and mass spectrometry-based imaging are promising in this research because the structure of plant cells, tissues and organs can be better examined and detailed. But these techniques should be adopted by the centers responsible for drawing up the pharmacopoeia monographs. Innovative techniques are not necessarily the most difficult and expensive ones, but need training.

Poor taxonomic knowledge, probably due to the superficiality of botanical courses in the pharmaceutical formation, leads to difficulties in using the official scientific nomenclature. Scientific names of families and species remain outdated and incorrect in monographs and articles due to lack of knowledge about the systematic botany literature, such as taxonomic revisions, species descriptions found in papers or continental floras (see, for example, Flora Brasiliensis of Martius et al. 1840-1906, The Plant List, Flora do Brasil 2020, all available online) and Angiosperm Phylogeny Group works (especially APG III and APG IV [17, 32]). Examples of recurrent errors are to use (a) Asclepiadaceae as a family name instead of Apocynaceae (there is an Asclepiadoideae subfamily); (b) Bombacaceae as a family name instead of Malvaceae; (c) Mimosaceae, Papilionaceae and Caesalpiniaceae as family names instead of Fabaceae (= Leguminosae); (d) Malvaceae as comprising anise species (*Illicium*) instead of Schisandraceae (see APG IV [17]); (e) Moraceae as comprising marijuana (*Cannabis sativa* L.) instead of Cannabaceae (see APG IV [17]).

In addition, we draw attention to the use of a further comparative approach in monographs and papers by selecting exclusive features of the sampled plant group in order to improve the quality of the diagnosis of plant drugs. In most cases, comparisons are made between not closely related plant groups, aiming only the most common errors found at the moment of drug commercialization which makes the drug diagnoses artificial and too practical.

A good identification of a crude drug in order to prevent misidentification and adulterations should also be based on consultations of vouchers of a renowned herbarium for comparisons of samples with herbarium specimens properly identified by taxonomy experts. Taxonomic keys (see [33] as an example), widely found in papers of botanical systematics, could also be used as a tool for crude drug identification, if they were better known and disclosed among health professionals.

Finally, it is important to remember that new technologies should also be used in order to preserve the species and their natural environments, avoiding excessive extraction and searching for techniques of careful removal of bark, roots, rhizomes, latex, resins, and essential oils. Some studies with copaiba and Brazilian rosewood have wisely shown that some organs such as rhizomes, roots and barks could be replaced with other organs that, if removed, would not cause much damage to the plant, such as the leaves [34-35].

Acknowledgments

We thank Cristina Ribeiro Marinho and Thais Cury de Barros for providing some images, Edimárcio S. Campos for technical assistance and Elletra Greene for the English revision. S. P. Teixeira is the recipient of a CNPq fellowship (grant number 303493/2015-1).

References

[1] McNeill, J., F. R. Barrie, H. M. Burdet, V. Demoulin, D. L. Hawksworth, K. Marhold and J. H. Wiersema (2006). *International Code of Botanical Nomenclature* (Vienna Code). Regnum vegetabile, 146, 568.

[2] Paulino, Juliana. V., Elisangêla Pessine and Simone P. Teixeira (2010). Estudos morfoanatômicos da semente e da plântula de espécies de Anileiras (*Indigofera* L., Leguminosae). *Acta Botanica Brasilica* 24: 1-7.

[3] Oliveira, Fernando, Gokithi Akisue and Maria K. Akisue (1998). *Farmacognosia.* São Paulo: Ed. Atheneu.

[4] Lorenzi, Harri, and Francisco. J. A. Matos (2002). *Plantas medicinais no Brasil – nativas e exóticas.* Nova Odessa: Instituto Plantarum de Estudos da Flora Ltda.

[5] Hayashi, Adriana H., A. S. Penha, R. R. Rodrigues, and Beatriz Appezzato-da-Glória (2001). Anatomical studies of shoot bud-forming roots of Brazilian tree species. *Australian Journal of Botany* 49: 745–751.

[6] Apezzato-da-Glória, Beatriz (2003). *Morfologia de sistemas subterrâneos – histórico e evolução do conhecimento no Brasil.* Ribeirão Preto: Ed. A. S. Pinto.

[7] Raven, Peter. H., Susan. E. Eichhorn and Ray. F. Evert (2014). *Biology of Plants.* 8th Ed. New York: W H Freeman.

[8] Fahn, Abraham (1990). *Plant Anatomy.* 4th ed. Oxford: Pergamon Press

[9] Teixeira, Simone P., and Antonio C. Gabrielli (2006). Taxonomic value of foliar characters in *Dahlstedtia* Malme (Leguminosae, Papilionoideae, Millettieae). *Acta Botanica Brasílica* 20: 397-405.

[10] Baas, Pieter, Rudolf Schmid and Bertier J. van Heuven (1986). Wood anatomy of *Pinus longaeva* (bristlecone pine) and the sustained length-on-age increase of its tracheids. *IAWA Journal* 7: 221–228.

[11] Rao, R. V., T. R. Hemavathi, M. Sujatha, C. Luxmi, and R. Raturi (1998). Stemwood and rootwood anatomy of *Santalum album* L. and the problem of wood adulteration. *ACIAR Proceedings Series* 84: 93-102.

[12] Heady, Roger. D., J. G. Banks and P. D. Evans. (2002). Wood anatomy of wollemi pine (*Wollemia nobilis*, Araucariaceae). *IAWA Journal* 23: 339-357. http://florabrasiliensis.cria.org.br/opus.

[13] Endress, Peter. K. (1994). *Diversity and evolutionary biology of tropical flowers*. New York: Cambridge University Press.

[14] Lersten, Nels R. (2004). *Flowering Plant Embryology*. Iowa: Blackvell Publishing.

[15] Cocucci, Alfredo E., and José E. A. Mariath. (2004). Gametogênese, fecundação, seleção do gametófito mais apto, embriogênese e diásporo maduro. In *Germinação: do básico ao aplicado,* edited by Ferreira, Alfredo G. and Fabian Borghetti 15-30. Porto Alegre: Ed. Artmed.

[16] Bremer, Káre. (1994). *Asteraceae – Cladistics & Classification*. Portland: Timber Press.

[17] APG IV. 2016. An update of the Angiosperm Phylogeny Group classification for the orders and families of flowering plants: APG IV. *Botanical Journal of the Linnean Society* 181: 1–20.

[18] Judd, Walter. S., Christopher S. Campbell, Elizabeth A. Kellog, Peter F. Stevens, Michael J. Donoghue. (1999). *Plant Systematics – A phylogenetic approach*. Sunderland: Sinauer associates.

[19] Souza, Luiz Antonio (2006). *Anatomia do fruto e da semente*. Maringá: Ed. UEPG.

[20] Souza, Luiz Antonio, Ismar S. Moscheta, and Mathias K. S. Mourão. (2012). Fruto. In *Anatomia Vegetal,* edited by Beatriz Apezzato-Da-Glória and Sandra M. Carmello-Guerreiro. (2006). 347-368. 3rd ed. Viçosa: Editora UFV.

[21] Beltrati, Célia M. and Adelita A. S. Paoli. (2012). Semente. In *Anatomia Vegetal*, edited by Beatriz Apezzato-Da- Glória and Sandra M. Carmello-Guerreiro, 369-391. 3rd ed. Viçosa: Editora UFV.

[22] Caetano, Ana Paula S., Simone Pádua Teixeira, Eliana R. Forni-Martins and Sandra M. Carmello-Guerreiro, Sandra. M. (2013). Pollen insights into apomictic and sexual *Miconia* (Miconieae, Melastomataceae). *International Journal of Plant Sciences* 174: 760-768.

[23] Natesh, S., and M. A. Rau. (1984). The Embryo. In *Embryology of Angiosperms*, edited by B. M. Johri, 377-434. Berlin: Springer-Verlag.

[24] Lakshmanan, K. K., & Ambegaokar, K. B. (1984). Polyembryony. In *Embryology of Angiosperms,* edited by B. M. Johri, 445-474. Berlin: Springer-Verlag.

[25] Teixeira, Simone P. and Vani M. A. Corrêa. (2007). Morfoanatomia do envoltório seminal de espécies brasileiras de *Indigofera* L. (Leguminosae, Papilionoideae). *Rodriguésia* 58: 265-273.

[26] Fahn, Abraham. (1979). *Secretory tissues in plants*. New York: Academic Press.

[27] Fahn, Abraham. (1988). Transley Review No. 14. Secretory tissues in vascular plants. *New Phytologist* 108: 229-257.

[28] Fahn, Abraham. (2002). Functions and locations of secretory tissues in plants and their possible evolutionary trends. *Israel Journal of Plant Sciences* 50: S59 - S64.

[29] Wagner, George J. (1991). Secreting glandular trichomes: more than just hairs. *Plant Physiology* 96: 675-679.

[30] Vogel, S. (1990). *The role of scent glands in pollination: on the structure and function of osmophores*. Washington: Smithsonian Institution Libraries. Translated by S.S. Renner.

[31] Teixeira, Simone P., Sandra M. Carmello-Guerreiro and Silvia R. Machado (2004). Fruit and seed ontogeny related to the seed behaviour of two tropical species of *Caesalpinia* (Leguminosae). *Botanical Journal of the Linnean Society* 146: 57-70.

[32] APG III. (2009). An update of the Angiosperm Phylogeny Group classification for the orders and families of flowering plants: APG III. *Botanical Journal of the Linnean Society* 161: 105-121.

[33] Castro, Marília M., Hermógenes F. Leitão-Filho and Walkyria R. Monteiro. (1997). Utilização de estruturas secretoras na identificação dos gêneros de Asteraceae de uma vegetação de cerrado. *Brazilian Journal of Botany* 20: 163-174.

[34] Milani, Juliana F., Joecildo F. Rocha and Simone P. Teixeira. (2012). Oleoresin glands in copaiba (*Copaifera trapezifolia* Hayne: Leguminosae), a Brazilian rainforest tree. *Trees* 26: 769–775.

[35] Fidelis, Carlos H. V., Fabio Augusto, Paulo T. Sampaio, Pedro Krainovic and Lauro E. S. Barata. (2012). Chemical characterization of rosewood (*Aniba rosaeodora* Ducke) leaf essential oil by comprehensive two-dimensional gas chromatography coupled with quadrupole mass spectrometry. *The Journal of Essential Oil Research* 24: 245-251.

In: Recent Developments in Phytomedicine Technology ISBN: 978-1-53611-977-0
Editors: L. A. Pedro de Freitas et al.

Chapter 2

RECENT DEVELOPMENTS IN PHARMACOGNOSTIC EVALUATION

Jairo K. Bastos*[1,*]*, PhD and Caroline Arruda*[1]*, MD

[1]School of Pharmaceutical Sciences of Ribeirão Preto–University of São Paulo, Ribeirão Preto, SP, Brazil.

ABSTRACT

The use of plants for medicinal purposes has been reported since ancient civilizations, as a part of their cultures, and usually in a mystic way. With the technological advances in the last century, there has been a demand enforced by legislation to provide security, efficacy and quality for medicines derived from plants. Many studies over the past few years have provided technical innovations on extraction, isolation, analysis, detection and quantification of biologically active compounds found in plants. These methods are extremely important to assure the quality regarding the chemical composition and concentrations of active compounds in plant products, in all phases of its production chain. It includes cultivation, harvesting, processing, as well as stability and shelf life studies of final products, among others. Some of the most common problems related to medicinal plants are the lack of knowledge of its chemical components, adulteration and incorrect identification of plant material, among others. In order to ensure the quality, and consequently, the efficacy and safety of drugs derived from plants, there are several tools that can be used, such as: a) Gas chromatography coupled with Flame Ionization Detector (FID); b) High Performance Liquid Chromatography coupled with diode array detector. The use both equipments allow the development of reliable and simple methods with high sensitivity; c)HPLC tandem mass spectrometry (HPLC-DAD-MS/MS); d) GC/MS (gas-chromatography-mass spectrometry). The use of c and d allows not only obtaining the mass spectra of the

* Corresponding Author: jkbastos@fcfrp.usp.br.

compounds, but also to study their fragments and propose their full chemical structures. Additionally, chemical reactions can be used to characterize the presence of different class of compounds not only in plant extracts, but also in plant tissues by histochemical analysis and chemical color reactions using specific reagents to detect compounds, such as: alkaloids, steroids, terpenes, saponins, tannins, flavonoids, anthraquinones, among others. Additionally, the use of thin layer chromatography analysis continues to be an important tool for the quality assurance of plant materials. There are also innovative tools for specific purposes, such as electronic system (e-nose) to differentiate volatile organic compounds. The tests to monitor the microbiological contamination, content of insecticides, herbicides and heavy metals are not the subjects of this chapter. We expect that the techniques and methods presented in this chapter would be useful for enhancing the skills of anyone in charge of doing quality control of plants raw material and their products, aiming to ensure safety, efficacy and quality of herbal drugs.

Keywords: medicinal plants, quality control, plant compounds analysis, extraction, quantification

INTRODUCTION

The use of plants for medicinal purposes has been reported since the ancient civilizations as a part of their cultures. In the last century with the technological advances and the need to provide security, efficacy and quality for medicines, which have been enforced by legislation in several countries, it is mandatory to apply a scientific methodology for the use of herbal medicines. Recent studies have shown that between 1981 and 2010, most of the compounds, majority low molecular weight, which became pharmaceuticals have natural origins: natural compounds are usually employed without any molecular modification, as a semi synthetic or synthetic derivative, as well as by mimicking their natural precursor [1]. Therefore, the importance of the research in the field of natural biologically active compounds and its extraction and analysis is clear.

Therefore, to get a better use of plant material and to improve the tools of quality control, over the past few years, many studies have provided technical innovations on extraction, isolation, analysis, detection and quantification of biologically active compounds. These methods are extremely important to assure the quality regarding the chemical composition and its concentration in all phases of drug development, including cultivation, harvesting, storaging, processing and in the final products stability [2].

In this chapter it is reported and discussed the currently methods of extraction and characterization of natural products, as well as the main tools employed in detection, quantification, analysis and identification of organic compounds obtained from plant sources, since these methods are essential for the development of novel drugs, as well as for the quality control of plant material and its compounds. It is also important in the food chain, not only in the identification and quantification of the chemical composition of fresh plants consumed daily, but also to ensure the safety before consuming these products, as drugs, dietary supplements, phytotherapeutics and nutraceuticals.

The analysis to monitor the microbiological contamination, insecticides, herbicides and heavy metals in plant materials and its products, are also very important for safety, but they are not the subjects of this chapter. We expect that the techniques and methods presented in this chapter would be useful for enhancing the skills of anyone in charge of doing quality control of plants raw material and their products, to ensure safety, efficacy and quality of herbal drugs, nutraceuticals and phytochemicals.

HISTOCHEMICAL AND CLASSICAL TECHNIQUES

Several Pharmacognostic analysis methods as visual examination, microscopic inspection and histochemical analysis are already well studied and are established in numerous pharmacopoeias. These are not very recent techniques, but still constitute important tools for the analysis of herbal drugs, since they provide key information for the identification of both the analyzed plant and the class of compounds, and are constantly optimized [3].

The 5th edition of the Brazilian Pharmacopoeia describes a lot of procedures used for quality control of medicinal plants, including several histochemical reactions that can be performed with either fragmented fresh material or sectioned in microtome or after adding paraffin or macrogol: it can be verified the presence of hydroxyanthraquinones, saponins and tannins by adding potassium hydroxide (5%), sulfuric acid and ferric chloride (10%) plus sodium carbonate, respectively. The presence of compounds of these classes is indicated by red color (1,8-di-hydroxyanthraquinones), violet or blue-green and blue-green (hydrolysable tannins), respectively [3].

A current example of the use of histochemical analysis is reported by Mamoucha et al. 2016 [4]. They report the reactions to detect flavonoids, steroids and tannins in epidermal vegetable cells, as well as terpenes, phenols, and others, in different leaf structures (Table 1). The use of these tests allowed the detection of alkaloids and phenolic compounds in laticifers and vacuoles of the epidermal cells of *Ficus carica* (Moraceae), respectively. It shows that histochemical assays are still of utmost importance for determining the secondary metabolites produced by plants and to correlate amounts of these compounds with the biological activities of each plant species. Another example is shown in Figure 1: the presence of phenolic compounds in the secretory idioblasts of *Indigofera suffruticosa* and *Indigofera sabulicola*, respectively, is indicated by staining, after its reaction with ferric chloride.

Table 1. Reagents to reveal secondary metabolites from plants [4]

Compounds investigated	Reagent used
Terpenes	Concentrated H_2SO_4
Flavonoids	Vanilin/HCl
Steroids	Antimony trichloride
Alkaloids	Wagner's reagent
	Dittmar's reagent
Tannins	Potassium bichromate
Phenols	Ferric chloride
	Vanillin test
	4-Nitrosophenol
Phenolic tannin precursors	Dimethoxy-benzaldehyde

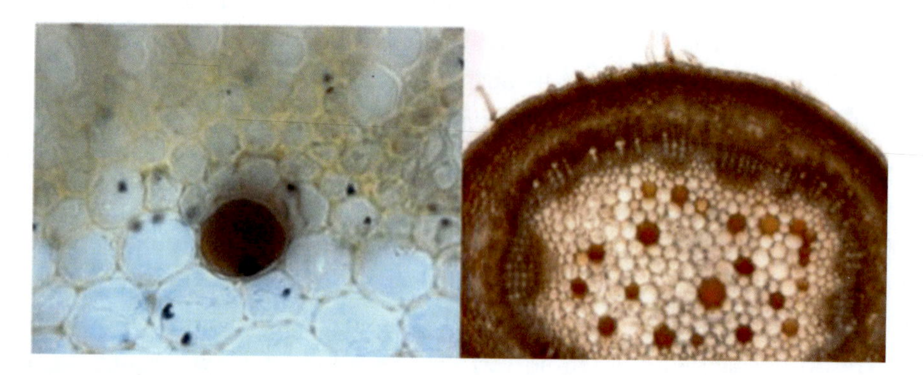

Figure 1. *Indigofera suffruticosa*' idioblast foliole and *Indigofera sabulicola*' branch observed in a microscope after reaction with ferric chloride: the staining indicates the presence of phenolic compounds. By Drª Simone de Pádua Teixeira.

Stesevi'c et al. 2016 [5] applied histochemical tests to investigate the presence of essential oils, alkaloids, steroids and flavonoids in *Chaerophyllum coloratum*, an endemic species of the Western Balkans: it was employed similar reagents to those shown in Table 1 in different plant tissues, such as: leaves, flowers, roots, stems and sectioned flowers. These tests allowed the authors to show that there are essential oils in the epithelial cells of the secretory ducts of the roots, leaves and fruits. It was detected in the cells and in the secretion of the larger secretory ducts of the stem. Also, it was possible to observe the presence of flavonoids by adding $AlCl_3$ to sectioned plant structures. The prominent staining observed by fluorescence microscopy in two different UV filters indicates the presence of these secondary metabolites in the stems and in the leaves.

Histochemical tests can be complementary to other analysis, and are valuable for determining the chemical composition of vegetables and the location of the secondary metabolites in plant tissues, therefore, improving the isolation of the target compounds and its analysis. It is also important to determine the compounds responsible for the biological activities described for each part of the plant.

Besides histochemical tests, many other protocols for assessing the quality and chemical composition of plant materials are available: a great number of simple and inexpensive methods can be used for this purpose reliably and are really useful, especially when daily analysis must be performed. One example is the analysis of dried capitula of *Matricaria chamomilla*, a plant that shows anti-inflammatory and antispasmodic activity due to the presence of the sesquiterpenes bisabolol, bisaboloxides A and B and the sesquiterpene lactone matricine (Figure 2) in its essential oil. It is used as herbal medicine in the US and Europe; in Brazil, it is widely used in cosmetics and it is also commercially available to prepare tea. Part of its quality control can be performed by using chromogenic reagents: after adding the reagent (4-dimethylaminobenzaldehyde + acetic acid + phosphoric acid + water) in M. *chamomilla's* extract, followed by the addition of concentrated sulfuric acid and heating, the presence of proazulene is indicated by the appearance of blue-green color [6].

A complementary method to the *M. chamomilla's* analysis uses Thin Layer Chromatography (TLC), in which a bisabolol standard solution and its essential oil are applied on a silica plate and, after development of the chromatographic run using toluene and ethyl acetate in a ratio of 93:7 as a mobile phase, the retention factors of each constituent and color observed, after revealing with vanillin and sulfuric acid can be compared to table 2, indicating the presence of these compounds in the essential oil [6].

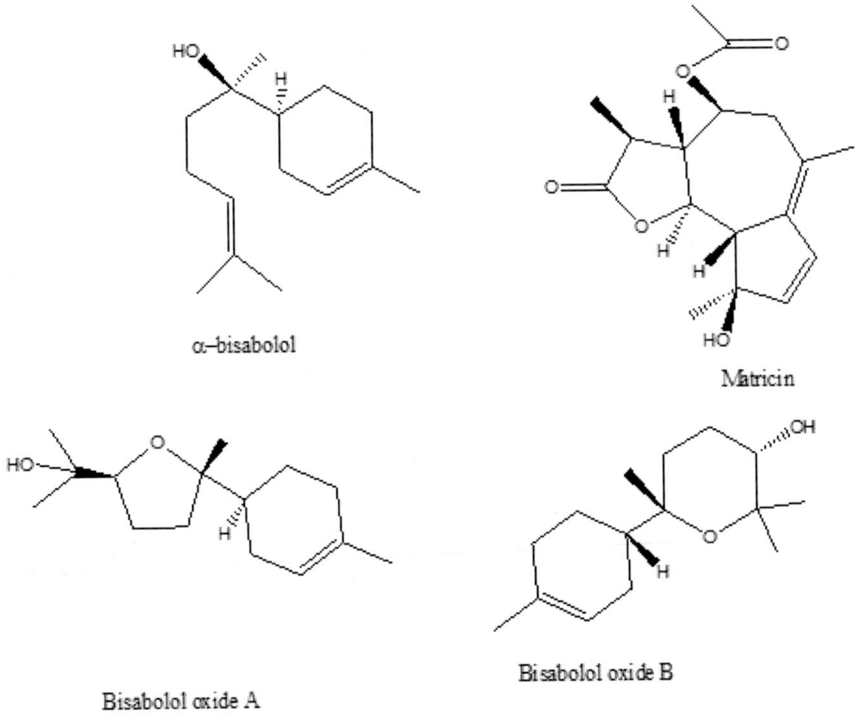

α-bisabolol

Matricin

Bisabolol oxide B

Bisabolol oxide A

Figure 2. Chemical structures of *M. chamomilla's* main bioactive compounds [6].

Table 2. Parameters for comparison of TCL's essential oil of *Matricaria chamomilla*

Rf*	Detection	Colour	Compounds
0,2	Vanillin-Sulfuric	Yellow Green	Bisabolol Oxides A/B
0,25	Vanillin-Sulfuric	Violet	Spathulenol
0,35	Vanillin-Sulfuric	Violet	Bisabolol
0,5-0,6	Vanillin-Sulfuric	Brown	Polyines
0,95	Vanillin-Sulfuric	Red-violet	Azulene
0,99	Vanillin-Sulfuric	Blue-violet	Farnesene, THC

*Rf: retention factor.

A well-established technique applied reliably in the quantification of medicinal plant compounds is spectrophotometry: Stesevi'c et al. 2016 [5] used it to perform the quantification of total phenols in *Chaerophyllum coloratum*'s extracts: after constructing an analytical curve, it can be performed a chromogenic reaction of phenols with Folin-Ciocalteu reagent and, after the addition of sodium bicarbonate, the total phenols can be measured by the absorbance of the extract at 725 nm.

Quantification of total flavonoids, saponins and other compounds may also be performed by spectrophotometry and it is well described in the scientific literature: Cheok et al. 2014 [7] quantified total steroidal saponin susing a colorimetric reaction in order to increase the wavelength of absorption of these compounds and consequently enable its quantification. The steroidal saponins react with vanillin or anisaldehyde, sulfuric acid and ethyl acetate to give a compound that its absorbance can beread at 430 nm and it is quantified by applying this value in the analytical curve.

Extraction, Isolation and Purification of Natural Compounds

The extraction of drugs from its plant sources has been performed since the eighteenth century, when some compounds, including morphine, a drug with unquestionable relevance to medicine today, were isolated [8]. However, the versatility and improvement of extraction techniques occurred with the development of chromatography in 1906 by a Russian botanist Mikhael Semenovich and the improvement of this technique by Martin and Synge in 1941 [9]. Nowadays, chromatographic methods are undoubtedly some of the most important in the analysis, isolation and purification of plant compounds.

Usually, the first step of isolation is to obtain the plant's extract, which can be done using some of the numerous existing techniques. A few of the conventional ones are maceration, infusion, decoction, boiling under reflux and steam distillation, among others [10].

Wang et al. 2014 [11] applied maceration with ethanol 70% acidified with 0.1% HCl for 24 h to extract anthocyanins and monomers from wild blue-berry fruits (two consecutive extractions). Sangmalee et al. 2016 [12] also used maceration, but with methanol as extractor solvent to get a *Derris scandens* extract that contains flavonoids. One of the main advantages of using maceration as extracting method is that it does not use heating. Then, the solvent can be selected according to the polarity of the target compounds. Usually, it allows to get a good yield of extraction, but it should be performed several extractions consecutively of the same plant material to accomplish this purpose, spending a lot of time and solvent.

Stodt et al. 2015 [13] obtained a black tea extract by decoction of its leaves and subsequent extraction with ethyl acetate at room temperature on a shaking bath. The main disadvantage of decoction is the use of heat for extracting the compounds, not allowing its use when thermolabile compounds are the targets.

An alternative is applying unconventional techniques, such as extraction assisted by microwave, by ultrasound, supercritical fluid, with pressurized fluid, hydrotropic, assisted by enzymes, among others. The development and improvement of these techniques occurred in an attempt to solve problems related to the extraction time, amount of solvent, use and control of temperature, in order to increase the yield, etc. Several papers recently published describe microwave-assisted extraction (MAE), since this process promotes the extraction by the microwave energy and allows a better control of the extraction conditions, resulting in higher yield, shorter time of extraction and less amount of solvent [10].

Upadhyay et al. 2012 [14] have used this method to extract chlorogenic acid (Figure 3) from green coffee beans. Furthermore, they optimized the process conditions and obtained results that corroborate with the potential of this technique as an alternative to traditional methods of extraction of phenolic compounds, such as chlorogenic acid.

Another technique currently employed is ultrasound assisted extraction: the molecules of interest migrate to the liquid in a lower temperature and in a shorter time compared to other traditional methods due to cavitations promoted by ultrasound that culminates in cell disruption, releasing to the extractor solvent the compounds that were inside plant cells [15]. Celli et al. 2015 [16] have optimized an anthocyanin extraction from haskap berries using ultrasound assisted extraction and have demonstrated that it is an efficient way to obtain a mixture of these substances with good yields in a short time and low temperature. Moreover, these authors also established, by experimental design, the main factors that are statistically related to the efficiency of the extraction and, therefore, were able to set an optimum condition for extraction of these compounds applying ultrasound.

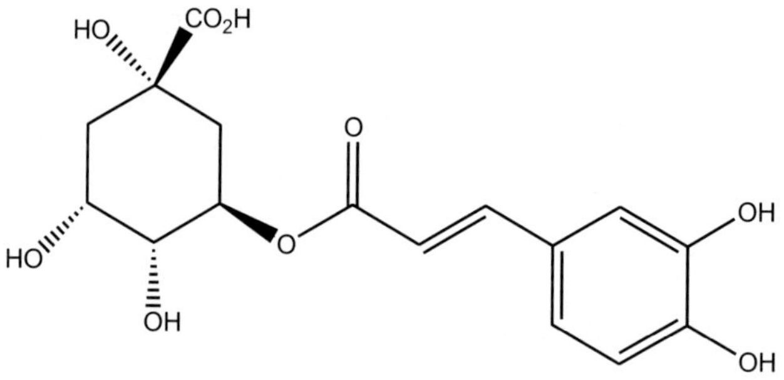

Figure 3. Chemical structure of chlorogenic acid [14].

The extraction by supercritical CO_2 has also been increasingly applied: Domingues et al. 2013 [17] employed it to extract triterpenic acids from *Eucalyptus globules* bark, since this technique is efficient and considered a Green Technology because it employs less or no toxic solvents, aiming to reduce the emission of these products to the environment and its contact with humans and animals. Currently, this is extremely important from both laboratorial and industrial perspective, considering that law requirements regarding safety, working conditions, emission and discharge of pollutants, besides the current situation of the planet (high greenhouse effect, warming global, pollution, etc.). Moreover, this technique is extremely versatile, because of the properties of supercritical CO_2. Its low cost makes it even more interesting. The authors also used a co-solvent (ethanol) since its addition increases the yield of extraction.

Regarding the extraction of essential oils, it is usually performed by hydro-distillation (Clevenger apparatus) on a small scale. However, this technique can lead to the formation of artifacts due to the high temperature. Besides, the essential oil should be dried with anhydrous Na2SO2, for example, after extraction [9]. By employing supercritical CO_2 such problems do not occur and the essential oil obtained is generally more pure than the ones obtained by other methods [18].

Frequently, after obtaining the crude extract, the next step of purification is fractioning it via liquid-liquid chromatography (partition), classical column chromatography or vacuum liquid chromatography. Sangmalee et al. 2016 [12] partitioned the methanolic extract of Derris scandens with ethyl acetate and water to give three fractions of different polarities. Then, the fraction in ethyl acetate, the one that contains the compound of interest, was fractionated by vacuum liquid chromatography: silica gel as stationary phase and different ratios of hexane and ethyl acetate in an increasing gradient of polarity as mobile phase. They obtained new seven fractions. Since the target compounds were in fraction 4, this was fractionated by column chromatography to finally yield the purified compound of interest (Figures 4 and 5). These steps of isolation are classics and have been used for years with efficiency in the isolation of natural compounds.

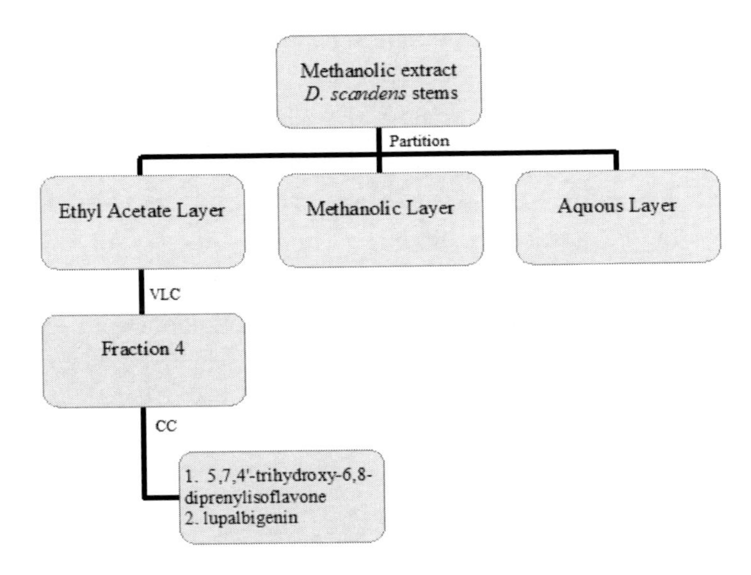

Figure 4. Steps of purification used by Sangmalee et al. 2016 to isolate two flavonoids [12].

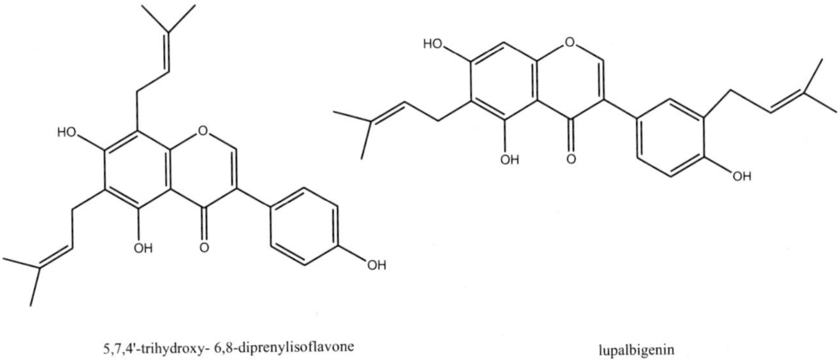

HO OH O OH

HO O OH O OH

5,7,4'-trihydroxy- 6,8-diprenylisoflavone

lupalbigenin

Figure 5. Chemical Structures of the isoflavones isolated by by Sangmalee et al. 2016 [12].

Shafaat-Al Mehedi et al. 2015 [19] used another separation mechanism for isolation of flavonoids from the bark of *Entadarheedii Spreng*: initially the extract was fractionated in a similar way to Shangmalee et al. 2016 by partitioning it to obtain fractions in petroleum ether, dichloromethane, ethyl acetate and water. After, the ethyl acetate fraction was fractionated by size exclusion chromatography: Sephadex LH-20 was the stationary phase and dichloromethane-methanol in a ratio of 1: 1 was the mobile phase. Fifty fractions were collected and analyzed by Thin Layer Chromatography: fractions 12-15 had similar chromatographic profile and were combined in one fraction. Then, this new fraction was submitted to separation by preparative thin layer chromatography to obtain pure epicatechin. The dichloromethane fraction was also fractionated by exclusion chromatography, and then the similar fractions were combined and purified by preparative thin layer chromatography too, affording liquiritigenin, glabridin, 4'-O-methylglabridin, isoliquiritigenin, and hispaglabridin A, and shinflavanone (Figures 6 and 7).

Also, there are other methods used in the isolation of natural products such as Countercurrent Chromatography (CCC): a liquid-liquid chromatography employing solvents that are immiscible, one as stationary phase and the other as mobile phase (partition). Some of the advantages of this technique are: use of small amounts of solvents, possibility of application of a large volume of the sample dissolved, versatility of mobile and stationary phase and the irreversible adsorption does not occurs with liquid stationary phases as it happens with silica, for example. Nowadays, one of Countercurrent chromatography techniques most used is the High-Speed Countercurrent chromatography, because of its efficiency and speed in the isolation [13].

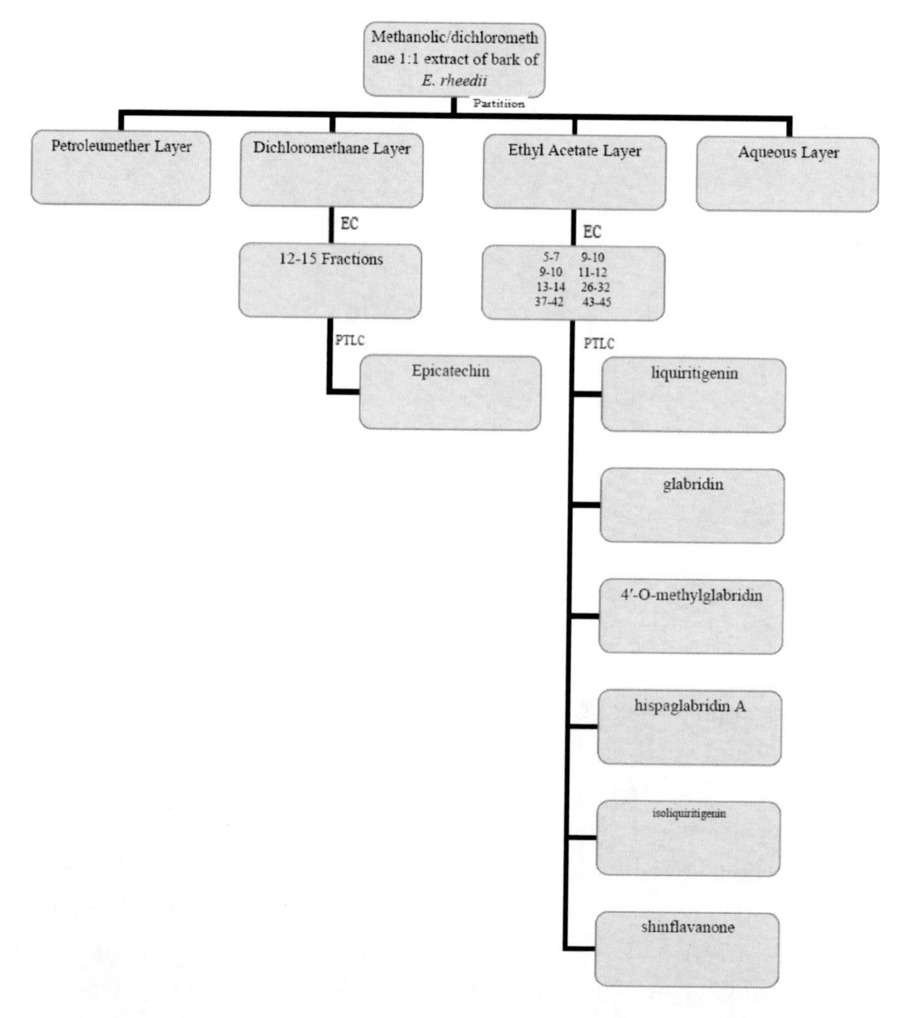

Figure 6. Isolation and purification of flavonoids. Shafaat-Al-Mehdi et al. 2015 [19].

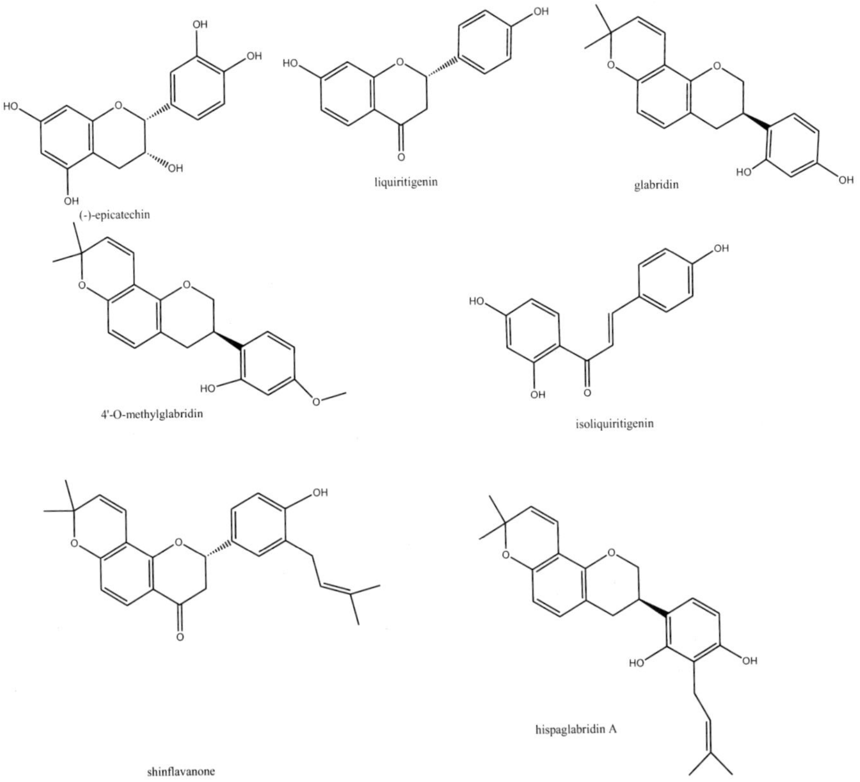

Figure 7. Chemical structures of the isolated flavonoids by Shafaat-Al-Mehdi et al. 2015 [19].

Stodt et al. 2015 [13] used this process after cleaning their extract using XAD-7 resin for purification of the arubigins from black tea. After comparative studies between other methods and CCC, the authors found that if the goal is the isolation of the arubigins with high purity, the CCC is an excellent choice. The results obtained by Nogueira et al. 2015 [20] reinforce it: they isolated the flavonoids quercitrin, afzelin, 3-O- (3-O-methyl-galloyl) quinic acid, 3,4-O- (3-O-methyl-galloyl) quinic acid, 3,5-di-O- (galloyl) -4-O- (3-O-methyl-galloyl) quinic acid, and 3,5-di-O- (3-O-galloyl-methyl) - 4-O- (galloyl) quinic acid (Figure 8) by HSCCC methods, which proved to be selective for these flavonoids. The subfractions containing the two first compounds contained more than 90% of these compounds, showing the efficiency and relevance of this technique. The authors also employed other chromatographic techniques such as Preparative High Performance Liquid Chromatography for purification of the compounds.

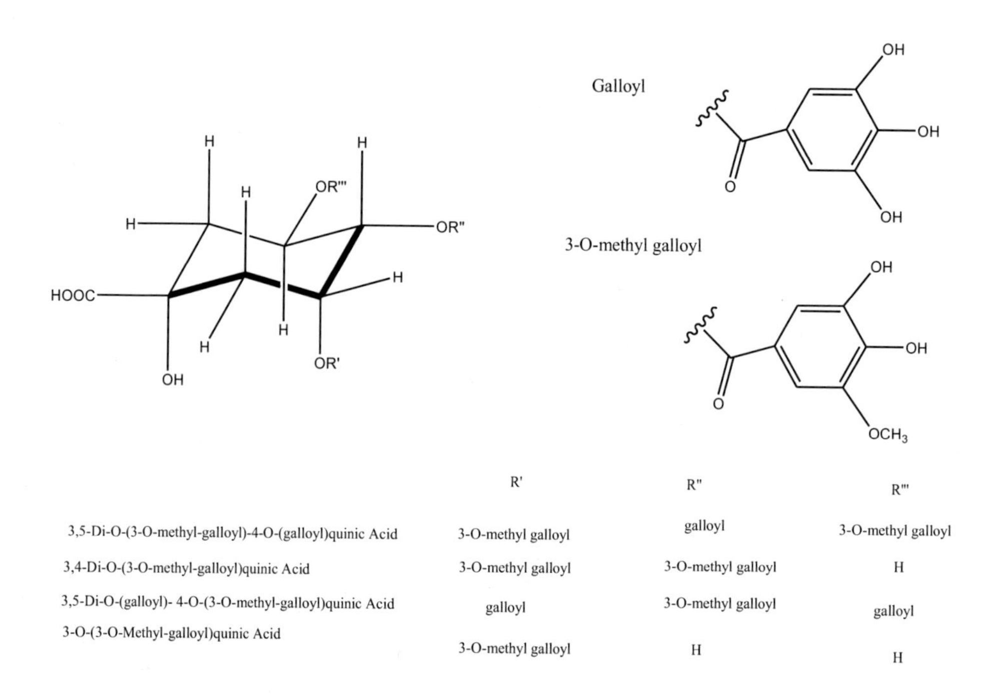

quercitrin

afzelin

Figure 8. Flavonoids isolated by Nogueira et al. 2015 [20].

High Performance Liquid Chromatography can also be used with a chiral stationary phase, allowing the isolation of enantiomers often found in natural compound mixtures: Wu et al. 2016 described the separation of racemic mixtures of lignans, neolignans, norlignans and sesquineolignans from *Phyllanthus glaucus* Wall. (Euphorbiaceae) using Daicel chiral-pak IA column as stationary phase, and n-hexane, ethanol and formic acid in different proportions as mobile phase. They isolated novel compounds and described their absolute configurations, which is important to establish the chemical composition of this plant species and for chemical structure- biological activity relationship studies of these compounds [21]. Two pairs of the isolated enantiomers are displayed in Figure 9.

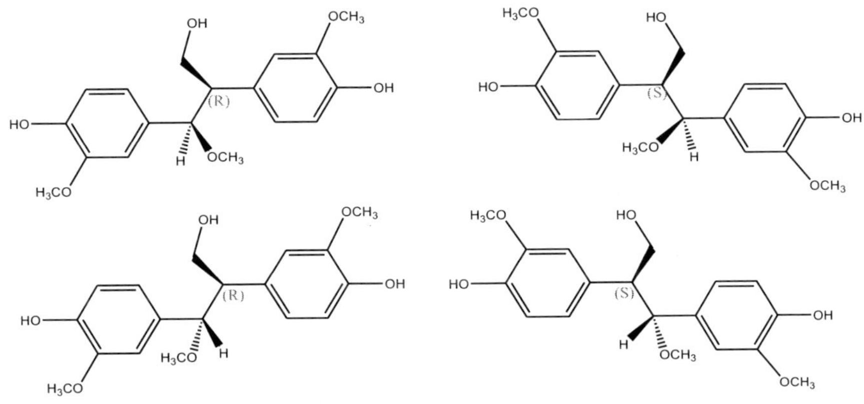

Figure 9. Two pairs of the enantiomers isolated by Wu et al. 2016 [21].

Analysis and Quantification of Secondary Metabolites in Natural Matrixes and Its Products

Gas-Chromatography and Liquid Chromatography

Currently, there is a great number of methods for analysis and quantification that are suitable for compounds found in plants, and these can be chosen according to the characteristics of the samples to be analyzed. Most of the analysis and quantification techniques, as well as methods for extraction and isolation, results from the enhancement of existing tools [10].

For volatile compounds like monoterpenes, sesquiterpenes, some alkaloids, some lignans, coumarins, furanocoumarins, among other compounds from secondary metabolism of plants and micro-organisms, gas chromatography is an excellent tool for analysis and quantification due to its high resolution capacity, low detection limits, and when it is used with flame ionization detector (FID), it can detect virtually any organic compound with excellent response [22, 23, 24, 25].

Sousa et al. 2011 [22] have established a method in GC-FID for quantitation of the sesquiterpenes β-caryophyllene, α-humulene and α-copaene (Figure 10) in *Copaifera* oleoresins, since it can be used in quality control of samples of *Copaifera* oleoresin obtained both from natural and commercial sources. This method is important because this oleoresin is widely used in pharmaceutical and cosmetic products. Therefore, it is necessary to confirm their identity and composition to guarantee its effectiveness and safety. To ensure the reliability of this method, the authors validated the method according to guides provided by regulatory agencies and showed that this is selective, accurate, precise, reproducible and robust in the range of defined concentrations.

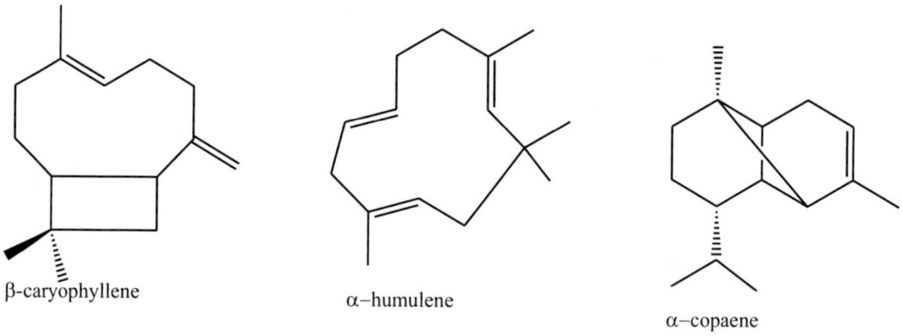

β-caryophyllene α–humulene α–copaene

Figure 10. Sesquiterpenes quantified by a GC method in *Copaifera* oleoresin [22].

McDougal et al. 2015 [23] also used GC-FID to quantify natural compounds: they quantified the alkaloids ammodendrine, anagyrine, cytisine, dehydrolupanine, lupanine, matrine, N-methyl cytisine, sparteine (Figure 11) in *Sophora* species from New Zealand. It is Important for the phytochemical study of these species, its quality control, as well as to correlatethe compounds with the biological effects caused by these species.

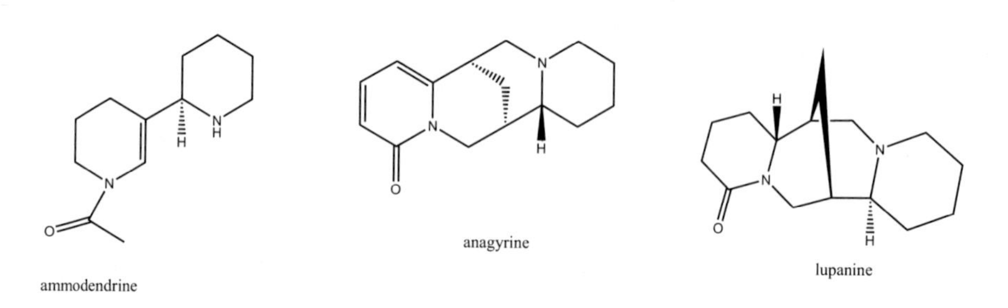

Figure 11. Some alkaloids quantified by McDougal et al. 2015 [23].

By observing these examples and others available in the scientific literature, it is clear that it is possible to develop simple, sensitive and reliable methods using gas chromatography able to analyze complex matrixes of natural products with excellent resolution and quantitation capabilities. It can be used for quality control of raw materials, in the evaluation of extraction processes efficiency, to verify the amount of target compounds in pharmaceutical forms and its degradation products, etc.

Another technique, which was developed in the twentieth century, and has been improved up to the present day, is High Performance Liquid Chromatography (HPLC): there is no need for the sample to be volatile for analysis. It only should be soluble in the mobile phase. HPLC has good preparative capability and excellent resolution and detection. However, there is a problem related to the main detectors used in HPLC, PDA and UV: compounds need to have chromophores to be detected. There are other detectors in the market, such as fluorescence, refractive index, light scattering, electrochemical, corona, among others: it presents several disadvantages and their use is more complex than the conventional ones. An excellent alternative that has being increasingly employed is the use of mass spectrometers coupled to HPLC [9].

Regarding the analysis of natural compounds by HPLC-DAD-UV technique, are very useful, since many of the natural products have chromophores. Souza et al. 2012 [26] analyzed *Copaifera* species oleoresin and observed that only the diterpene copalic acid is present in the nonvolatile fraction of all analyzed *Copaifera* species, allowing this compound to be considered its chemical marker. Copalic acid (Figure 12), such as other diterpenes, are not volatile, and to be analyzed by GC it must be derivatized before analysis, requiring an additional step.It makes the analysis by HPLC more interesting, sincediterpenes, such as copalic acid can be detected and quantified by simple, fast, reliable and sensitive methods by PDA-HPLC or UV-HPLC. Regarding to the stationary phase, the use of reverse phase HPLC was excellent for analysis of *Copaifera* oleoresin and this method is indeed relevant to quality control of this material. Furthermore, the identity of the *Copaifera* species is represented by the presence of copalic acid in the non-volatile fraction and its concentration is directly related to the biological effects caused by this compound.

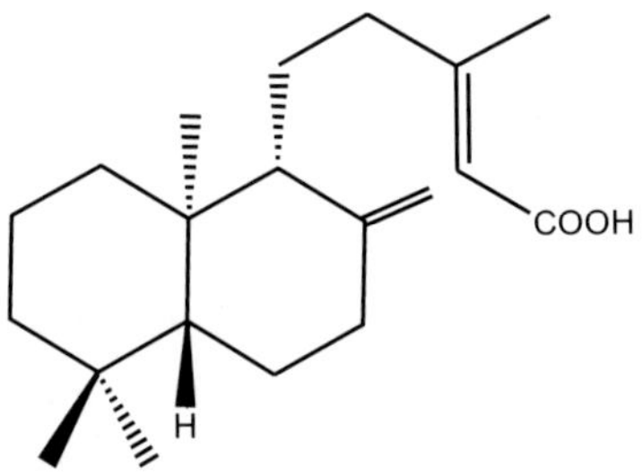

copalic acid

Figure 12. Chemical structure of copalic acid [26].

Another example of the efficiency of RP-HPLC-PDA for quantification of secondary metabolites in plants was reported by Tiossi et al. 2012 [27]: A reliable RP-HPLC-PDA method was developed for the quantitative analysis of glycoalkaloids solasonineand solamargine in accordance with the guidelines of ANVISA and ICH [28, 29]. The developed method allows the analysis of these glycoalkaloids in different plant tissues of *Solanum lycocarpum* and in pharmaceutical formulations. These compounds display several biological activities, such as: antifungal, antiparasitic, and cytotoxicity against several tumor cell lines.

In recent years, an improvement in high-performance liquid chromatography led to the development of Ultra High Performance Liquid Chromatography: it employs smaller particle sizes in the stationary phase, thereby reducing the analysis time and solvent consumption and improving selectivity, sensitivity and resolution of the analysis [30]. Bernart, 2015 [30] used the UHPLC to analyze limonene, a monoterpene with several biological activities and industrially important in *Citrus sinensis* oil: the developed method takes 1.2 minutes, while several methods in Gas Chromatography for this analysis takes around 30 minutes. The method is sensitive to nanogram of limonene, is linear in the working range established by the author, is precise and accurate, according to the parameter defined by the United States Pharmacopoeia (USP). Hence, the many advantages of this technique allowed the development of excellent methods to analyze natural products, which are being enhanced every day due to its importance to quality control of plants and their products.

Usually, the quantification and analysis of organic compounds extracted from plants can be efficiently and reliably performed by Reverse-Phase High Performance Liquid Chromatography. However, a problem may arise: the presence of enantiomers. One way to analyze and to isolate enantiomers is by using chiral high performance liquid chromatography columns, in which the stationary phase is selective for one of the enantiomers to be analyzed and / or quantified. It is not possible by using normal or reverse phase chromatography, since these compounds have the same physical properties, with the exception of the deviation of the polarized light, and the same polarity [9]. The chiral chromatography is an extremely significant advance because some of the enantiomers in the mixture can lead to different biological effects, such as toxicity and other side effects. Therefore, to the development of drugs and medicines and quality control of medicinal plants, it is indispensable to have an analytical method able to identify and quantify these compounds reliably.

Sayre and Davies, 2013 [31] developed three methods in Chiral-HPLC to quantify the flavonoids liquiritigenin, pinocembrin, and pinostrobinin in products and plants that claimed to contain these compounds. Its presence is relevant due to its many beneficial effects to the organism. The authors found variation in the quantities of these, and in some samples none of the compounds were available: the methods used in quality control are mandatory to confirm and quantify the target compounds, which reflect on the safety and efficacy of the product.

Hyphenated Techniques

Hyphenated techniques are widely employed in the isolation and quantification of organic compounds originated from plants, and also in its chemical structure characterization. FID (gas chromatography) and PDA (liquid chromatography) detectors are part of these hyphenated techniques: HPLC-PDA is a very useful detector for natural products bearing chromophores: UV spectrum is an indicative of the chromophores present in the analyzed compound. However, for confirmation of the compound's chemical structure, it is necessary to compare its retention time and UV spectrum with an authentic chromatographic standard. GC-FID presents a similar problem, also requiring standards for comparison between the retention time of the compound of interest and the standards. In an attempt to solve these problems, many papers have described the use of HPLC and GC coupled to detectors such as mass spectrometers or nuclear magnetic resonance because it is possible to quantify and also identify the compound without its isolation. It is a huge advantage to natural compounds' research and to industries, since it is possible to do the dereplication [10] studies. This technique allows the identification of compounds of interest without wasting time isolating know compounds, thus getting faster and better results in the search for novel drugs.

Carvalho et al. 2013 [32], after verifying several folk uses of the essential oil of *Vernonia crotonoides*, undertook its analysis by GC-MS by comparing the mass spectra of each compound to libraries. It was identified 40 different constituents in this oil, totaling 91.7% of the compounds, without its isolation. The authors used a mass spectrometer in which the ionization method is by electronic impact, because the fragmentation by this technique is reasonably reproducible and the sample has the properties to be analyzed by this technique. Furthermore, the available libraries are helpful to the structural identification of the compounds. However, a major limitation of this technique is the use of heating: it can only be used when the compounds are thermally stable, but sometimes the properties of the analytes are unknown, which difficult the use of this ionization method. Moreover, since volatilization of the sample is done by heating, EI-MS cannot be coupled to High Performance Liquid Chromatography, further limiting its use.

Another way to ionize the sample is by electrospay: it has been extensively employed because it does not use heating to ionize the sample, and it can be coupled to HPLC or UHPLC. However, it has its limitations too. One is the lack of reproducibility of fragmentation: it is possible to obtain two different spectra of the same compound at different analysis and / or different equipment. Then, the fragments obtained, shall be proposed rationally, always considering the basic principles of organic chemistry. Some of the main features of this technique, which are attractive, are: the analyte does not need to have chromophores, by employing MS tandem, and it is possible to obtain the fragment of the fragment, which is of immense importance for structural elucidation, as well as the excellent sensitivity of mass spectrometers [33].

Zhou et al. 2014 [34] used this features to develop and validate an analytical UHPL-TQ / MS2 method to determine 26 compounds extracted from *ginkgo* seeds. Due to the chromatographic system consisting of an UHPLC, the method has a good resolution and efficiency, allowing identifying and quantifying these 26 compounds in 15 minutes. The detector, because a tandem mass spectrometer is used to this purpose, has the capability to fragment the fragments, which provides important structural information of the analytes.

The mass spectrometers of high resolution have its analyzers with the ability to detect the mass of a compound up to three or four decimal digitsand have been widely used in recent years because it allows the differentiation of compounds with very close molecular weights [33]. Braunberger et al. 2013 [35], by using LC-MS and other techniques, identified flavonoids and ellagic acid derivatives in *Drosera peltata*: the detector was a 3D quadrupole ion trap ESI mass spectrometer. This detector allowed the authors to acquire the mass of each of the 13 compounds with high resolution and accuracy. The authors also used LC-NMR, liquid chromatography coupled to a nuclear magnetic resonance, to determine the chemical structures of the phenolic compounds: the data acquired by mass spectrometry, along with the nuclear magnetic resonance allowed the total structural elucidation of these 13 compounds. For quantification, as phenolic compounds have chromophoric groups, they employed LC-PDA to quantify it in plant biomass.

Another ionization method is Matrix Assisted Laser Desorption Ionization (MALDI), which allows acquiring images: Pina et al. 2016 [36] used it to locate 22β-hydroxy-maytenin and maytenin in root tissue of *Peritassa laevigata*, and quinonemethide triterpenoids, which are responsible for several biological activities. The presence of these two compounds was confirmed by MALDI-TOF/TOF in root cultures of the plant and its outermost location close to the vascular cylinder suggests a role of these compounds in the plant chemical defense against microorganisms and in exudation processes.

In addition to these techniques, there are specific ones to certain purposes, such as the innovative tool for essential oil analysis: the application of an electronic system (e-nose) that mimics the biological sense of smell through gas sensors which interact with the odor molecules and produce electronic signals that are processed in a computer (multivariate statistical analysis), allowing the differentiation of the volatile organic compounds: a recent study showed that this technology allows distinguishing the following species: *Vitexnegundo* (Lagundi) *Mentha arvensis* (Yerba Buena), *M. piperita* (Peppermint), *Artemisia dracun-culus* (Taraggon), *Blumeabalsa fimera* (Sambong) *and Plectranthus amboinicus* (Cuban Oregano) [37].

CONCLUSION

Several simple methods are described in detail in recent issues of pharmacopoeias, books and other references for medicinal plants analysis, comprising histochemical analysis, thin layer chromatography, colorimetric reactions, among others, allowing the analysis of a wide range of plants.

Among the main extraction methods currently employed, there are the classics ones, such as maceration, decoction and distillation, among others. However, new unconventional techniques have been developed, such as: microwave assisted by ultrasound, supercritical fluid with pressurized liquid, etc. For the isolation methods, the well established chromatographic methods are the most used.

For analysis, detection and quantification of natural products, some of the tools commonly used are: HPLC or UHPLC coupled to a diode array detector (when the analyte has chromophores) and/or coupled to mass spectrometry; Gas Chromatography (for volatile compounds) coupled to FID detector or Mass Spectrometer.

The mass spectrometry is one of the tools that has been highlighted due to information on the chemical structure of the analyte that it provides, in addition to be useful when coupled with HPLC or UHPLC, for developing reliable analytical methods that are able to identify and quantify compounds of natural origin. Regarding the structural elucidation, in addition to mass spectrometry, Nuclear Magnetic Resonance has unquestionable applicability.

Among these techniques, several can be employed in the isolation, identification and quantification of organic compounds, each one with its advantages and disadvantages and, depending upon the compound (s) to be isolated, analyzed and/or quantified, the most appropriate technique(s) can be chosen. Moreover, it can be seen that the techniques used complement each other, thereby improving the process.

Therefore, it is observed that the most used techniques are currently the optimized ones from previous processes: methods for detection, quantification and isolation of natural products, have been improved. Thus, every day new chromatographic methods have been available, culminating in the production of non-ambiguous studies, as well as faster and better resolution of the analysis. These features are essential to quality control of plant compounds and derivatives, showing the importance of implementation of the existing and development of new techniques. It also contributes to the studies on the application, advantages and disadvantages of each technique.

REFERENCES

[1] Pferschy-Wenzig, Eva-Maria, and Rudolf Bauer. (2015). “The relevance of pharmacognosy in pharmacological research on herbal medicinal products.” *Epilepsy & Behavior* 52:344:62. Accessed May 27, 2016.doi: 10.1016/j.yebeh.2015.05.037.

[2] Wu, Haifeng, Jian Guo, Shilin Chen, Xin Liu, Yan Zhou, Xiaopo Zhang, and Xudong Xu. (2013). "Recent developments in qualitative and quantitative analysis of phytochemical constituents and their metabolites using liquid chromatography–mass spectrometry." *Journal of Pharmaceutical and Biomedical Analysis* 72: 267-91. Accessed May 27, 2016. doi:10.1016/j.jpba.2012.09.004.

[3] Simões, Cláudia M. O., Schenkel, Eloir P., de Mello, João C. P., Mentz, Lilian A., and Pedro Ros Petrovick. (2017). Farmacognosia: do produto natural ao

medicamento, 69-105. Porto Alegre: Artmed. [Pharmacognosy : from natural product to the medicament, 69-105. Porto Alegre : Artmed].

[4] Mamoucha, Stavroula, Nikolas Fokialakis, and Nikolaos S. Christodoulakis. (2016). "Leaf structure and histochemistry of *Ficuscarica* (Moraceae), the figtree." *Flora* 218:24-34. Accessed May 27, 2016.doi: 10.1016/j.flora.2015.11.003.

[5] Stešević, Danijela, Mijat Božović, Vanja Tadić, Dragana Rančić, and Zora Dajić Stevanović. (2016). "Plant-part anatomy related composition of essential oils and phenolic compounds in *Chaerophyllum coloratum*, a Balkan endemic species." *Flora* 220:37-51. Accessed May 27, 2016. doi:10.1016/j.flora.2016.01.006.

[6] Wagner, Hildebert and Sabine Bladt. (1996). Plant drug analysis. A thin layer chromatography. 1-384. Berlín: Springer-Verlag.

[7] Cheok, Choon Yoong, Hanaa Abdel Karim Salman, and Rabiha Sulaiman. (2014). "Extraction and quantification of saponins: A Review." *Food Research International* 16:40-59. Accessed May 27, 2016.doi: 10.1016 /j.foodres.2014.01.057.

[8] Pinto, Angelo C., Dulce H. S. Silva, Vanderlan S. Bolzani, Norberto P. Lopes and Rosângela A. Epifânio. (2002). "Produtos naturais: atualidade, desafios e perspectivas." *Quimica Nova* 25:45-61. Accessed May 27, 2016. doi: 10.1590/S0100-40422002000800009. [Natural products : present, challenges and perspectives. *Novel Chemistry* 25:45-61].

[9] Collins, Carol H., Gilberto.L. Braga, and Pierina S. Bonato. (2006). Fundamentos de Cromatografia, 1-436. Campinas: Editora UNICAMP.[Chromatography fundamentals, 1-436. Campinas: UNICAMP Editor].

[10] Brusotti, G., I. Cesari, A. Dentamaro, G. Caccialanza, and G. Massolini. (2013). "Isolation and characterization of bioactive compounds from plant resources:The role of analysis in the ethnopharmacological approach." *Journal of Pharmaceutical and Biomedical Analysis*.Article in Press.doi:10.1016/j.jpba.2013.03.007.

[11] Wang, Erlei, Yongguang Yin, Caina Xu, and Jingbo Liu. (2014). "Isolation of high-purity anthocyanin mixtures and monomers from blueberries using combined chromatographic techniques." *Journal of Chromatography A* 1327:39-48. Accessed May 27, 2016. doi:10.1016/j.chroma.2013.12.070.

[12] Sangmalee, Suphattra, Areerat Laorpaksa, Boonchoo Sritularak, and Suchada Sukrong. (2016). "Bioassay-guided Isolation of Two Flavonoids from *Derris scandens* with Topoisomerase II Poison Activity."*Biological and Pharmaceutical Bulletin Advance Publication* 39 (2):631-35. Accessed May 27, 2016 doi:10.1248/bpb.b15-00767.

[13] Stodt, Ulf W., Janina Stark, and Ulrich H. Engelhardt. (2015). "Comparison of three strategies for the isolation of black tea thearubigins with a focus on countercurrent chromatography."*Journal of Food Composition and Analysis* 43:160-68. Accessed May 27, 2016. doi:10.1016/j.jfca.2015.07.002.

[14] Upadhyay, Rohit, K. Ramalakshmi, and L. Jagan Mohan Rao. (2012). "Microwave-assisted extraction of chlorogenic acids from green coffee beans." *Food Chemistry* 130:184-88. Accessed May 27, 2016.doi:10.1016/j.foodchem.2011.06.057.

[15] Rostagno, Mauricio A., and Juliana M Prado. (2013). Natural Product Extraction: Principles and Applications, 1-398. Cambridge: Royal Society of Chemistry.

[16] Celli, Giovana Bonat, Amyl Ghanem, and Marianne Su-Ling Brooks. (2015). "Optimization of ultrasound-assisted extraction of anthocyanins from haskap berries (Loniceracaerulea L.) using Response Surface Methodology." *Ultrasonics Sonochemistry* 27:449-55. Accessed May 27, 2016. doi: 10.1016/j.ultsonch.2015.06.014.

[17] Domingues, Rui M.a., Marcelo M.r. De Melo, Eduardo L.g. Oliveira, Carlos P. Neto, Armando J.d. Silvestre, and Carlos M. Silva. (2013). "Optimization of the supercritical fluid extraction of triterpenic acids from *Eucalyptus globulusbark* using experimental design." *Journal of Supercritical Fluids* 74:105-14. Accessed May 27, 2016.doi: 10.1016/j.supflu.2012.12.005.

[18] Fornari, Tiziana, Gonzalo Vicente, Erika Vázquez, Mónica R. García-Risco, and Guillermo Reglero. (2012). "Isolation of essential oil from different plants and herbs by supercritical fluid extraction." *Journal of Chromatography A* 1250:34-48. Accessed May 27, 2016.10.1016/j.chroma.2012.04.051.

[19] Mehedi, Md. Shafaat -Al-, Choudhury Mahmood Hasan, and Mohammad Rashedul Haque. (2015). "Isolation of flavonoids from the bark of *Entada rheedii* Spreng." *Oriental Pharmacy and Experimental Medicine* 15:347-51. Accessed May 27, 2016.10.1007/s13596-015-0201-y.

[20] Nogueira, Mauro S., Ricardo.A. Furtado, and Jairo Kenupp Bastos. (2015). "Flavonoids and Methoxy-galloylquinic Acid Derivatives from the Leaf Extract of *Copaifera langsdorffii* Desf." *Journal of Agricultural Food Chemistry* 63:6939-945. Accessed May 27, 2016.doi: 10.1021/acs.jafc.5b01588.

[21] Wu, Zhaodi, Yongji Lai, Lei Zhou, Ye Wu, Hucheng Zhu, Zhengxi Hu, Jing Yang, Jinwen Zhang, Jianping Wang, Zengwei Luo, Yongbo Xue, and Yonghui Zhang. (2016). "Enantiomeric Lignans and Neolignans from *Phyllanthus glaucus*: Enantioseparation and Their Absolute Configurations." *Nature: Scientific Reports* 6:24809. Accessed May 27, 2016.doi: 10.1038/srep24809.

[22] Sousa, João Paulo B., Ana P.S. Brancalion, Ariana B. Souza, Izabel C.C. Turatti., Sérgio R. Ambrósio, Niege A.J.C., Furtado, Norberto P., Lopes and Jairo K. Bastos. (2011). "Validation of a gas chromatographic method to quantify sesquiterpenes in copaiba oils." *Journal of Pharmaceutical and Biomedical Analysis* 54:653-59.Accessed May 27, 2016.doi:10.1016/j.jpba.2010.10.006.

[23] Mcdougal, Owen M., Peter B. Heenan, Peter Jaksons, Catherine E. Sansom, Bruce M. Smallfield, Nigel B. Perry, and John W. Van Klink. (2015). "Alkaloid variation

in New Zealand kwhai, *Sophora* species." *Phytochemistry* 118:9-16. Accessed May 27, 2016.doi: 10.1016/j.phytochem.2015.07.019.

[24] Huang, Zhongping, Yilei Huang, Shiqiang Xu, Wenxia Dong, Zaifa Pan, and Lili Wang. (2015). "Discrimination of the Traditional Chinese Medicine from *Schisandra* Fruits by Flash Evaporation-Gas Chromatography/Mass Spectrometry and Fingerprint Analysis." *Chromatographia* 78:1083-1093. Accessed May 27, 2016.doi: 10.1007/s10337-015-2917-8.

[25] Tabanca, Nurhayat, Maia Tsikolia, Gulmira Ozek, Temel Ozek, Abbas Ali, Ulrich R. Bernier, Ahmet Duran, K. H. C. Baser and Ikhlas A. Khan. (2016). "The Identification of Suberosin from *Prangos pabularia* Essential Oil and Its Mosquito Activity Against *Aedes aegypti.*" *Records of Natural Products* 10:311-25. Accessed May 27, 2016. https://www.researchgate.net/publication/283825430_The_identification_of_suberosin_from_prangos_pabularia_essential_oil_and_its_mosquito_activity_against_aedes_aegypti.

[26] Souza, Ariana B., Monique R. Moreira, Carly H. G. Borges, Marília R. Simão, Jairo K. Bastos, João Paulo B. de Sousa, Sérgio R. Ambrosio and Rodrigo Cassio Sola Veneziani. (2013). "Development and validation of a rapid RP-HPLC method for analysis of (-)-copalic acid in copaíba oleoresin." *Biomedical Chromatography* 27:280-83.doi: 10.1002/bmc.2788.

[27] Tiossi, Renata F. J., Mariza A. Miranda, João Paulo B. de Sousa, Fabíola S. G. Praça, Maria Vitória L. B. Bentley, James D. McChesney and Jairo Kenupp Bastos. (2012). "A Validated Reverse Phase HPLC Analytical Method for Quantitation of Glycoalkaloids in *Solanum lycocarpum* and Its Extracts." *Journal of Analytical Methods in Chemistry* Article ID 947836 8 pages.Accessed May 27, 2016 doi:10.1155/2012/947836.

[28] ANVISA- Sanitary Surveillance Agency. (2003). Resolution No. 899, Guide for validation of analytical and bioanalytical methods. Accessed May 27, 2016.http://www.anvisa.gov.br/legis/resol/ 2003/re/899 03re.htm.

[29] ICH—International Conference on Harmonization of Technical Requirements for registration of Pharmaceuticals for Human Use Topic Q2 (R1). (2005). Validation of Analytical Procedures: Text and Methodology, Geneva, Switzerland. Accessed May 27, 2016.http://www.ich.org/fileadmin/Public_Web_Site/ICH_Products/Guidelines/Quality/Q2_R1/Step4/Q2_R1__Guideline.pdf.

[30] Matthew W. Bernart. (2015). "Ultra-High Performance Liquid Chromatography (UHPLC) Method for the Determination of Limonene in Sweet Orange (*Citrus sinensis*) Oil: Implications for Limonene Stability." *Journal of AOAC International* 98: 94-7.Accessed May 27, 2016.doi: 10.5740/jaoacint.14-157.

[31] Sayre, Casey L., and Neal M. Davies. (2013). "Quantification of Three Chiral Flavonoids with Reported Bioactivity in Selected Licensed Canadian Natural

Health Products and US Marketed Dietary Supplements."*Journal of Pharmacy and PharmaceuticalSciences* 16(2):272-78. Accessed May 27, 2016. http://ejournals.library.ualberta.ca/index.php/JPPS/article/view/19511/15277.

[32] Carvalho, Cintia C., Izabel C. C. Turatti, Norberto P. Lopes and Andrea M. do Nascimento. (2013). "Chemical composition of the essential oil of *Vernonia crotonoides*." *Chemistry of Natural Compounds* 49:761-62. Accessed May 27, 2016 http://link.springer. com/article/10.1007%2Fs10600-013-0734-6.

[33] Demarque, Daniel P., Antonio E. M. Crotti, Ricardo Vessecchi, João L. C. Lopes and Norberto P. Lopes. (2016). "Fragmentation reactions using electrospray ionization mass spectrometry: an important tool for the structural elucidation and characterization of synthetic and natural products." *Natural Product Reports* 33:432-55. Accessed May 27, 2016.doi: 10.1039/c5np00073d.

[34] Zhou, Guisheng, Xin Yao, Yuping Tang, Dawei Qian, Shulan Su, Li Zhang, Chun Jin, Yong Qin, and Jin-Ao Duan. (2014). "An optimized ultrasound-assisted extraction and simultaneous quantification of 26 characteristic components with four structure types in functional foods from ginkgo seeds." *Food Chemistry* 158:177-85. Accessed May 27, 2016. doi:10.1016/j.foodchem. 2014.02.116.

[35] Braunberger, Christina, Martin Zehl, Jürgen Conrad, Sonja Fischer, Hamid-Reza Adhami, Uwe Beifuss, and Liselotte Krenn. (2013). "LC–NMR, NMR, and LC–MS identification and LC–DAD quantification of flavonoids and ellagic acid derivatives in *Drosera peltata*." *Journal of Chromatography B* 932:111-16. Accessed May 27, 2016.doi:10.1016/j.jchromb.2013.06.015.

[36] Pina, Edieidia S., Denise B. Silva, Simone P. Teixeira, Juliana S. Coppede, Maysa Furlan, Suzelei C. França, Norberto P. Lopes, Ana Maria S. Pereira, and Adriana A. Lopes. (2016). "Mevalonate-derived quinone methide triterpenoid from *in vitro* roots of *Peritassa laevigata* and their localization in root tissue by MALDI imaging." *Scientific Reports* 6:22627. Accessed May 27, 2016.doi: 10.1038/srep22627.

[37] Kiani, Sajad, Saeid Minaei and Mahdi Ghasemi-Varnamkhasti. (2016). "Application of electronic nose systems for assessing quality of medicinal and aromatic plant products: A review." *Journal of Applied Research on Medicinal and Aromatic Plants* 3:1-9. Accessed May 27, 2016.doi:10.1016/j.jarmap.2015.12.002.

In: Recent Developments in Phytomedicine Technology ISBN: 978-1-53611-977-0
Editors: L. A. Pedro de Freitas et al.

Chapter 3

THE QUALITY BY DESIGN (QBD) APPROACH TO THE DEVELOPMENT OF MODERN PHYTOMEDICINES

Luis Arthur D. Freitas, Luis Victor D. Freitas, Ana Carolina R. Montes and Luis Alexandre P. Freitas*

Faculdade de Ciências Farmacêuticas de Ribeirão Preto,
Universidade de São Paulo-USP, São Paulo, Brasil

ABSTRACT

Using medicines derived from plants is as old as the history of mankind, dating back thousands of years and properly registered in ancient folk medicine systems, such as Ayuerveda and Sinica in Asia, and Unani-Tibb in Arabic and North African civilizations. Today plant based medicines, or phytomedicines, have evolved technologically and play important roles in popular medical systems both in developed and developing countries. Physicians and patients have become increasingly demanding in terms of ensuring that industrialized phytomedicines bring about proper therapeutical effects, based on solid scientific and technological foundations concerning efficacy, safety and quality. Furthermore, recent technological booming and globalization press phytomedicines development into international standardization and harmonisation, providing users with worldwide acceptable technological and quality level. In this chapter, recent international policies and guidelines for pharmaceutical product development will be presented and discussed. Guidelines from the International Conference on Harmonisation (ICH) and some concepts that should be adopted in the development and manufacturing of phytomedicines worldwide, such as Quality by Design (QbD) will also be introduced citing two examples of QbD application for phytopharmaceutical technology studies, specifically extraction and drying.

* Corresponding Author address, Email:lapdfrei@fcfrp.usp.br.

Keywords: process development, harmonisation, unit operations, ICH, QbD, extraction, drying

INTRODUCTION

Manufacturing high quality phytomedicines involves various steps of quite distinct areas of technology, such as selection, reproduction and crop of the plant specimen, post-harvest processing, storage, industrial manipulation and finally the distribution and dispensation [1, 2]. The quality of the final product depends on each of all these steps, which must be managed with the most modern production, supervision and quality control principles [1-6].

Nowadays, physicians and patients expect herbal medicines to have the same degree of technological sophistication found in allopathic medicine [3]. The most reliable modern medicines are strongly based on the "quality, safety and efficacy" [6]. The industrial manufacturing step is of utmost importance to the quality of herbal medicines, providing consumers with the much-desired assuredness of health restoration [1, 2]. The industrial process must be technically developed to provide the phytomedicines with the composition, purity, stability and constancy required for its use, avoiding any risk to patients. Furthermore, compliance with official regulatory standards is essential, assuring that quality batch to batch and throughout the production process is fully reproducible [3, 6, 7]. The current concept is to treat phytomedicines no longer as second class pharmaceutical products, but as therapeutic options having the same modern technologies applied to allopathic drugs [3]. Cutting-edge technologies originating from allopathy such as bioadhesion, modified release, microencapsulation and nanotechnology among others, will be increasingly expanded to phytomedicines [3, 8, 9].

However, this will bring about very rapid changes to the level of technological sophistication for herbal medicines, increasing the need to understand in-depth what happens in industrial manufacturing practices [2], especially considering the unit operations of comminution, solid-liquid extraction, liquid-liquid extraction, crystallization, filtration, distillation/ evaporation, drying [1-3] and the production into final dosage form by encapsulation, mixture, granulation, compaction and coating [10]. All these processes should not only be optimized from the physical-chemical and economical point of view, but they should also be studied and known in detail to preserve bioactives and avoid any risks to medicine quality.

Recently, guidelines for the development of pharmaceuticals in the USA, Europe and Japan were redefined by the ICH - International Conference on Harmonisation, 2009 [7]. Although the ICH monographs are meant for allopathic drugs, the concepts contained therein should be extrapolated to herbal medicines, as physicians and patients expect herbal medicines to have the same level of technological sophistication imposed by the quality, safety and efficacy as allopathic medicines. In other words, the quality throughout the production process and batch by batch should be fully reproducible. It is also expected that the latest technologies applied to allopathic drugs, such as bioadhesion, microencapsulation, nanoencapsulation, among others, will be expanded to herbal medicines [3, 11] and will update the technological sophistication of herbal medicines.

Due to the fact that phytomedicine manufacturing is a long and complex process including various steps [1, 2] from raw plant material to the end product, using sophisticated techniques brings more credibility to these medicines. Unit operations such as extraction and drying, for example, should be specified using a reduced number of steps or even in a single step, thus reducing costs and risk to the quality of the final product [7]. Another very important point nowadays is adopting less polluting techniques that are eco-friendly using less toxic or non-toxic solvents with low energy consumption, as recommended by Green Chemistry principles [12-14]. However, among the various modern unit operations and techniques used to develop herbal medicines, none are used with unanimity, since the choice of a particular technique depends very much on the characteristics of the plant material and the purpose of its use [1, 2]. For instance in recent years, advances in some of the new techniques, such as Microwave Assisted Extraction (MAE) [15] or Ultrasound Assisted Extraction (UAE) [16], have expanded their range of applications from small scale analytical to full industrial. These techniques are usually reproducible, safer, economic viable, scalable and eco-friendly, allowing for the production of reliable herbal medicines.

How to Develop Phytomedicines Ensuring Internationally Harmonized Quality?

The long history of worldwide tragedies on launching and usage of medicinal products has driven the continuous upgrading of regulatory standards and practices [17]. The historic Food and Drug Administration (FDA) "American Chamber of Horrors, 1930-1933" exhibited a series of misfortune medicines and medical devices, including an eyelash dye that blinded women, a hair remover that caused baldness, mercury or lead poisoning lotions, creams and hair dyes and a deadly weight-loss product, among others [17, 18]. Very famous tragedies were related to sulfa anti-infective using diethylene glycol, in an oral "elixir of sulfanilamide," resulting in 107 people dead [19], to phenobarbital, polio vaccines, acetaminophen and the European catastrophe of thalidomide. In the 1960s, approximately 10,000 children were born with severe deformities linked to thalidomide. Since then, there has been a rapid increase in laws, regulations and guidelines worldwide, seeking for the safety, quality and efficacy of new medicinal products [19]. However, regulatory guidelines depend on government policies and, therefore, technical standards and requirements still vary according to the country. The need for international harmonisation on regulatory issues became overt with the advent of globalization [7].

The first movements in terms of harmonisation initiatives began with the creation of the European Union (EU) and the consequent single market for pharmaceuticals, shared policies and regulatory guidelines [7]. The success of the EC stimulated bilateral discussions between Europe, the US and Japan leading to the idea of a joint conference with representatives from regulatory agencies and industry. This was the beginning of the International Conference on Harmonisation (ICH) in 1990. The ICH Steering Committee (SC) divided the discussion on harmonisation into three major guidelines that set out the new medicinal product international standards: Safety, Quality and Efficacy.

"The current ICH Terms of Reference (ICH, 2000a) are:

1) To maintain a forum for a constructive dialogue between regulatory authorities and the pharmaceutical industry on the real and perceived differences in the technical requirements for product registration in the EU, USA and Japan in order to ensure a more timely introduction of new medicinal products and their availability to patients;
2) To contribute to the protection of public health from an international perspective;
3) To monitor and update harmonized technical requirements leading to a greater mutual acceptance of research and development data;
4) To avoid divergent future requirements through harmonization of selected topics needed as a result of therapeutic advances and the development of new technologies for the production of medicinal products;
5) To facilitate the adoption of new or improved technical research and development approaches which update or replace current practices, where these permit a more economical use of human, animal and material resources, without compromising safety;
6) To facilitate the dissemination and communication of information on harmonized guidelines and their use such as to encourage the implementation and integration of common standards" [7].

Regarding phytopharmaceutical technology developments, most of the concerns in manufacturing aspects of herbal medicines are addressed in the "Quality Guidelines" [7]. This section brings harmonization landmarks for stability studies, impurities testing and a roadmap to improving risk management in pharmaceutical industry based on Good Manufacturing Practice (GMP) [19], as well as new concepts such as Quality by Design (QbD). Guidelines Q1A to Q1F deal with the *stability* of medical products, Q2 provides references for *analytical validation*, Q3A to Q3D discuss *impurity* thresholds, Q4 and Q4B give recommendations about *pharmacopoeial texts*, Q5A to Q5E provide frameworks for the *quality of biotechnological products*, Q6A and Q6B address the process of selecting tests and methods and setting *specifications* for testing drug substances and dosage forms, Q7 focuses on the need to formalize *GMP requirements* for the pharmaceutical product components - both active and inactive [20], Q8 provides guidance on the development of pharmaceutical products before the clinical research stages of *pharmaceutical development* [21], Q9 establishes principles and tools for *Quality Risk Management* (QRM) applied to development, manufacturing, distribution, inspection and submission/review processes throughout the lifecycle of products [22], Q10 discusses the *Pharmaceutical Quality Systems* (PQS) for all product lifecycle stages [23], Q11 harmonizes scientific and technical principles of the *development and manufacturing of drug substances* (Active Pharmaceutical Ingredients - APIs), Q12 provides guidance to facilitate the post-approval changes considering the *product lifecycle management*, promoting innovation, continual improvement and complementing ICH Q8 to Q11 Guidelines.

Specifically, the Q7 to Q10 guidelines are closely related to the manufacturing of pharmaceutical products [24] and their principles can be extended to industrial aspects of herbal medicines and as a change to the way the phytopharmaceutical technology works. The ICH also indicates that guideline Q8 might also be appropriate for other types of products, such as phytomedicines, but local regulatory authorities should be asked about their applicability for a particular type of product. However, regardless of submission requirements by local authorities, the key concepts proposed in Q8, such as using QbD [25-30] in product development should be universalized in the development of all dosage forms [29], including the area of phytopharmaceutical technology [31,32]. The choice of adhering to the ICH-Q8 document brings companies the timeliness of continuously enhancing scientific and technological basis of their processes by implementing QbD, QRM and PQS.

One of today´s premises of herbal medicine quality from an industrial perspective is controlling risks concerning product specifications or assuring product reproducibility [1-3]. This can only be achieved by an in-depth understanding of the steps or stages of industrial manipulation of the vegetal material. QbD provides a framework to gain all the necessary knowledge and assure quality needs [27]. The ICH-Q8 defines QbD as: "A systematic approach to development that begins with predefined objectives and emphasizes product and process understanding and process control, based on sound science and quality risk management." Proper application of QbD principles should provide an assured high level of product quality, cost-efficient industrial operations, optimal manufacturing process, reduced compliance interventions, room for continual improvement and innovation, increased affinity with authority's actions such as pre-approval inspection (PAI), regulatory surveillance, post approval cGMP inspections and changes [20-30].

QbD Principles

QbD principles are a modern vision of Quality Management [7, 24, 26]. Quality Management is a concept that dates back to old craftsman work and apprentice inspection by more experienced workers in the Middle Ages [17-19]. In the early 20th century, several pioneers, such as Deming and Juran [33, 34], started to forge the modern quality control fundamentals. Since then, the concepts of control, assurance and Quality Management have evolved significantly. Joseph M Juran (1902-2008) was an electrical engineer at the Western Electrical Company. After the II World War, he worked as a consultant in industrial quality improvement and started to format the concepts of Quality Management. In 1951, he wrote the Quality Control Handbook, now called Juran´s Quality Handbook (McGraw-Hill Education) which is in its 7th Edition (2016) [33]. While Dr Juran established the basis of Quality Management in the administrative aspects, William E Deming (1900-1993) developed the principles of statistical analysis applied to quality control [34]. His work in Japan´s automotive industry from 1947 was recognized worldwide and he worked as a consultant for many companies. His four-step management method, PDCA or OPDCA (observe-plan-do-check-act), applied to quality management became famous in the control and continuous improvement of processes and products.

The systematic approach to attaining quality proposed by QbD is an evolution of modern concepts and proposes the full evaluation of all product essential attributes from the beginning of the development stage and continuously throughout its entire lifecycle [24]. The development of pharmaceutical products should be based on solid scientific knowledge and methodology, e.g., on hypothesis-driven experiments and obtaining experimental proof [7]. Studies to establish dosage forms, formulations, process conditions and an acceptable range of quality attributes should apply all pertinent scientific tools [20-30]. These tools determine the parameters that are essential for the product´s safety, efficacy and quality, such as formulation, process and operational conditions [21]. The QbD approach is now accepted and stimulated by the FDA to fill the New Drug Application, NDA. FDA authorities describe QbD as "a maximally efficient, agile, flexible pharmaceutical manufacturing sector that reliably produces high-quality drug products without extensive regulatory oversight. (J. Woodcock; FDA's Center for Drug Evaluation and Research - CDER)" [24] and "the desired state will be realized upon the implementation of Quality by Design to product and process design and development and establishing robust quality systems. (M. Nasr, FDA's Office of New Drug Quality Assessment – NDQA)" [24]. The differences between regular and QbD approaches to product development are illustrated in Table 1, based on the comparative framework created by ICH and presented in ICH-Q8R2 [21].

Table 1. Summary illustrating main characteristics of conventional and QbD approaches to pharmaceutical development

Activity	Conventional approach	QbD approach
Pharmaceutical Development	• Empirically based planning • Univariate experimental procedures	• Scientific and GMP driven inventory of material/process relation to CQAs • DOE - Design of experiments (multivariate) • Ascertainment of design space • PAT tools preferably utilized
Manufacturing	• Fixed conditions • Validation primarily based on initial full-scale batches • Focus on optimization and reproducibility	• Conditions adjustable within design space • Lifecycle approach to validation and, ideally, continuous process verification • Focus on control strategy and robustness • Use of SPC - statistical process control methods
Process Controls	• In-process tests primarily for go/no go decisions • Off-line analysis	• PAT tools, on-line and in-line supervisory • Supervisory control and continual improvement efforts post approval
Product Specifications	• Primary means of control • Based on batch data available at time of registration	• Part of the overall quality control strategy • Based on desired product performance with relevant supportive data
Control Strategy	• Drug product quality controlled primarily by intermediates (in process materials) and end product testing	• Drug product quality ensured by risk-based control strategy for well understood product and process • Quality controls shifted upstream, with the possibility of real-time release testing or reduced end-product testing
Lifecycle Management	• Reactive to problems (i.e., solving and corrective action)	• Preventive action • Continual improvement facilitated

Source: ICH-Q8R2 [21].

Table 1 clearly shows that the conventional approach is based on final product quality testing, which is known in the pharmaceutical area as Quality by Testing (QbT) [21]. On the other hand, QbD is a knowledge and risk-based approach to pharmaceutical development and proactive product and process improvement during lifecycle [24]. According to recommendations, QbD development begins by defining the product profile, moves to processes understanding and control. Identifying quality characteristics that are critical for product performance in therapy and process parameters that are essential for obtaining a product with the desired characteristics are essential in QbD development [21, 27]. The main elements of QbD were described elsewhere and their definitions are shown in Table 2.

QbD Development

Figure 1 depicts the comprehensiveness of QbD work evolution [27-36]. The development of a phytomedicine should begin by defining the product desired characteristics or Quality Target Product Profile (QTPP) defined in Table 2 which includes the product´s physical, chemical, microbiological and therapeutic properties, focusing on the patient needs, but also on other productive chain issues, such as raw material availability, purity, cost, transportation, market, local laws and many others [21-24]. After defining the QTPP, knowledge space on manufacturing of this kind of products should be gained from all sources, including company staff training and experience, internal cGMP history and documentation, scientific and technology literature, patents, consulting companies, supplier´s capabilities, regulatory issues and others [34-36]. The knowledge space information should be filtered to define the design space, where manufacturing aspects such as civil installations, energy supply, utilities available, equipment to be used, raw materials and their specifications, analytical methodologies and instrumentation [35] and staff qualification among others should be carefully defined, as in this design space the qualitative and quantitative relationships between the many formulation and process variables and the product quality requirements should be determined.

In the design space stage, the equipment and materials for each of the unit operations should be defined and studied. For example, in phytomedicine manufacturing [1, 2], the size of the drug is of upmost importance in the bioactives extraction [37], therefore comminution plays an important role in process reproducibility. In the design space stage, comminution apparatus and raw materials should be already defined to allow for a multivariate study on what and how process conditions affect the final size of the drug. In this case, the size can be considered a critical quality attribute of the intermediate product as it may influence the bioactive content considering the plant extract [21, 37]. Thus, in the design space steps, the most important product characteristics or Critical Quality Attributes (CQAs) should be listed and their relationships with the Critical Process Parameters (CPPs) should be studied experimentally with sound scientific basis. This relationship is determined by the multivariate experimental approach [38]. Much better than the univariate approach, multivariate analysis can identify linear, quadratic and interaction effects between independent and dependent variables, CPPs and CQAs, fitted to mathematical models which can be used to identify the control space region [38] (Figure 1). In the control space region, any variations of CPPs will result in a predictable change in CQA, but still within the technically acceptable range for quality requirements or specifications, allowing for the implementation of a flexible and robust manufacturing process adaptable over time.

Table 2. Terms and definitions used in QbD based product development

Term		Description
Quality by Design	QbD	A systematic approach to development that begins with predefined objectives and emphasizes product and process understanding and process control, based on sound science and quality risk management.
Quality Target Product Profile	QTPP	The full set of product characteristics that ensure the quality required for its efficacy and safety. This should be determined based on the team´s space of knowledge and using adequate quality risk tools.
Critical Quality Attribute	CQA	A product property or characteristic, whether physical, chemical, biological or microbiological, which is critical to product quality and should be strictly controlled during manufacturing.
Critical Process Parameter	CPP	A process or equipment parameter that exerts critical influence on the product CQA and must be monitored and controlled to reduce or eliminate risks to product quality.
Design of Experiments	DOE	A statistical technique often applied to determine, with less effort and high reliability, the relationship between independent and dependent variables in a process. Also known as multivariate analysis, it provides researchers with models (response surfaces) revealing mathematical relationships between inputs (CPPs) and outputs (CQAs) in a QbD development.
Space of knowledge		The combination or full set of all sources of information on the product, process, equipment, procedures involved in the manufacturing of the desired product, including internal cGMP documentation, books, papers, theses, staff experience and others. Used to define CQAs and CPPs.
Design Space		The region of risk based control determined by DOE analysis, which provides assurance of quality. Working within the design space is not considered a change and does not initiate a regulatory post approval change process. The multidimensional region (design space) is obtained from the DOE model for input (CPPs) and output (CQAs). Design space is proposed by the applicant and is subject to regulatory assessment and approval (ICH Q8).
Proven acceptable range		The proven range of variation of one CPP, when other CPPs are maintained fixed, that allow the achievement of product meeting relevant quality criteria (CQA).
Process Analytical Technology	PAT	An approach to designing, analyzing, and controlling the manufacturing process or unit operation by measuring CPPs and CQAs, using preferably on-line and in-line tools to ensure product quality.
Quality risk management	QRM	An approach to adequately implementing perennial assessment, control, communication and review of risks to the quality of a product across its lifecycle.
Lifecycle		All phases in the life of a product from the initial development through marketing until the product's discontinuation (ICH Q8).

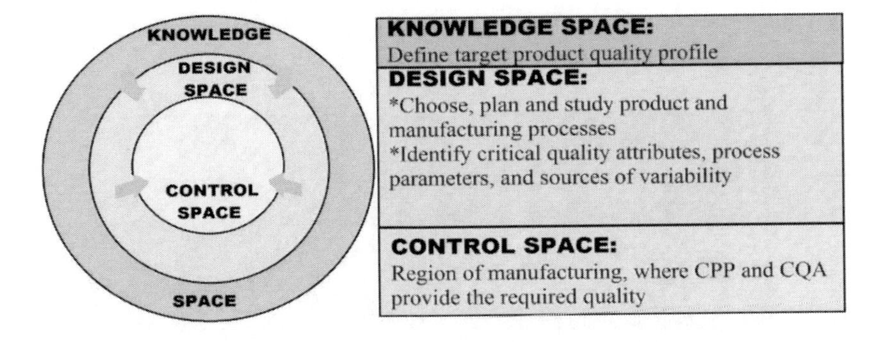

Figure 1. Relationships diagram for QbD development: moving through different stages.

It is important to note that the application of multivariate analysis, or DOE [38], is an essential part of QbD development and completely understanding complex information such as formulation and process relationship is not feasible using traditional univariate analysis. In fact, the gateway that enables migration from design space to control space is the multivariate analysis and modeling [21, 22]. Figures 2 and 3 show a series of plots that help to understand crucial differences between the two methods. Suppose in the development of the extraction of compounds from a vegetal material, the researcher wants to study the influence of solvent, pH and temperature on the % of bioactive extracted. In Figure 2A, the researcher decides to study first the pH aiming to find the best extraction condition to move to the temperature experiments. According to the results in Figure 2 A, the best % Extracted was obtained at pH 7.5. In the next runs, the researcher fixes the best pH and start to vary temperature in a series of runs, as shown in Figure 2B. The maximum %Extracted value is observed at 32°C, as can be seen in Figure 2C. This is a common approach even today when varying one variable at a time which is called univariate experimental design. By applying this design the investigator is not able to verify if temperature influences how pH affects the %Extracted. In DOE nomenclature, these cross-effects are called "interactions" and they commonly occur between factors in complex phenomena, such as extraction of plant materials. However, when investigators use a DOE for multivariate analysis, all the factors are varied in two or more levels simultaneously, allowing for building response surfaces such as the one in Figure 3.

The response surface gives a representation of the phenomena in a region corresponding to the whole range of factors studied. As can be seen in this response surface (Figure 3) the optimum extraction condition is not pH 7.5 and 32°C, as indicated by the univariate approach, but it is observed for the lowest temperature (25°C) and the highest pH (12).

Under QbT, a product specification is often set by observing data from a small number of batches believed to be acceptable [20-22]. End product testing only confirms the quality of the product and is not part of the manufacturing consistency or process control. Considering the QbD paradigm, pharmaceutical quality for generic drugs is assured by understanding and controlling formulation and manufacturing variables [21-23].

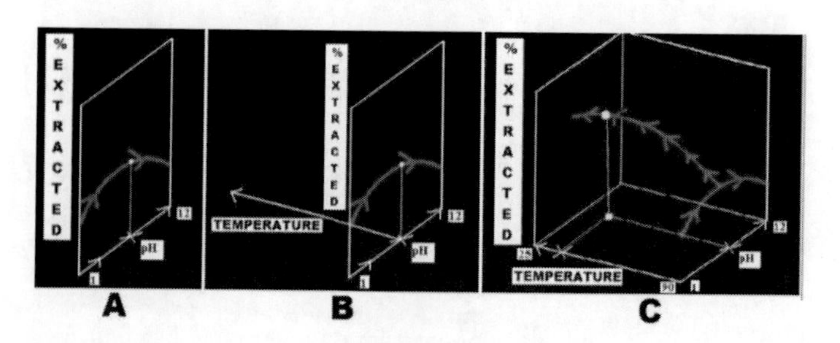

Figure 2. Plots showing univariate experimental approach to determine the best extraction condition: A - first varying pH; B now varying T(°C) and C: the best condition.

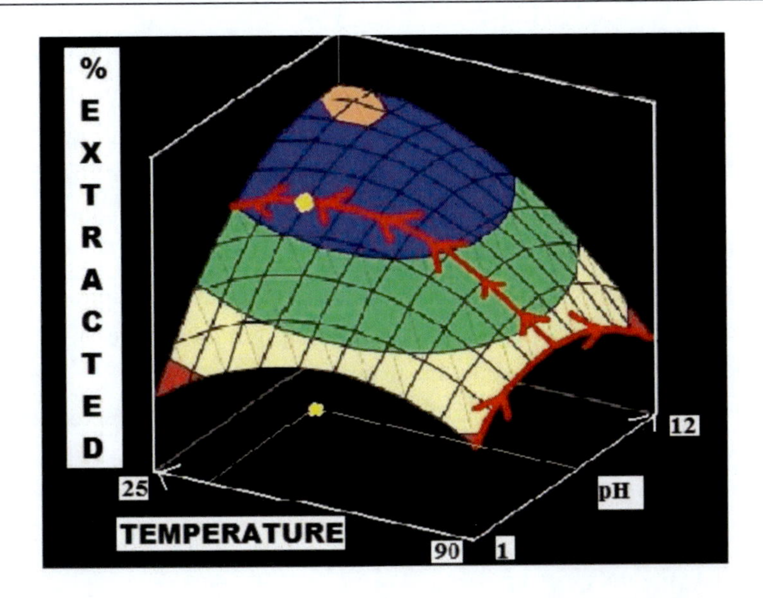

Figure 3. Plot showing multivariate experimental approach (DOE) to determine best extraction condition: simultaneous variation of pH and T(°C) and modeling into a response surface.

QbD Application to Phytopharmaceuticals

The first step in developing a systematic knowledge inventory is to determine what information will be most useful to catalog. Generally, the information components necessary to determine facility requirements are the same ones needed to address a review dialog. The basic flowcharts for processing phytopharmaceuticals or manufacturing herbal medicines were presented by a few authors [1, 2]. The main unit operations consistently belong to the same categories, resulting in similar process flowcharts that provide a good overview of the manufacturing system. A common flowchart for the production of standardized dried extracts from medicinal plant material is shown in Figure 4. In this flowchart, unit operations related to post-harvesting processing are not shown, as this is usually done at the agricultural site. Post-harvesting operations usually include vegetal part selection, drying and grinding, aiming to give better stability to the plant material until it reaches the industrial site and during its storage in hoppers (#1, Figure 4). Industrial processing begins with milling the vegetable raw material, as shown in item 5 (Figure 4). Milling is one of the most important unit operations in plant drug processing because it can cause bioactive loss due to temperature increases, but certainly the final degree of comminution of the drug influences the subsequent extraction operation. After reducing the size, the material is subjected to extraction (#6, Figure 4), which can be followed by steps of enrichment, such as filtration or centrifugation or concentration of the extract by evaporation or distillation (#8, Figure 4). Finally, the concentrated extract moves on to the step of totally eliminating the solvent by drying (#9, Figure 4). Other important components of an industrial plant, such as solvent storage and recovery by distillation, energy or steam generation, water treatment facility and residue treatment/disposal facility are not described in detail here, but it should be noted that they play an important role in industrial design. After the standardized dried extract is obtained, other typical operations to prepare the final herbal medicine form, whether liquid, semi-solid or solid form, are subsequently carried out, such as granulation and tablet compression.

However, comprehensive descriptions of techniques and equipment for grinding, milling, extraction, purification, concentration, drying, granulation, compression or other typical unit operations in herbal medicine manufacturing is not within the scope of this chapter. Otherwise, examples of application of QbD approach on selected unit operations will be given, with highlight to the use of multivariate techniques like DOE.

The extraction and drying of *Curcuma longa* L, also known as turmeric, will be used to illustrate the QbD approach.

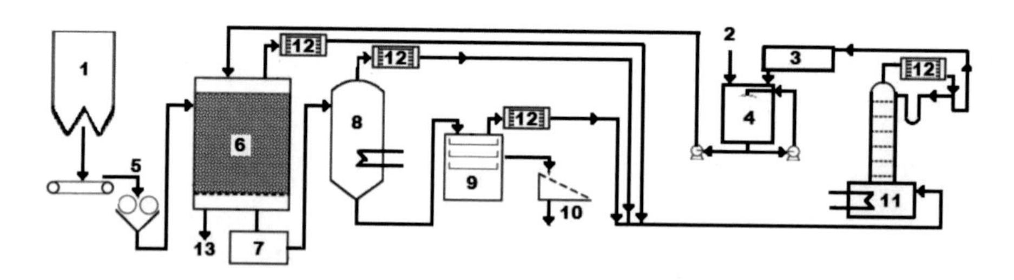

Figure 4. Flowchart of a typical sequence for preparing the standardized dried extract. 1) Hopper; 2) Solvent 1; 3) Solvent 2; 4) Mixing tank; 5) Mill; 6) Extractor; 7) Extract tank; 8) Evaporator; 9) Dryer; 10) Sieves; 11) Distillation column; 12) Condenser and 13) Extraction residues.

EXTRACTION

Extracting curcumin adopting the QbD approach will be used as an example of modern phytopharmaceutical technology development. Curcumin is a polyphenol from *Curcuma longa* L roots, a plant native to Asia. It is popularly known as turmeric and it has spread worldwide due to its food-colouring properties [39]. As an ancient Ayurvedic medicine, turmeric and its extracts were studied for their therapeutic properties [39]. Curcumin is the main curcuminoid isolated from Curcuma *longa* L and there is scientific proof that it possesses anti-inflammatory, hepatoprotective, antiviral, antibiotic, anticholesterolemic, antioxidant, neuroprotective and antitumoural properties [41-43]. Moreover, curcumin and other curcuminoids are regarded as safe, and turmeric products are widely used in the food industry as a major ingredient of curry, as a food color additive in cheese, pickles, mustard, soups, cereals and other foodstuffs to replace artificial food coloring [39]. Due to the wide range of biological activities and the safety of curcumin, many projects are currently investigating its effectiveness on age-related cognitive impairment as a dietary supplement, especially for the treatment of Alzheimer´s disease [39-43].

Curcumin has already been tested as a chemopreventive agent for cancer and Alzheimer's disease in a few short-term clinical runs [42-43]. Curcumin demonstrated no or very low toxicity in a single dose of up to 12 g and in doses of 8 g/day for 3 months. However, the combination of the lipophilic nature of curcumin, its relative insolubility in aqueous solutions, and its short half life leads to low bioavailability following oral administration, which has limited its therapeutic application [11, 44]. Additionally, curcumin is unstable at alkaline pH which interferes with the therapeutic activity of the plant and may explain non-conclusive clinical trials [44].

Extracting curcumin by dynamic maceration [45] was studied using DOE and will be used as an example of the QbD approach for drug extraction [46]. For instance, the first decision an investigator should make is to choose the solvent and the method of extraction [47]. The solvents must be chosen by the chemical characteristics of the substance of interest [48], but a contemporary view should also include solvent environmental and toxicity properties, e.g., solvents should be preferably GREEN [12-14] and GRAS (generally regarded as safe) [37]. Concerning the extraction method, traditional extraction techniques, such as Sohxlet [49,50], maceration [37, 51] percolation, dynamic maceration [45, 52, 53] and high pressure [54, 55] should compete with the modern Ultrasound Assisted extraction (UAE) [56-60] and the Microwave Assisted Extraction (MAE) [61-64], turbolysis or supercritical and Subcritical Fluid Extraction (SFE) [65-68]. The possibilities and limitations for future use of techniques such as ultrasound and microwaves, as well as the main drying techniques used for plant products such as lyophilization, nebulization and fluidized bed driers will be discussed further in Chapters 5 and 6.

The extraction method presented here [45], the dynamic maceration, consists of extracting bioactives from the powdered drug suspended by the extracting solvent in a tank or vessel with continuous agitation by a propeller [1, 2]. Usually there is no renewal of the extracting liquid, but the agitation makes the powdered drug and solvent contact very efficient due to the convective mass transfer, enabling it to reach the bioactive concentration equilibrium between the two phases [1]. The dynamic maceration method is described in detail in Chapter 5 of this book. It is one of the most used industrially due to its favorable operating costs, high extraction efficiency and moderate extraction time [1, 37, 45, 52, 53]. Various factors may influence the results of plant drug dynamic maceration [1, 37], such as the tank and impeller geometric details, agitation speed, ratio of plant drug to solvent volumes, solvent properties, drug powder density and granulometry, temperature, extraction time and others [37,53]. The whole QbD process to develop an extraction process is illustrated in Figure 5.

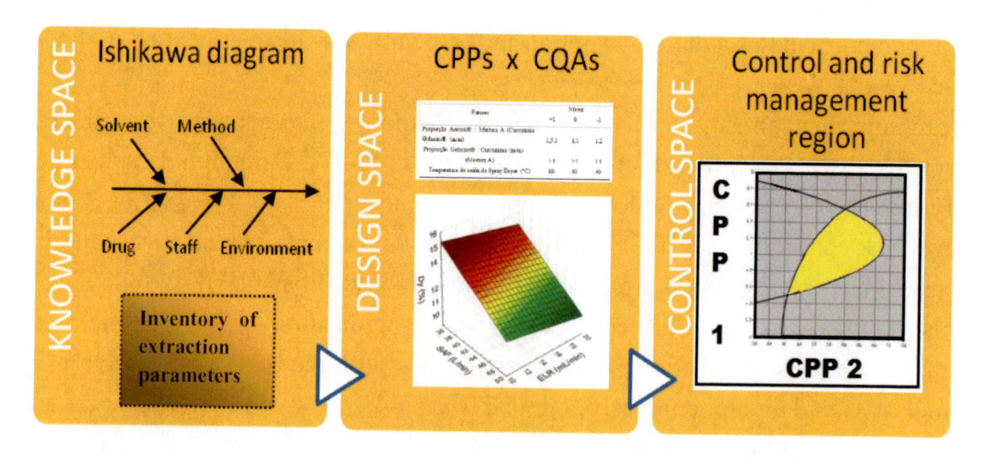

Figure 5. QbD approach scheme of process development for phytopharmaceutical extraction.

The QbD approach first entails depicting an inventory of important factors considering this extraction method, collecting information from papers, books, manuals, patents and internal company knowledge. One of the most used techniques to organize and show the expected effects is the Ishikawa diagram [69], also called Fishikawa or fishbone diagrams, cause-and-effect diagrams or herringbone diagrams. These diagrams were proposed by Kaoru Ishikawa in 1968 and are used to identify cause-effect relationships in product and process design, preventing risks to quality defect [69]. Factors of different types may be included in Ishikawa diagrams, such as groups of people or the staff involved, a set of methods or techniques, equipment, analytical tools and whole environmental conditions such as location, time, temperature and even local cultural aspects. Figure 6 shows an example of an Ishikawa diagram for dynamic maceration of plant material. The factors listed include: 1) solvent: polarity, pH, density, surface tension, viscosity; 2) bioactive: pKa, logP, polarity, stability to oxygen, light and heat; 3) drug powder: granulometry, bulk density, swelling index, solvent uptake, 4) dynamic maceration conditions: equipment geometry, volume in tank, agitation speed, temperature, drug to solvent mass ratio, pressure, duration (time); 5) environment: temperature, humidity, light, pressure; and 6) staff: training and commitment.

Many factors such as the extractive method, solvent composition, extraction time, extraction temperature, solvent to drug ratio and extraction pressure, among others, are assumed to significantly influence the efficiency of curcumin extraction [45, 65]. In the study presented herein, published by Paulucci and others [45], curcuma samples with moisture content of 9.82±0.15% (w/w), total ash content 7.4±0.05% (w/w), swelling index of 4.72 ± 0.07 and moderately coarse size (37% of the particles passed through the sieve with mesh 1mm) were extracted by following a 2^5 full factorial statistical design in 100 ml borosilicate flasks. The factors studied, which in this case represent the chosen

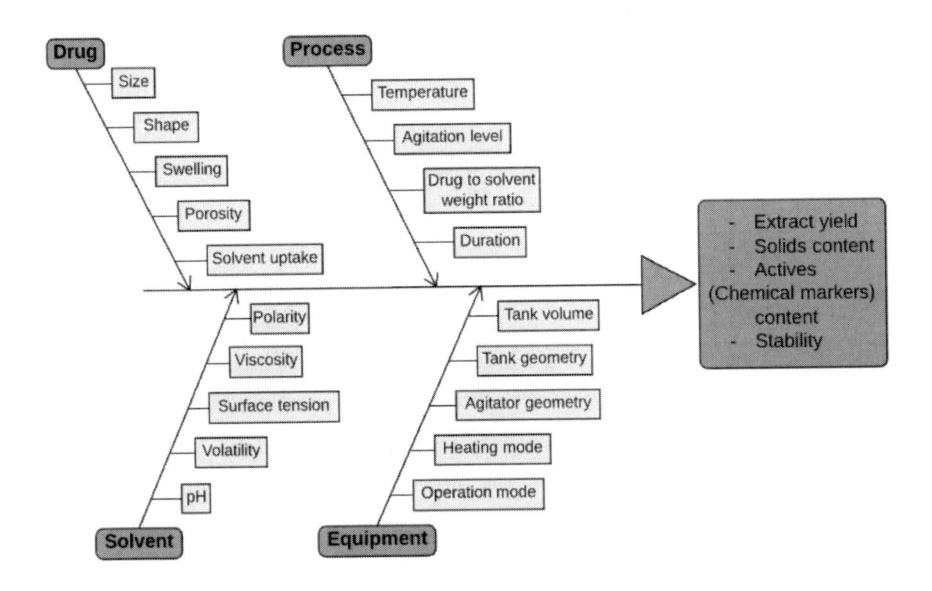

Figure 6. Example of Ishikawa diagram for dynamic maceration of plant drug.

Critical Quality Attributes (CQAs), were selected based on the CPP inventory shown in the Ishikawa diagram and in the literature of the most influential ones. The chosen factors were also based on preliminary experiments and they included: extraction time, Et (12 and 24 h), agitation speed, As (30 and 70 rpm), drug to solvent weight ratio in dry basis, DSr (1/6 and 1/4, g/g), extraction temperature, T (50 and 80ºC) and ethanol strength, ES (70 and 96%, v/v). The factors were codified to carry out the analysis of variance (ANOVA) by the Response Surface Methodology (RSM) using the software Design Expert® 7.0 (Stat-Ease® Inc., Minneapolis, MN, USA). The mathematical models for each response were evaluated using a multiple regression method. The response function used was a linear polynomial equation, given by Equation (1):

$$Y = \beta_0 + \sum_{i=1}^{k} \beta_i x_i + \sum \beta_{ij} x_i x_j \quad (1)$$

In Equation (1), Y is the dependent variable; β_0 is the constant term; k is the number of variables; β_i represents the coefficients of linear parameters; βii represents the coefficients of quadratic terms; β_{ij} represents the coefficients of interaction parameters.

The curcumin contents, CS, in extracted samples were quantified by a validated HPLC method. The solid contents ranged from 0.8 to 3.4%, while CS ranged from 0.1 to 1.8%. These values correspond to soluble solid yields ranging from 4.1 to 14.1% and curcumin yields ranging from 2.0 to 62.6%. The curcumin yield was higher in the present study as compared to a previous work [70], in which curcumin yields ranging from 4.5 to 12.9% were obtained.

The RSM analysis showed that neither the soluble solid contents (SSc) nor the curcumin contents (CS) were affected by the agitation speed or drug to solvent ratio, DSr. However, the Extraction Temperature (ET) and Ethanol Strength (ES) exerted a strong impact on the SSc, with a 0.01% significance level. The ET and ES accounted for 38.9 and 45.2% of SSC variation, respectively. The surface response plot of SSc as a function of the ET and ES is presented in Figure 7, where an increase in the ET had a positive effect on SSC, while ES had a negative effect. The response surface for curcumin contents (CS) can be seen in Figures 8 and 9 and show that CS depended on ET and ES at significance levels of $p<0.01$ and $p<0.05$, respectively. Furthermore, the DOE and response surface analysis could demonstrate the complex relationships among CPPs and CQAs, as all linear terms had a negative influence on CS, but the interactions ET x ES and DSr x ES, had a positive influence at significant levels of 0.1 and 5%, respectively. RSM analysis also showed that ES contributed to 74.3% of the response variability, indicating that this factor is the main CPP to quality risk and should be strictly supervised on an industrial scale. Other terms, such as ET, ET x ES and DSr x ES accounted for 3.0%, 5.0% and 3.0% of CS variability, respectively, and must also be part of a robust process of quality management. It is clear from the results that the alcoholic proportion is the main factor involved in the extraction by dynamic maceration of curcumin from turmeric. The trends observed concerning the influence of ES on the curcumin contents match the trends observed for the SSc, which emphasizes the predominance of curcumin within the curcuminoids found in the sample. The expressive extraction of curcumin using ethanol 70% in the solvent mixture may be due to the higher dielectric constant of this solvent, when compared to the other proportion used (96%) [48]. It is also noteworthy to mention that longer extraction times led to a decrease in the efficiency of the process. A plausible explanation for this behavior may be the occurrence of degradation of the curcumin during extraction.

When developing a QbD, it is important to obtain fitted mathematical models from the RSM analysis. These models are polynomial equations of the dependent variables, CQAs, as a function of the studied factors, CPPs, to predict the quality indicators. The model adequacies were checked accounting for the coefficient of determination, R^2, which is the proportion of variation in the response, attributed to the model rather than random errors and was suggested that for a well fitted model, R^2 should not be less than 80%, or 0.8000. A study on the effect of four factors on curcuma extraction using central composite rotatable design reported R^2 of 0.7800 [70, 38].

Another important fact to comment on is the significance level, α. The value of α should be chosen by the investigator before the data collection and is usually set to 5% ($p<0.05$) or lower. The significance level represents the probability of rejecting the null hypothesis, given that it is true [38]. When the authors decided to study the effect of ET on curcuma extraction, they assumed the hypothesis that this factor has an influence on CS, while the data and ANOVA analysis will confirm if the hypothesis is null or not. For example, the experimental data confirms that ET affects CS at 5% significance level, which means that the probability ($p<0.05$) of being wrong in their assumption (hypothesis) is 5% or only 1 chance in 20. Although from the statistical point of view, significance levels are typically 5% or much lower from the perspective of evaluating the risks to quality in a process, the investigator may choose higher values of α. For instance a probability of 1 chance in 10, or $p<0.10$ (10%), that a specific CPP affects the CQAs may be important in quality risk evaluation.

As well as identifying the main influential CPPs on CQAs, the multivariate approach provides the models and tools to determine the "control space" and also finds the optimal condition. The control space is the region where all CQAs are within their acceptable ranges or within specification limits. One of the techniques that can be adopted for optimization is the Desirability Functions (DF). In the example discussed herein, curcumin extraction from Curcuma *longa* L was carried out by DF using Design Expert 7.0 software. The authors used this technique to show the best operational condition, e.g., to maximize the total soluble solids and curcumin content in the extracts. Among the 30 solutions found by the authors [45], one with 69.0% overall desirability provided the total SSc of 2.9% (w/w) in dry basis and curcumin content of 1.0% (w/w) in dry basis. The extraction in this optimal condition gave "*extracta fluida*" with 12.6% and 35.8% of soluble solid and curcumin yield, respectively. The work provided a successful QbD approach using DOE and RSM for the extraction of curcumin from C. longa rhizomes by dynamic maceration. The critical extraction factors, CPPs, such as extraction time, agitation speed, drug to solvent weight ratio in dry basis, extraction temperature and ethanol strength were identified and their effects were quantified by ANOVA, modeled by RSM and optimized by DF. The solid scientific approach recommended by ICH-Q8 allowed the uncovering effects of in-process parameters on the extraction of curcumin from C. longa rhizomes.

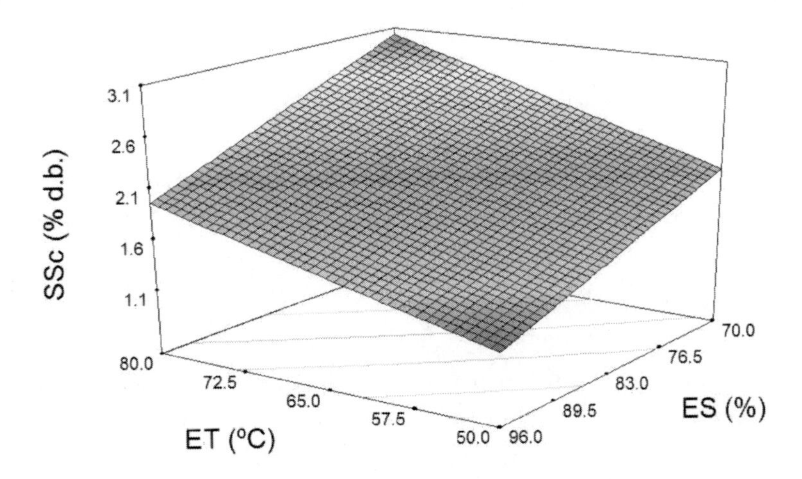

Figure 7. Surface response plot of soluble solid content as a function of the Extraction Temperature and Ethanol Strength in the solvent mixture [45]. (With permission from Rev.Bras. Farmacogn., Elsevier).

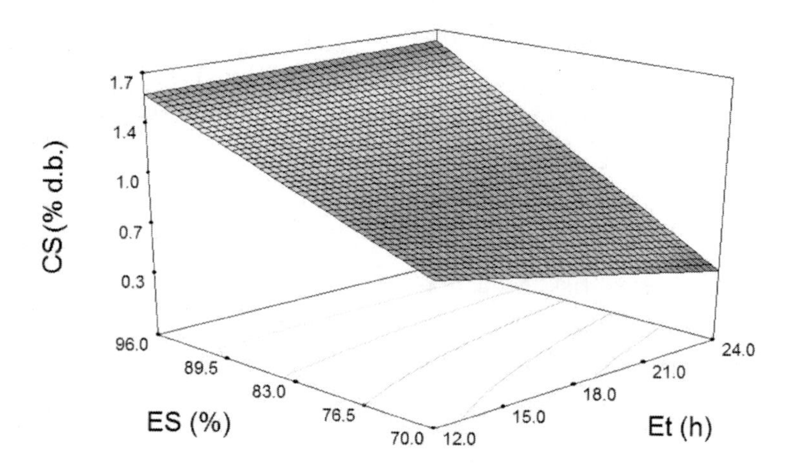

Figure 8. Surface response plot of curcumin content as a function of Extraction Time and Ethanolic Strength in the solvent mixture [45]. (With permission from Rev.Bras. Farmacogn., Elsevier).

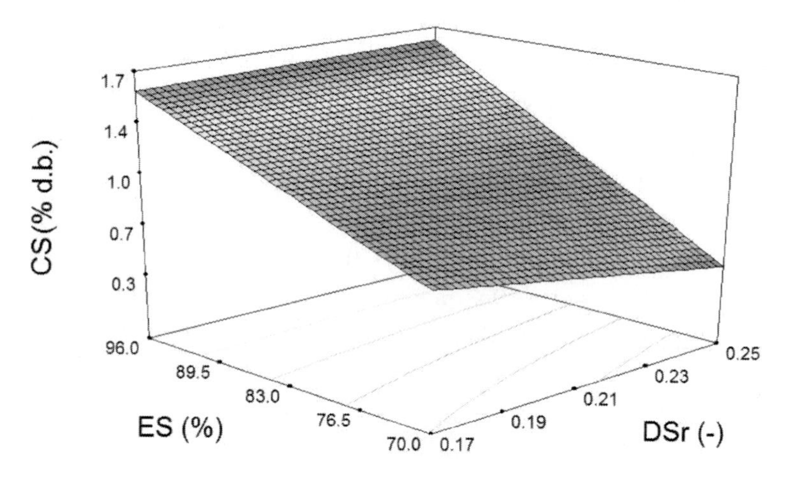

Figure 9. Surface response plot of curcumin content as a function of the weight of the drug to the weight of the solvent ratio and Ethanol Strength in the solvent mixture [45]. (With permission from Rev.Bras. Farmacogn., Elsevier).

DRYING

Liquid plant extracts or "*extracta fluida*" are commonly transformed into dry powders by spray drying or freeze drying for many reasons [71]. Dry plant extracts have the advantages of reduced volume and consequently smaller storage room, easier transportation, increased stability in solid state [72-81] and the possibility of standardizing the bioactive content by combined drying with proper diluents or drying adjuvants [71]. These very positive aspects of dried extracts make drying one of the most important unit operations in the manufacturing of phytomedicines, but at the same time one of the most complex. There are several options of drying methods and equipment available for drying plant extracts and choosing the most suitable one can be a challenging task. Among the most used are freeze drying and spray drying, but the details of each method and criteria for selecting a drying method are discussed in detail in Chapter 6 of this book. The text herein will discuss the application of the QbD principles in the development of a drying process in a spray dryer. First of all, the CPPs and CQAs for a spray drying process should be raised and selected for the study, considering the characteristics of the drying technique chosen and also the main specifications of the final product. The characteristics of the final product, which is a dried powder, will obviously depend on its application and, therefore, many questions arise, such as: Is this the powder a final product? Will it be incorporated into semi-solid formulations such as cream or gel? Will it be used in direct compression? Should it be granulated before compression? Will it be filled in gelatin capsules? Will it be necessary to use drying adjuvants? How can drying adjuvants be chosen? Details in main aspects of drying and spray drying will be discussed in Chapter 6. For now, the focus will be an example of the QbD approach to develop functionalized spray dried plant extracts with the help of a hydrophillic carrier to increase the actives' solubility and bioavailability.

An application of QbD principles to plant extract was presented by [73] and aimed at obtaining dry forms of curcuma extract by spray drying [73] a ternary solid dispersion containing standardized curcumin content. The final form intended was a powder containing a solid dispersion [74] of a lipid carrier with curcumin and a drying adjuvant. The aim was to improve curcumin solubility and achieve better biological activities from curcumin. The lipid carrier chosen was Gelucire® 44/14, a surface-active carrier, consisting of a mixture of glyceril and PEG 1500 esters of long-chain fatty acids [74], thus making the powder obtain a third generation solid dispersion. Finally, the drying adjuvant was a colloidal silicon dioxide, Aerosil®, which is common filler in pharmaceutical preparations and is also a lubricant for solid forms. A schematic diagram showing the main CPPs and CQAs for this case study can be seen in Figure 10.

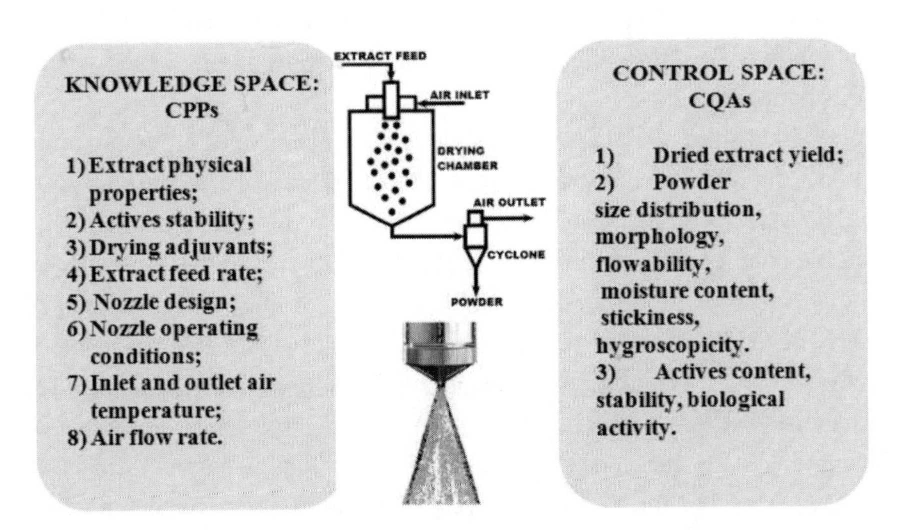

Figure 10. Schematic diagram showing the main Critical Process Parameters, CPPs and Critical Quality Attributes (CQAs) for spray drying of a plant extract using a hydrophilic carrier.

The solid dispersions were prepared by adding a solution of curcumin in ethanol:water (1:1) in molten Gelucire® 44/14 under high shear mixing at 14,000 to 18,000 rpm and slowly adding Aerosil for subsequent drying in a lab scale spray dryer model MSD 0.5 (*Labmaq do Brasil Ltd*, Ribeirão Preto, Brazil) equipped with a two fluid pneumatic atomizer. Drying was performed at a dispersion feed rate of 5 mL/min, atomization air pressure 4.0 kgf/cm2, drying air flow rate 1.5m^3/min, extract solids content 7.5% (w/w). Aiming at using the QbD approach for their development, the authors [73] studied the effect of the Curcumin/Gelucire® ratio - CG, the ratio of Aerosil® - AE, and the outlet temperature – T, on bulk and tapped densities, Hausner ratio and Carr index, angle of repose, water activities and curcumin solubility - CS, following a Box Behnken design with three factors at three levels. The data was analyzed by the surface response methodology, using Statistica 9 (Statsoft, Inc. USA). The authors also adopted 5% as a significance level. Dry extract bulk density varied from 0.14 to 0.21 g/cm3, the Hausner factor varied from 1.08 to 1.63 and Carr indexes from 7.0 to 22.0%. Only three conditions studied led to powders with poor flow and compressibility. The powder water activity was always below 0.5, which is adequate for proper stability. All the relationships between the three CPPs studied and the CQAs were modeled by polynomial fittings and represented by response surfaces. CPPs significantly affected the bulk density and Carr index. As an example, Gelucire® increasing content in composition contributes to the improvement of the powder compressibility characteristics, which may be related to the plastic behavior of this excipient at room temperature. Unexpected influences were also observed, such as the higher angles of repose with increasing Aerosil® content and outlet temperature. This drying adjuvant is widely recognized for its lubricant and excellent flow properties, but in the ternary solid dispersion, had complex interactions with Gelucire, resulting in different particle morphological and flow properties. However, the most important result is related to curcumin solubility. This substance´s low solubility in water is one of the most limiting factors for its therapeutical use.

The spray dried solid dispersions promoted an enhancement of curcumin solubility in water to 1.312 mg/ml, which represented a 1,750 fold increase when compared to the pure drug. The analysis by response surface methodology showed that although there was a huge increase in curcumin solubility in the solid dispersion and that Aerosil® is needed to make the powdered solid dispersion feasible by spray drying, the increase in Aerosil® content has a negative effect on the solubility. The mathematical relationship between Curcumin Solubility, (CS) and the significant factor is shown in Equation 2, fitted with a correlation coefficient R = 0.9834. The ANOVA confirmed the hypothesis that Aerosil® ratio influences CS, as its linear and squared terms had negative influences at the significance levels of 1% and 5%, respectively. The highly hygroscopic character of the type of Aerosil® used, capable of forming a gel in outer layers the microparticles, thus acting as a barrier and negatively affecting drug solubility may explain the AE negative effect on CS.

$$C_s = 0.41 - 0.57\left(\frac{AE:CG-1}{0.5}\right) + 0.26\left(\frac{AE:CG-1}{0.5}\right)^2 \quad (2)$$

This equation, together with all the other relationships for CPPS and CQAs can be used to determine the control space and also the optimal condition to obtain curcumin solid dispersions with high yield, good flow/compression properties, adequate hygroscopicity and the highest solubility enhancement. The authors [73] concluded that the best solid dispersions were obtained with Aerosil® to Gelucire® ratio of 1:5, the lowest ratio of Gelucire® to curcumin, and the lowest drying temperature, 40ºC. Considering these CPP values, the optimal CQAs were: angle of repose of 39.6º, Carr índex of 8% and Hausner ratio of 1.05, the curcumin solubility was 3,200 fold larger than pure drug. Only as complimentary information, the CS in solid dispersion was 6.7 fold higher than its solubility in the physical mixture, which shows that the solubility enhancement was not only due to the formulation itself, but was also a consequence of the process chosen (spray drying) and the operational conditions.

The surface plot of CS as a function of AE and temperature is shown in Figure 11, where there is an evident effect of Aerosil® content, but no influence of temperature on CS.

Differential Scanning Calorimetry (DSC), Hot Stage Microscopy (HSM), Infra Red Spectroscopy (FT-IR), X-ray Powder Diffraction (XRPD) and microparticles morphology by Scanning Electron Microscopy (SEM) complemented the study of solid dispersion characterization. Besides the curcumin solubility in water, CS, the dissolution rate is also important for the bioavailability of the drug. The dissolution profile, according to the Pharmacopoeia (USP, 1995), of curcumin from solid dispersion inserted in membrane bags in HCl (pH 1.2) and phosphate buffer (pH 5.8 and 7.4) solutions are shown in Figure 12. The Figure also shows the dissolution rate of pure curcumin. After 10 minutes of dissolution assay, 90% of curcumin from DS was released in pH 1.2 and 5.8. Furthermore, 75% of the curcumin was released in 10 minutes in phosphate buffer pH 7.4, while for the pure drug the amount released was not detectable by liquid chromatography (HPLC). The maximum curcumin released was 95% for solid dispersion and 20% for pure curcumin. The data provided is a good example of how the QbD approach may lead to robust and efficient processes.

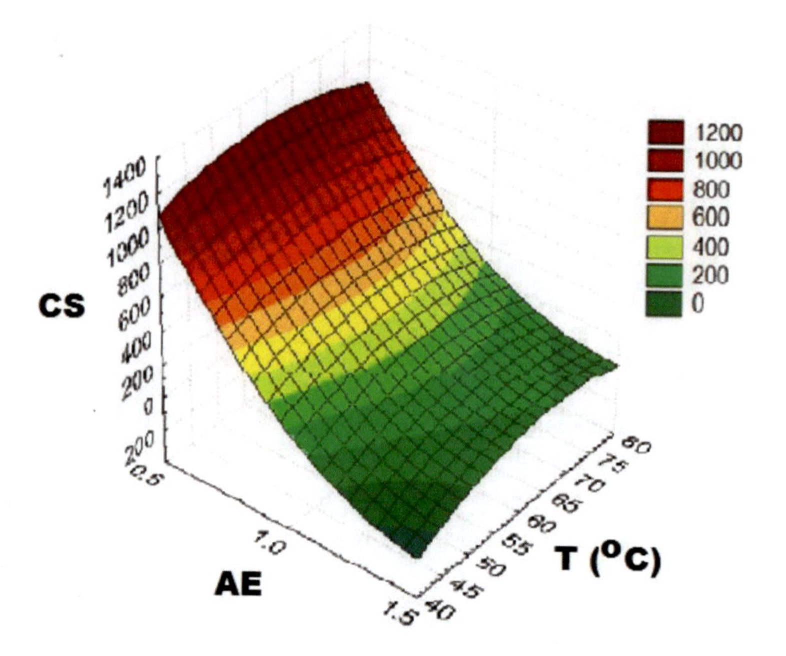

Figure 11. Surface response plot of curcumin solubility as a function of outlet spray air temperature and Aerosil® ratio in solid dispersion [73]. (With the permission of Drying Technology Journal, Taylor & Francis Inc.).

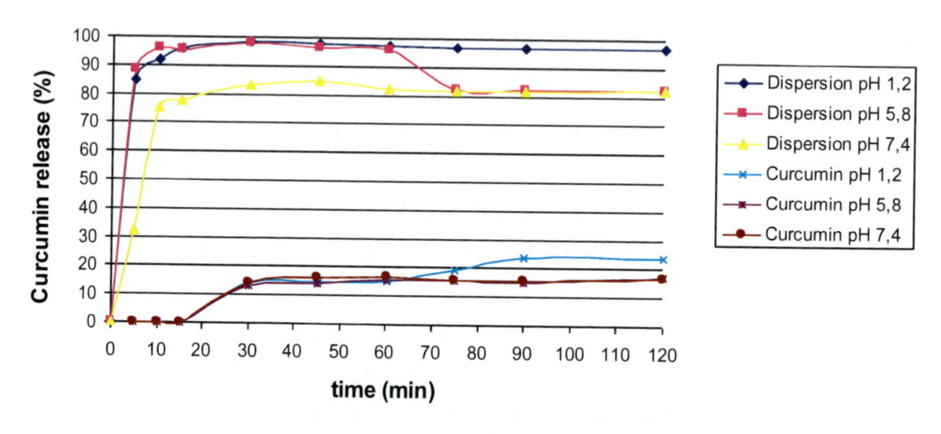

Figure 12. Dissolution of curcumin from solid dispersions in pH 1.2, 5.8 and 7.4 [73]. (With the permission of Drying Technology Journal, Taylor & Francis Inc.).

References

[1] List, P.H., Schmidt, P.C. Phytopharmaceutical Technology. *CRC Press,* Boca Raton, Fl, USA, 374 p., 1984.

[2] Wijesekera, R.O.B. The Medicinal Plant Industry. *CRC Press*, Boca Raton, Fl, USA. 2000.

[3] Musthaba, S.M.; Baboota, S.; Ahmed S.; Ahuja A.; Ali, J. Status of novel drug delivery technology for phytotherapeutics. *Expert Opin Drug Deliv.* 6(6):625-37, 2009.

[4] Gurib-Fakim, A. Medicinal plants: traditions of yesterday and drugs of tomorrow. *Mol Aspects Med.* 27(1):1-93, 2006.

[5] Tyler, V.E. Phytopmedicines: back to the future. *Journal of Natural Products.* 62: 1589-1592, 1999.

[6] Calixto, J.B. Efficacy, safety, quality control, marketing and regulatory guidelines for herbal medicines (phytotherapic agents). *Braz J Medical & Biol Research.* 33: 179-189, 2000.

[7] International Conference on Harmonisation, ICH. 2000. Quality Guidelines, Q1 to Q12. http://www.ich.org/products/guidelines/ quality/article/quality-guidelines. html.

[8] Ansarim S.H.; Islam, F.; Sameem, M. Influence of nanotechnology on herbal drugs: A Review. *J Adv Pharm Technol Res.* 3(3): 142–146, 2012.

[9] Bonifácio, B.V.; Silva, P.B.; Ramos, M.A.; Negri K.M.; Bauab, T.M.; Chorilli, M. Nanotechnology-based drug delivery systems and herbal medicines: a review. *Int J Nanomedicine.* 9:1-15, 2014.

[10] Jiang, W.; Yu, L.X. Modern Pharmaceutical Quality Regulations: Question-based Review. Chap 38, p. 885-901. In: Qiu, Y.; Chen, Y.; Zhang, G.G.Z.; Liu, L; Porter, W.R. *Developing Solid Oral Dosage Forms: Pharmaceutical Theory and Practice.* Academic Press/ Elsevier, New York, NY, USA, 943 p.; 2009.

[11] Sun, M.; Su, X.; Ding, B.; He, X.; Liu, X.; Yu, A.; Lou, H.; Zhai, G. Advances in nanotechnology-based delivery systems for curcumin. *Nanomedicine.* 7(7):1085-100, 2012.

[12] C. Capello, U. Fischer, K. Hungerbuhler, What is a green solvent? A comprehensive framework for the environmental assessment of solvents, *Green Chem.,* 9(2007) 927-934.

[13] F. Chemat, N. Rombaut, A.S. Fabiano-Tixier, J.T. Pierson, A. Bily, Green extraction: from concepts to research, education and economical opportunities, In: *Green Extraction of Natural Products: Theory and Practice,* 1st edition, Eds F Chemat & S Struhe, Wiley-VCH Verlag GmbH & Co, Berlin, 2015, pp 1-36.

[14] F. Chemat, M.A. Vian, G. Cravotto, Green extraction of natural products: concept and principles, *Int J Mol Sci.,* 13(2012) 8615-8627.

[15] Mandal, V.; Mohan, Y.; Hemalatha, S.; Microwave Assisted Extraction – An Innovative and Promising Extraction Tool for Medicinal Plant Research. *Pharmacognosy Reviews*, 1: 7-18, 2007.

[16] Shirsath, S.R.; Sonawane, S.H.; Gogate, P.R. Intensification of extraction of natural products using ultrasonic irradiations-A review of current status. *Chemical Engineering and Processing,* 53: 10-23, 2013.

[17] Immel, B.K. "A Brief History of the GMPs for Pharmaceuticals." *Bio Pharm.* 13(8): 26-36, 2000. Revised version: GMP News. http://gmpnews.ru/wp-content/uploads/2010/05/History-gmp.pdf, accessed in 01/18/2017 15:30h.

[18] Office of Women's Health, FDA Milestones in Women's Health: Looking Back as We Move into the New Millennium (FDA, Rockville, MD, 2000), www.fda.gov/womens/milesbro.html.

[19] FDA. Food and Drug Administration. U.S. Department of Health and Human Services. Guidance for Industry. Process Validation: General Principles and Practices. 2011. http://www.fda.gov/Drugs/Guidance Compliance Regulatory Information/Guidances/default.htm. Acessed 01/28/2017 at 9:58h.

[20] Q7-ICH, International Conference on Harmonization of Technical Requirements for Registration of Pharmaceuticals for Human Use. Q7 Good Manufacturing Practice. ICH Expert Working Group, 2009. http://www.ich.org/products/guidelines /quality/article/quality-guidelines.html.

[21] Q8-R2-ICH, International Conference on Harmonization of Technical Requirements for Registration of Pharmaceuticals for Human Use. Q8(R2) Pharmaceutical Development. ICH Expert Working Group, 2009.

[22] Q9-ICH, International Conference on Harmonization of Technical Requirements for Registration of Pharmaceuticals for Human Use. Q9 Pharmaceutical Quality Risk Management. ICH Expert Working Group, 2009. http://www.ich.org /products/guidelines/quality/article/ quality-guidelines.html.

[23] Q10-ICH, International Conference on Harmonization of Technical Requirements for Registration of Pharmaceuticals for Human Use. Q10 Pharmaceutical Quality System. ICH Expert Working Group, 2009. http://www.ich.org/products/guidelines /quality/article/quality-guidelines.html.

[24] Somma, R.; Signore, A.A. Embracing Quality by Design: Applying QbD concepts can help CMOs create value. *Contract Pharma*, pg October 2008.

[25] Li, M. Implementation of Quality by Design Case Study. *Chemistry Today*. 31(5): 64-68, 2013.

[26] Van Buskirk, G.A.; Asotra, S.; Balducci, C.; Basu, P.; DiDonato, G.; Dorantes, A.; Mark Eickhoff, W.; Ghosh, T.; González, M.A.; Henry,T.; Howard, M.; Kamm, J.; Laurenz, S.; MacKenzie, R.; Mannion, R.; Noonan, P.K.; Ocheltree, T.; Pai, U.; Poska, R.P.; Putnam, M.L.; Raghavan, R.R.; Ruegger, C.; Sánchez, E.; Shah, V.P.; Shao, Z.J.; Somma, R.; Tammara, V.; Thombre, A.G. Best Practices for the Development, Scale-up, and Post-approval Change Control of IR and MR Dosage Forms in the Current Quality-by-Design Paradigm. *AAPS Pharm Sci Tech.* 15(3):665-692, 2014.

[27] Yu, L.X. Pharmaceutical Quality by Design: Product and Process Development, Understanding, and Control. *Pharmaceutical Research,* 25(4): 781-790, 2008.

[28] Neeway, J.O. Process Excellence: The five critical elements of Quality by Design. *Bioprocess International*. Pg. 18-22, 2008.

[29] Rathore, A.S. A Roadmap for implementation of Quality by Design (QbD) for biotechnology products. *Trends in Biotechnoloogy*. 27(9): 546-553, 2009.

[30] Huang, J.; Kaul, G.; Cai, C.; Chatlapalli, R.; Hernandez-Abad, P.; Ghosh, K.; Nagi, A. Quality by design case study: An integrated multivariate approach to drug product and process development. *International Journal of Pharmaceutics* 382 (2009) 23–32.

[31] Xu, B.; Shi, X.; Qiao, Y.; Wu, Z.; Lin, Z. Establishment of design space for production process of Chinese traditional medicine preparation. *China Journal of Chinese Materia Medica*. 38(6): 924-929, 2013.

[32] Yan, B.; Li, Y.; Guo, Z.; Qu, H. Quality by Design for Herbal Drugs: a Feedforward Control Strategy and an Approach to Define the Acceptable Ranges of Critical Quality Attributes. *Phytochem. Anal.* 2014, 25, 59–65.

[33] Juran, J.M. Quality Control Handbook. 6th Edition. McGraw Hill, NY, USA, 2010.

[34] Deming, W.E. The new economics: for industry, government, education. 2nd Edition. *MIT Press,* Cambridge, MS, USA, 2000.

[35] Aksu, B.; De Beer, T.; Folestad, S.; Ketolainen, J.; Lindén, H.; Lopes, J.A; Matas, M.; Oostra, W.; Rantanen, J.; Weimer, M. Strategic funding priorities in the pharmaceutical sciences allied to Quality by Design (QbD) and Process Analytical Technology (PAT). *European Journal of Pharmaceutical Sciences*. 47:402–405, 2012.

[36] Lebrun, P.; Krier, F.; Mantanus, J.; Grohganz, H.; Yang, M.; Rozet, E.; Boulanger, B.; Evrard, B.; Rantanen, J.; Hubert, P. Design space approach in the optimization of the spray-drying process. *European Journal of Pharmaceutics and Biopharmaceutics* 80 (2012) 226–234.

[37] Mello, P.M.; Thorat, B.N.; Lanchote, A.; Freitas, L.A.P. Green extraction of glycosides from Stevia rebaudiana (Bert) with low solvent consumption. *Res Effic Technol,* 2(4): 247-253, 2016.

[38] Box, G.E.; Hunter, J.S.; Hunter, W.G. Statistics for experimenters: Design, innovation and discovery. 2nd Edition. John Wiley & Sons Inc, 2005.

[39] Gupta SC, Patchva S, Koh W, Aggarwal BB 2012. Discovery of curcumin, a component of golden spice, and its miraculous biological activities. *Clin. Exp. Pharmacol. Physiol.* 39 (3): 283-299.

[40] Aggarwal BB, Harikumar KB 2009. Potential therapeutic effects of curcumin, the anti-inflammatory agent, against neurodegenerative, cardiovascular, pulmonary, metabolic, autoimmune and neoplastic diseases. *The International Journal of Biochemistry & Cell Biology* 41: 40-59.

[41] Ahmed T, Enam SA, Gilani AH 2010. Curcuminoids enhance memory in an amyloid-infused rat model of Alzheimer's Disease. *Neuroscience* 169: 1296-1306.

[42] Jurenka JS 2009. Anti-inflammatory Properties of Curcumin, a Major Constituent of Curcuma longa: A Review of Preclinical and Clinical Research. *Alternative Medicine Review* 14 (2): 141-153.

[43] Wilken R, Veena MS, Wang MB, Srivatsan ES 2011. Curcumin: A review of anti-cancer properties and therapeutic activity in head and neck squamous cell carcinoma. *Molecular Cancer*, 10(12): 1-19.

[44] Teixeira, C.C.C.; Mendonça, L.M.; Bergamaschi, M.M.; Queiroz, R.H.C.; Souza, G.E.P.; Antunes, L.M.G.; Freitas1, L.A.P. Microparticles Containing Curcumin Solid Dispersion: Stability, Bioavailability and Anti-Inflammatory Activity. *AAPS Pharm Sci Tech,* 17(2): 252-261, 2016.

[45] Paulucci, V.P.; Couto, R.O.; Teixeira, C.C.C.; Freitas, L.A.P. Optimization of the extraction of curcumin from Curcuma longa rhizomes. *Rev Bras Farmacogn*, 23(1): 94-100, 2013.

[46] Noriega P, Mafud DF, Souza B, Soares-Scott M, Rivelli DP, Barros SBM, Bacchi EM 2012. Applying design of experiments (DOE) to flavonoid extraction from Passiflora alata and P. edulis. *Revista Brasileira de Farmacognosia* Aop02812.

[47] Ong ES 2004. Extraction methods and chemical standardization of botanicals and herbal preparations. *Journal of Chromatography B* 812: 23-33.

[48] Jouyban A, Soltanpour S, Chan HK 2004. A simple relationship between dielectric constant of mixed solvents with solvent composition and temperature. *International Journal of Pharmaceutics* 269: 353-360.

[49] Luque de Castro, M.D.; Garcia-Ayuso, L.E. Soxhlet extraction of solid materials: an outdated technique with a promising innovative future. *Analytica Chimica Acta* 369 1-10, 1998.

[50] Zarnowski, R.; Suzuki, Y. Expedient Soxhlet extraction of resorcinolic lipids from wheat grains. *Journal of Food Composition and Analysis,* 17: 649–664, 2004.

[51] Siqueira, S.; Falcão-Silva, V.S. Agra, M.F.; Dariva, C.; Siqueira-Júnior, J.P. Fonseca, M.J.V. Biological activities of Solanum paludosum Moric. extracts obtained by maceration and supercritical fluid extraction. *The Journal of Supercritical Fluids*, 58: 391–397, 2011.

[52] Tacon, L.A.; Freitas, L.A.P. Box-Behken design to study the bergenin content and antioxidant activity of Endopleura uchi (L) Bark extracts obtained by dynamic maceration. *Rev Bras Farmacogn,* 23(1): 67-71, 2013.

[53] Costa-Machado, A.R.M.; Freitas, L.A.P. Dynamic maceration of Copaiba langsdorffii leaves: a technological study using fractional factorial design. *Rev Bras Farmacogn.* 23(1): 79-85, 2013.

[54] Kaufmann, B., & Christen, P. Recent extraction techniques for natural products: Microwave-assisted extraction and pressurized solvent extraction. *Phytochemical Analysis,* 13: 105–113, 2002.

[55] Rostagno, M.A. Palma, M. Barroso, C.G. Pressurized liquid extraction of isoflavones from soybeans. *Analytica Chimica Acta,* 522: 169–177, 2004.

[56] Costa FSO, Araújo Júnior CA, Silva EJ, Bara MTF, Lima EM, Valadares MC, Marreto RN 2011. Impact of ultrasound-assisted extraction on quality and photostability of the Pothomorphe umbellata extracts. *Ultrasonics Sonochemistry* 18: 1002-1007.

[57] Chemat, S.; Lagha, A.; AitAmar, H.; Bartels, P. V.; Chemat, F. Comparison of conventional and ultrasound-assisted extraction of carvone and limonene from caraway seeds. *Flavour and Fragrance Journal,* 19: 188–195, 2004.

[58] Gu, X.; Cai, J.; Zhu, X.; Su, Q. Dynamic Ultrasound-Assited Extraction of Polyphenols in Tobacco. *J. Sep. Sci.,* 28: 2477-2481, 2005.

[59] Mason, T.J.; Paniwnyk, L.; Lorimer, J.P. The uses of Ultrasound in Food Technology. *Ultrasonics and Sonochemistry*, 3: S253-S260, 1996.

[60] Patist, A.; Bates, D. Ultrasonic Innovations in the Food Industry: From the Laboratory to Commercial Production. *Innovative Food Science & Emerging Technol.,* 9:147-154, 2008.

[61] Mandal V, Mohan Y, Hemalatha S 2008. Microwave assisted extraction of curcumin by sample–solvent dual heating mechanism using Taguchi L9 orthogonal design. *Journal of Pharmaceutical and Biomedical Analysis* 46: 322-327.

[62] Brachet, A., Christen, P.; Veuthey, J.L. Focused microwave-assisted extraction of cocaine and benzoylecgonine from coca leaves. *Phytochemical Analysis,* 13, 162–169, 2002.

[63] Pan, Y.; He, C.; Wang, H.; Ji, X.; Wang, K.; Liu, P. Antioxidant activity of microwave-assisted extract of Buddleia officinalis and its major active component. *Food Chemistry,* 121: 497-502, 2010.

[64] Talebi, M.; Ghassempour, A.; Talebpour, Z.; Rassouli, A.; Dolatyari, L. Optimization of the Extraction of Paclitaxel from Taxus baccata L. by the Use of Microwave Energy. *J.Sep. Sci.,* 27: 1130-1136, 2004.

[65] Wakte PS, Sachin BS, Patil AA, Mohato DM, Band TH, Shinde DB 2011. Optimization of microwave, ultra-sonic and supercritical carbon dioxide assisted extraction techniques for curcumin from Curcuma longa. *Separation and Purification Technology* 79: 50-55.

[66] Brunner, G., Gas Extraction. An Introduction to Fundamentals of Supercritical Fluids and the Application to Separation Processes. Springer, New York, NY, 1994.

[67] Reverchon, E.; Senatore, F. Supercritical Carbon Dioxide Extraction of Chamomile Essential Oil and Its Analysis by Gas Chromatography-Mass Spectrometry. *J. Agric. food Chem.* 42: 154-158, 1994.

[68] Costa, A.R.M.; Freitas, L.A.P.; Mendiola, J.; Ibanez, E. Copaifera langsdorffii supercritical fluid extraction: chemical and functional characterization by LC/MS and in vitro assays. *J Supercritical Fluids*. 100: 86-96, 2015.

[69] Ishikawa, K.; Loftus, J.H. Introduction to quality control. 3rd Edition. Tokyo 3A Corporation, Tokyo, Japan, 1990, 435 pages.

[70] Sogi et al. extração de curcuma.

[71] Marreto, R.N.; Freire, J.T.; Freitas, L.A.P. Drying of Pharmaceuticals: The Applicability of Spouted Beds. *Drying Technology* 2006, 24: 327-338.

[72] Muzzio, F.J.; Shinbrot, T.; Glasser, B.J. Powder Technology in the Pharmaceutical Industry: The Need to Catch up Fast. *Powder Technology* 2002, 124: 1-7.

[73] Araújo, R.R.; Teixeira, C.C.C.; Freitas, L.A.P. The preparation of ternary solid dispersions of an herbal drug via spray drying of liquid feed. *Drying Technology*, 28, 412–421, 2010.

[74] Serajuddin, A.T. Solid dispersion of poorly water-soluble drugs: early promises, subsequent problems, and recent breakthroughs. *J. Pharm. Sci.* 1999, 88: 1058–1066.

[75] Souza, J.P.B.; Tacon, L.A.; Correia, C.C.; Bastos, J.K.; Freitas, L.A.P. Spray-dried Propolis Extract. II: Prenylated Components of Green Propolis. *Die Pharmazie* 2007, 62(7): 488-492.

[76] Couto, R.O.; Martins, F.S.; Chaul, L.T. Conceição, E.C.; Freitas, L.A.P. Bara, M.T.F.; Paula, J.R. Spray drying of Eugenia dysenterica extract: effects of in-process parameters on product quality, *Brazilian Journal of Pharmacognosy,* 23(1): 115-123, 2013.

[77] Endale, A.; Schmidt, P.C.; Gebre-Mariam, T. Standardization and Physicochemical Characterization of the Extracts of Seeds of Glinus lotoides. *Pharmazie,* 59: 34-38, 2004.

[78] Marquele, F.D.; Stracieri, K.M.; Fonseca, M.J.V; Freitas, L.A.P. Spray-dried Propolis Extract. I: Physico-chemical and Antioxidant Properties. *Die Pharmazie* 2006, 61(4): 325-330.

[79] Martins, R.R.; Pereira, S.V.; Siqueira, S.; Salomão, W.F.; Freitas, L.A.P. Curcuminoid content and antioxidant activity in spray dried microparticles containing turmeric extract. *Food Research International,* v. 50: 657-663, 2013.

[80] Murugesan, R.; Orsat, V. Spray Drying for the Production of Nutraceutical Ingredients—A Review. *Food Bioprocess Technol* 5: 3–14, 2012.

[81] Peixoto, M.P.G.; Freitas, L.A.P. Spray-dried extracts from Syzygium cumini seeds: physicochemical and biological evaluation. *Brazilian Journal of Pharmacognosy,* 23(1): 115-123, 2013.

In: Recent Developments in Phytomedicine Technology ISBN: 978-1-53611-977-0
Editors: L. A. Pedro de Freitas et al.

Chapter 4

THE IMPORTANCE OF EXPERIMENTAL DESIGN IN THE STANDARDIZATION FOR DEVELOPING ANALYTICAL METHODOLOGIES

Tatiana P. F. Cabral, Cristiane C. C. Teixeira, Aurea Donizeti Lanchote and Luis Alexandre P. Freitas*

Faculdade de Ciências Farmacêuticas de Ribeirão Preto,
Universidade de São Paulo-USP, Brasil

ABSTRACT

Experimental design is a development tool to validate and characterize methods and is an approach within the product and process development. Optimization of an analytic method is usually achieved by changing parameters one by one, which is commonly called the "one factor/variable at a time" methodology. On the contrary, the Design of Experiments (DoE) methodology investigates the effects of factors and the interactions between them by modifying multiple factors at a time. Combined with Design Space (DS), it leads to a powerful methodology (DoE-DS), which can identify optimal conditions to obtain robust analytical methods. It is also a key aspect of Quality by Design (QbD), which has the advantage of using method development for new methods or those that need improvement (seek to understand where critical process parameters are in the analytical method and to minimize their influence on accuracy and precision), method validation (validate the analytical method for a range of concentrations) and quantitation of the influence of analytical methods on product and process acceptance and out-of-specification. Consequently, using experimental design in QbD helps to obtain the maximum information from a minimum number of experiments. It also helps to study

* Corresponding Author Email: lapdfrei@fcfrp.usp.br.

effects individually by varying all operating parameters simultaneously and it takes into account variability in experiments, operators, raw materials or processes themselves.

Keywords: analytical method, analytical methodologies, experimental design, Quality by Design (QbD), Analytical Quality by Design (AQbD), validation

INTRODUCTION

A major obstacle encountered when dealing with natural products is separating and identifying their constituents. The structural diversity of their components is one of the reasons that make them interesting; however the same structural variability makes it difficult to quantify their constituents [1]. Aiming to reduce these limitations, increasingly more research has been conducted in an attempt to improve separation techniques, analysis and identification of these molecules. Analytical Quality by Design (AQbD) is used as a factorial design tool in this context. It is important as it helps to solve problems concerning methods of analysis of natural products.

Generic companies are implementing the QbD approach for formulation development and it is compulsory for the prospect of USFDA. There are still no specific requirements for QbD and PAT (Process Analytical Technology) in analytical development in regulatory agencies [2].

It should be mentioned that using the experimental design based on statistical principles one can obtain the maximum useful information by doing a minimum number of experiments [3]. Thus, data using statistical tools can select critical variables of the methods and then find the optimum condition of analysis [4].

By analyzing one variable at a time and keeping the others fixed, we have the univariate method of experimentation. Comparing this method with multivariate techniques (modifying all variables simultaneously), a considerable disadvantage can be observed as this method requires more time and precludes the study of the interaction between the variables. This study is extremely important because the optimal value of one of them may depend on the value of the others, a fact that is very common [5, 6].

In order to improve the process, decrease the variability of the results, as well as a reduction in time and costs analysis, proper planning is necessary because it is an essential tool [7].

Therefore, the main objective of this chapter is to show the use of this important quality tool found in the pharmaceutical industry to develop and validate analytical methods for natural products.

Location of Experimental Design within the Methodology to Develop and Standardize Analytical Methods

The pharmaceutical industry has been growing rapidly over the last decade, focusing on quality, safety and efficacy of the products. Taking this into account, it has invested in tools such as QbD and PAT, which can increase the number of developed products. Due to the fact that statistical analysis is included in analytical QDB is now called AQbD [2].

AQbD helps to develop a strong effective analytical method that is applicable throughout the life cycle of the product. It facilitates flexibility when regulating the analytical method. This means the freedom to change parameters within the experimental design method.

The development of traditional and scientific analytical methods is very different. The traditional approach does not use statistical calculations and risk assessment. The expression of the QbD and AQbD tools is different for process development and analytical development [4]. Figure 1 shows the steps for traditional and scientific approaches for the analytical development.

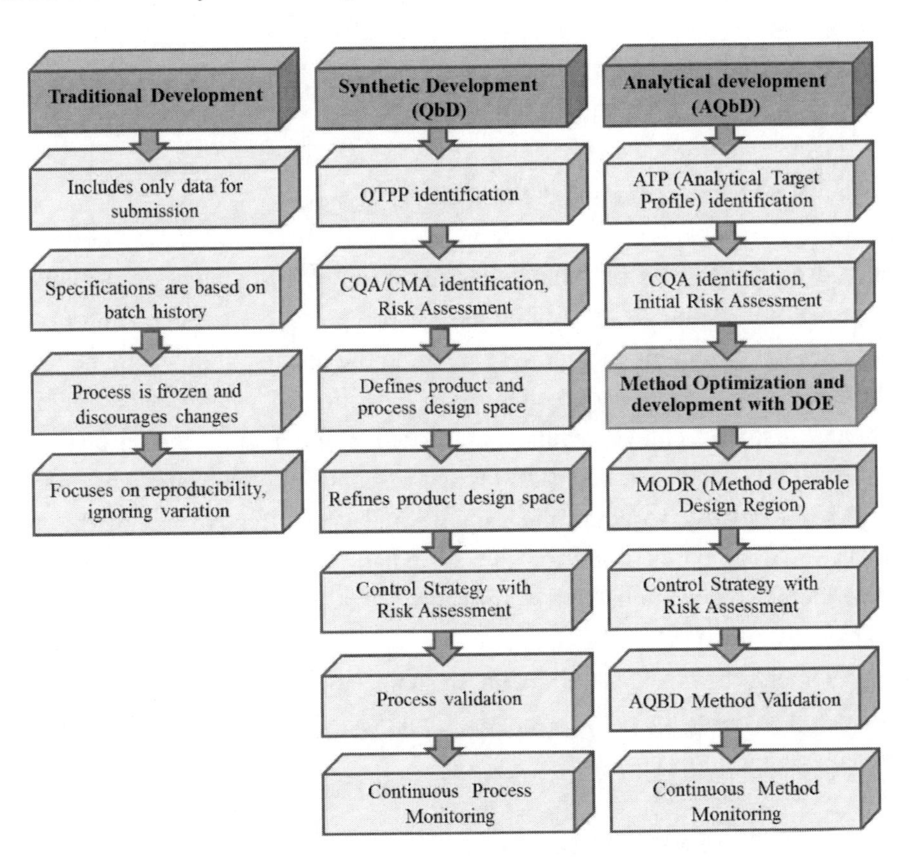

Figure 1. Difference between conventional method/QbD and AQbD [2, 4].

The conventional method consists of varying one variable at a time, keeping the others fixed (univariate method). In this method, many experiments are required and it does not allow for the study of the interactions between these variables. A single integrated project, which allows variations of more than one factor at a time and can determine the effects of interaction (multivariate method), facilitates and increases the chances of obtaining an effective analytical method, in terms of what is proposed.

Advantages of well-designed experiments are:

- Increased amount of information for experiments
- Improved efficiency and organization
- Reliability of information
- Assesssing interactions
- Reliable forecast

The main steps for the design of experiments (DOE) involve:

- Defining the goal,
- Selecting the variable process,
- Choosing an experimental design,
- Project execution,
- Analysing and interpreting the results.

It should be highlighted that implementing the DOE in the analytical method is not QbD, because DOE is one of the AQbD tools and represents the interaction between the input variables that affect the method response and the results. In this conjuncture, AQbD is the preferred and recommended strategy to be followed when developing analytical methods, and also to achieve regulatory flexibility and reduce the results of out-of-specification (OOS), out-of-trend (OOT), out-of-control (OOC) and out-of-statistical-control (OOSC), greatly reducing the strength and cost effectiveness of the analytical method. The six sigma is used for the systematic improvement of the process by eliminating defects with statistical significance (PUCC-Process of Understanding the Control and Capability) [8].

Using elements to manage the quality system, risk and statistical methods is more cost effective in terms of the process and the final product.

The main AQbD tools are:

- Analytical Target Profile (ATP)
- Critical Quality Attributes (CQAs)
- Optimization and Development Method with DOE

- Method operable design region (MODR)
- Control Strategy
- AQbD Method Validation
- Continuous Method Monitoring (CMM).

Analytical Target Profile (ATP)

The beginning of the AQbD process is called ATP, which aims to define the purpose of the process. ATP defines the analytes that are measured, the matrix, the concentration range and the criterion required for carrying out the method. All these features, as well as these specifications must be in accordance with the purpose of the analytical process. By being flexible, ATP enables the analytical methodology to be continuously improved [2, 9].

Critical Quality Attributes (CQAs)

The physical, chemical, biological or microbiological properties that are within a limit, range or distribution to ensure the desired product quality are called CQAs. The resolution criteria, separation, running time and accuracy can be related to CQAs [10].

The validation features (trueness, precision, accuracy, linearity range, limit of quantification) of the results obtained are the CQA keys, which need to be included with their respective values in the ATP [4, 11].

Optimization and Development Method with DOE

The purpose of a design of experiments is to identify the most important parameters for the result and define the minimum number of experiments. A parameter is considered important when its variation causes significant differences in the result [7].

The first step of the planning phase is to construct a table (screening design) with some combinations of the involved parameters. Calibrating the results with the observed values is important to check the possibility of reducing the parameter range variation and even exclude the uncalibrated events. The second step is to set a response surface for selected experiments; the surface is usually linear and with interaction between the parameters and verifies which terms actually contribute to the response [3].

It is worth mentioning that the choice of the type of planning to be used should take into account the objectives of the process and the experiment, as fractionated designs are performed to obtain a screening of variables, the complete designs to evaluate the influence of variables, modeling by least squares to build empirical models and the response surface for improvement [3].

The generation of experiments can be done using various techniques (Figure 2) [12]. Further details of these designs are described in chapter 3.

An important point in designing is the selection of variables and their levels. Process variables include both inputs and outputs, i.e., factors and responses. The most popular experimental design is relaying projected levels (tune level design) because it is ideal for simple and economical screening projects. It also provides most of the information needed to reach multilevel surface response experiments, if necessary [3].

Method Operable Design Region (MODR)

In addition to the validation method, the verification method can be performed through the junction of accuracy and precision assessment at different method factor points within the chromatographic separation (defining the MODR). Checking many points within MODR likely represents a high probability of the method's ability to meet the requirement of ATP [13, 14].

Validating and verifying the experiments should demonstrate the robustness across the parameter ranges from low to high through the target value of variable.

Control Strategy and Risk Assessment

Control strategy is a planned set of controls, derived from the analyte nature and understanding of MODR. Control strategy method can be established based on statistical data collected during the stages of DOE and MODR. Using these experimental statistical data, correlations can be drawn between the method and the analyte attributes for the ability to meet ATP criteria [15, 16].

The control strategy resolves the inconsistency of the method parameters (for example, reagent grade, trademark or instrument type and column type). The control strategy of the method does not dramatically seem different to the AQbD approach, compared to the traditional approach. However, the control methods are established based on CQA, DOE and the experimental data of MODR to ensure a stronger link between the purpose of the method and its performance.

AQbD Validation Method

The approach of the validation method by AQbD is the validation of the analytical method over a range of different batches of products. This uses both the DOE and MODR knowledge to conceive the validation method for all types of product manufacturing changes without revalidation [17].

The approach provides the validation elements mandatory ICH, as well as information about interactions, measurement uncertainty, control strategy and continuous improvement. This approach requires fewer resources than the traditional validation approach, without affecting the quality.

According to the ICH Q8 orientation process [18], robustness is defined as "the ability of a process to tolerate variability of materials and changes of the process and the equipment without a negative impact on the quality." The properties of the materials will affect the robustness of the substance in the synthetic process, impurity profile, the physico-chemical properties, capability and stability of the process.

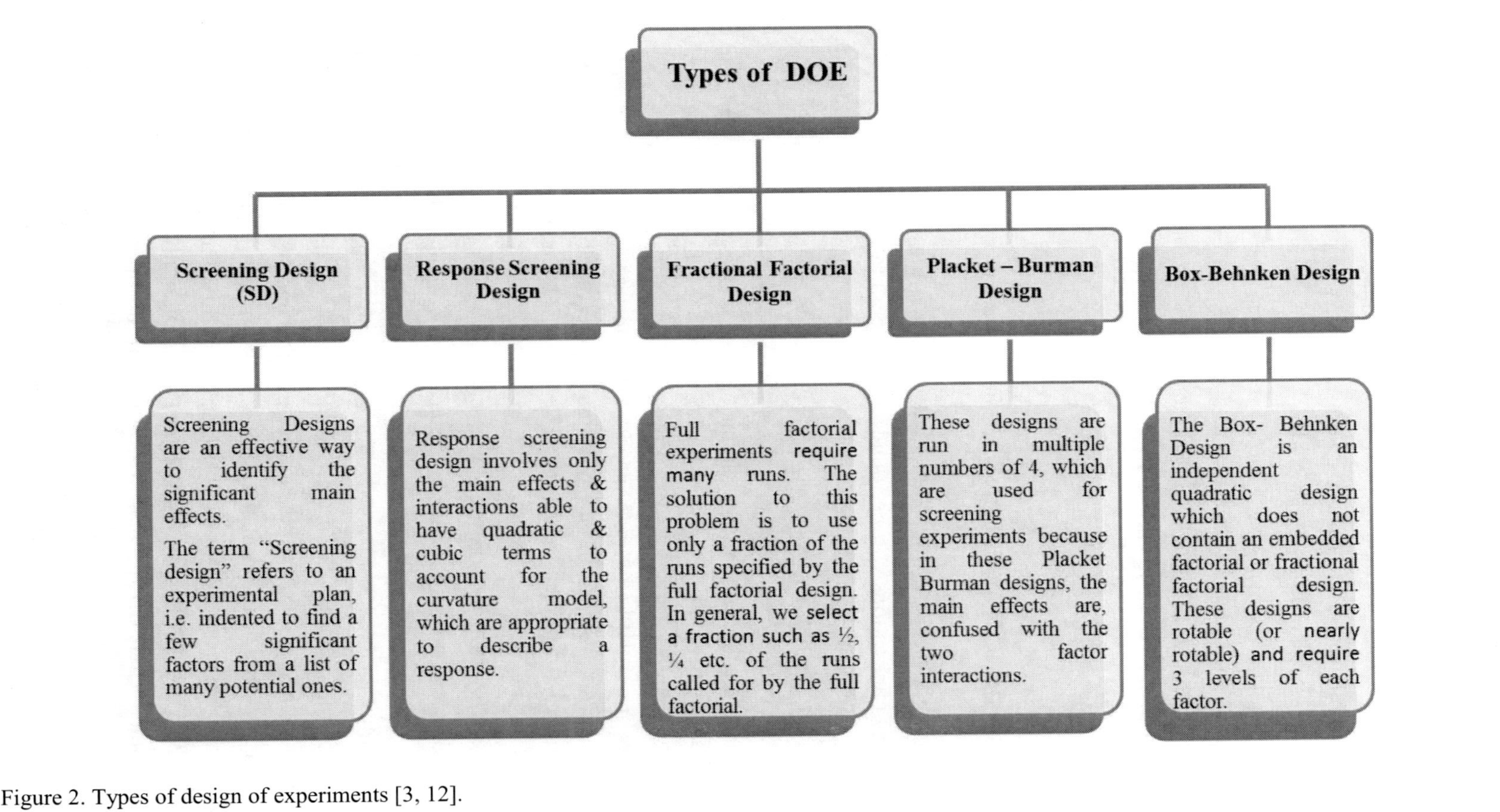

Figure 2. Types of design of experiments [3, 12].

Continuous Method Monitoring (CMM)

The last step of the AQbD cycle is called CMM. This process of sharing knowledge gained during the development and implementation of the production route can be used routinely, and the performance of the process is constantly monitored. This monitoring enables the analyst to detect, identify and address any defect or out-of-trend performance of the analytical method [2].

The success rate of AQbD depends on the right approach, planning, using tools and the performance of the work in a timely fashion. Applying the proper risk assessment tools at the right time can lead to preventing failure of the method and better understanding the designed strategy and its control.

Development of Analytical Methodologies

Various techniques, already consolidated, are widely used to characterize plant extracts [19]. Numerous publications can be found in the literature on this subject from technical fractionation and further analysis to spectroscopic techniques and high-performance liquid chromatography (HPLC) [20, 21]. Each analytical technique has a specific principle that can be selected based on the nature of the analytes.

Among the most modern analysis methods, chromatography occupies a prominent place, because it can separate, identify and quantify chemical species together with instrumental techniques, such as spectrophotometry or mass spectrometry [22].

Considering this, the use of HPLC, UPLC and GC can be mentioned, as well as various other methods of analysis and quantification: UV-visible, fluorescence, mass spectrometry, nuclear magnetic resonance (structure elucidation) and Corona CAD, among others.

Brief Observations on Chromatography

First used in 1906, chromatography was attributed to a Russian botanist, Mikhael Semenovich Tswett, who described his experiments of separating leaf extracts components. In this study, the passage of petroleum ether (mobile phase) through a glass tube filled with calcium carbonate (stationary phase), to which was added the extract led to the separation of components in colored bands. Despite this and several other previous studies, this technique was not used until the 1930s, when it was rediscovered. Since then, various studies have been carried out in an attempt to improve this technique [23].

The principle of this chromatography is to separate the components of a mixture by physico-chemical methods. Considering this, two phases are in intimate contact and the mixture will be distributed between the phases. One of the phases remains stationary and the other moves through it. During this passage, the mixture components are distributed among two phases, some components retained on the stationary phase and eluted together with other mobile phase [22].

Chromatographic methods are classified as illustrated in Figure 3.

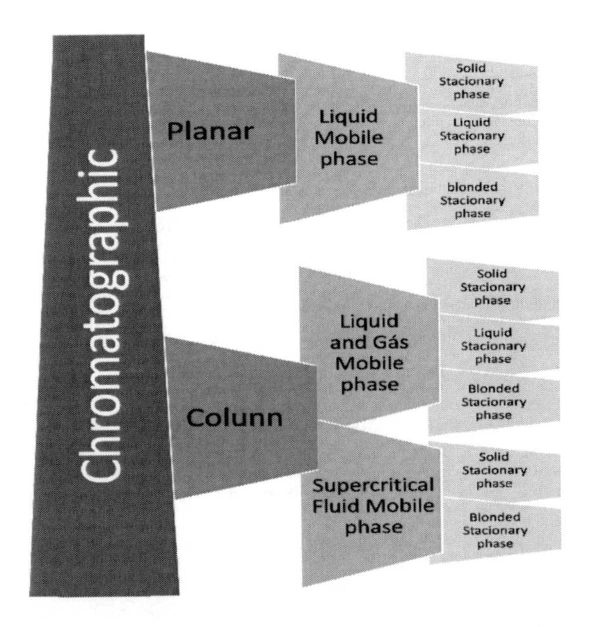

Figure 3. Classification of chromatographic methods [22].

It should be mentioned that in Figure 3, the chromatography can be classified according to the technique, mobile phase, stationary phase and type of chromatography. It is noteworthy that this technique can also be classified in relation to the separation method [24].

- Chiral
- Ion--exchange
- Ion--pair/affinity
- Normal phase
- Reversed phase
- Size exclusion

There are several different types of chromatography currently in use – i.e., paper chromatography; thin layer chromatography (TLC); gas chromatography (GC); liquid chromatography (LC); high performance liquid chromatography (HPLC) *and* Ultra Performance Liquid |Chromatography *(UPLC).* Among the various types of chromatography, the following can be highlighted when analyzing natural products: GC, HPLC and UPLC.

In addition to the various types of chromatography, there is also the supercritical fluid chromatography. This technique of separation is almost identical to that used in high performance liquid chromatography (HPLC). The most significant difference from HPLC is the replacement of most of the liquid mobile phase with a dense compressed gas, almost always carbon dioxide (CO_2) [25].

Technical Terms of Chromatography

Figure 4 shows a chromatogram obtained by planar chromatography. In this method, the mobile phase passes through the starting point of the sample and drags the components of the mixture. The distance traveled by the components is understood by d_r and the distance traveled by the mobile phase is understood by d_m [22].

In column chromatography, Gas Chromatography (GC), High Performance Liquid Chromatography (HPLC) and Ultra Performance Liquid Chromatography (UPLC), the obtained signals are recorded by an integrator or computer. In these techniques, retention is usually given in terms of retention time, instead of distance [22, 24].

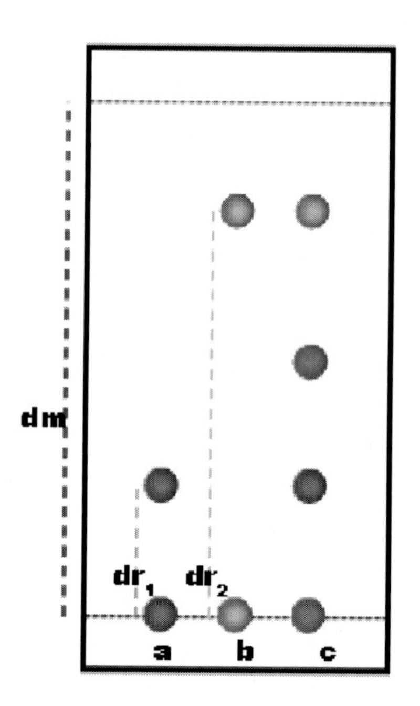

Figure 4. Thin-layer chromatography. Note: a and b were standards; c was a sample.

Figure 5 illustrates a chromatogram showing the retention time of a compound. The retention time, TR, refers to the time that the compound remains in the chromatographic system, either in the mobile phase or in the stationary phase and tm refers to the time spent by the mobile phase, or the time spent by the molecules of the mobile phase through the column [22, 24].

Considering these concepts, the time that the molecules of the substance to be separated are retained in the stationary phase can be calculated, Equation 1.

$$t\acute{}r = TR - tm$$

The relationship between the retention time of the stationary phase and the retention time in the mobile phase, k, is calculated using Equation 2.

$$k = \frac{TR - tm}{tm}$$

The separation factor, α, is calculated by the ratio of their retention factors, according to Equation 3. This factor always refers to the adjacent peaks.

$$\alpha = \frac{k2}{k1} = \frac{t\,'r2}{t\,'r1}$$

Another measure of separation refers to the resolution, Rs. In column chromatography, Rs is calculated by Equation 4:

$$Rs = 2\frac{(dr2 - dr1)}{(wb2 - wb1)} = 1{,}77\,\frac{(dr2 - dr1)}{(wh2 - wh1)}$$

In this equation, wb refers to the width of the base of the peak and wh the width in the half height, as shown in Figure 5. Rs value of 1.25 indicates good separation, sufficient for quantitative purposes, and a complete separation with Rs above 1.5 [22, 24].

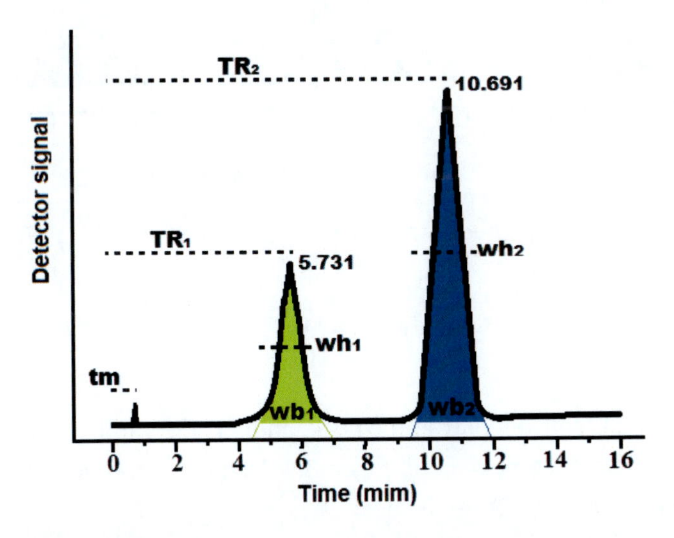

Figure 5. Chromatogram showing the retention time and w (width).

Another factor to be considered in the development of analytical methods by chromatography for quantitative purposes is the number of plates. Each plate is equivalent to an equilibrium stage, similar to the number of plates of a distillation column, thus with a greater number of plates, p, which is more efficient in the separation process [22, 24].

Several factors affect the number of plates [22, 24]:

- Condition Analysis
- Sample Size
- Column length

The peaks may appear symmetrically (optimal) or as having deformations (Figure 6), i.e., tailing peak, peak fronting, causing imprecisions in the data made by the software [26]. Tailing peaks are the most common chromatographic peak shape distortion.

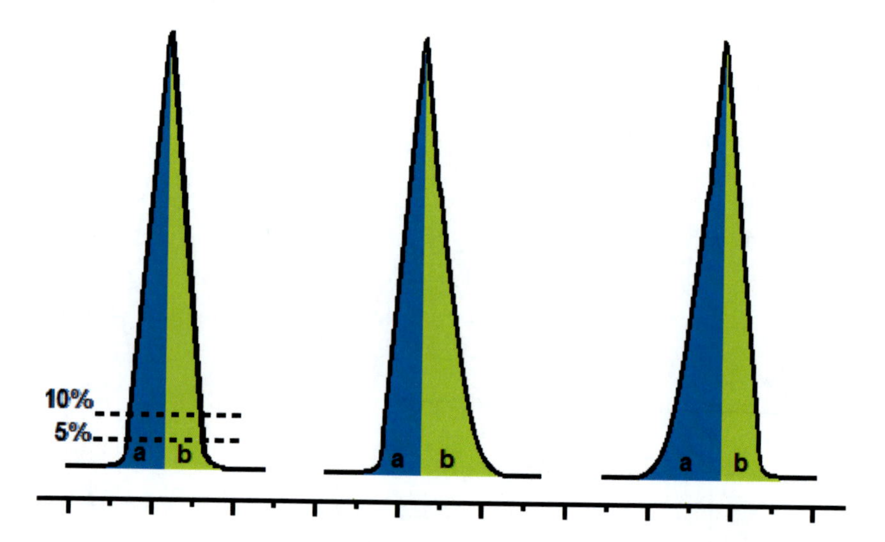

Figure 6. Chromatogram showing peak symmetry (A) and tailing peak (B), peak Fronting (C).

Peak Tailing is often measured by the peak asymmetry factor (A_s), Equation 5 [26]:

$$A_s = \frac{b}{a}$$

where a is the width of the front half of the peak, and b is the width of the back half of the peak measured at 10% of the peak height from the leading or trailing edge of the peak to a line dropped perpendicularly from the peak apex.

The asymmetry factor is frequently used in the pharmaceutical industry. However, the US Pharmacopeia use tailing factor (t_f), [26], Equation 6:

$$t_f = \frac{ac}{2ab}$$

where ac is the peak width at 5% of the peak height, and ab is the front half-width measured from the leading edge to a perpendicular dropped from the peak apex.

An asymmetry factor (As) of 0.9 to 1.2 is generally accepted. Several factors may be varied to optimize the chromatographic method, as shown in the Ishikawa diagram (Figure 7).

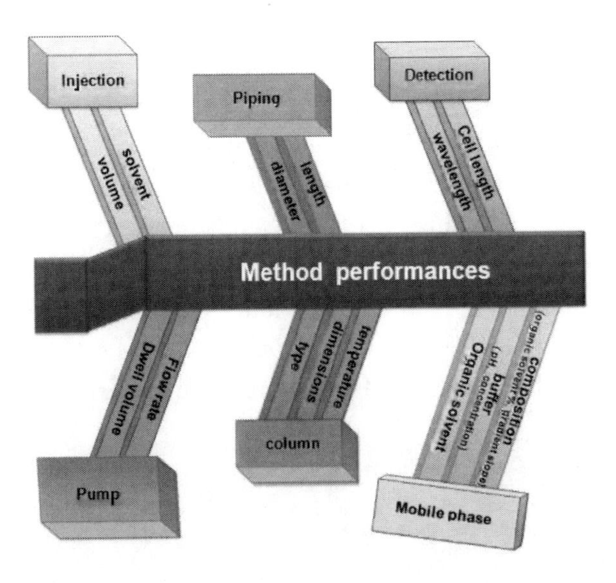

Figure 7. Ishikawa diagram.

The variables most commonly used for the optimization of the chromatographic method are:

- Number of theoretical plates
- Peak area
- Tailing factor
- Asymmetry factor
- Retention Time (RT)
- Separation factor, α
- Resolution, Rs

Experimental Design Applications to Standardize the Development of Analytical Methodologies

Applying AQbD and, consequently, using DOE to develop the analytical methodology to quantify actives in plant extracts is recent and there are few studies in the literature about this. There are many studies using DOE to optimize extraction and drying processes of herbal medicine [27, 28] and protease [29, 30], respectively.

It emphasizes that due to the complexity of the samples derived from plant extracts, the application of AQbD helps to develop and validate analytical methods, especially concerning sample preparation and separation of the compounds.

Below are some papers in which the authors used AQbD to develop analytical methodology and/or validation using plant extracts. Beringhset al. [31] developed a methodology for quantification by HPLC of Chlorogenic and caffeic acids, which are bioactive phenolic compounds found in *Cecropia glaziovii.* The previous methods described in the literature show the difficulty of separating chlorogenic acid from the interferents found in the samples. In this study, the authors rated the organic to aqueous content ratio, the acid content of the mobile phase and the elution method. These factors were analyzed using the Response Surface Methodology IV - optimal design. For atomization, the resolution between peaks, retention time tailing and retention factors, number of theoretical plates and peak widths were evaluated. The optimized methodology proved to be precise, fast, reliable, specific and a satisfactory resolution was achieved to separate the chlorogenic acid and an interfering compound.

Methods/ Design	Studied Factors	Responses	Substances	References
HPLC/3^3Full Factorial design	Flow rate (mL/min), wavelength (nm) and buffer pH	Peak area, tailing factor and number of theorical plates	Valsartan	[34]
UHPLC/ Placket Burman design	pH, Temperature, flow rate, gradient slope	Retention time, impurity efficiency, solvent comsumption	Dextromethorphan	[35]
HPLC/Box Behnken design	Mobile phase, pH and flow rate	Retention time	Anlodipine and valsartan C	[36]
GC-IT-MS/MS/ Plackett–Burman desgn and Central Composite Design (CCD)	Excitation voltage (EV), excitation time (ET), ion source temperature (IST) isolation time (IT), electron energy (EE)	Peak area	Organotin compounds	[37]
UPLC/ Fractional factorial	pH of the buffer, mobile phase and flow rate	Resolution	Robrepazole	[38]
HPLC-UPLC/two-level full factorial design	Flow rate, pH, mobile phase, column Oven temperature	Resolution	Omeprazole	[39]
HPLC / 2^5 full factorial design and Central composite design	Mobile phase, column temperature, flow rate and pH	Resolution, retention time, chromatographic optimization function (COF) and the capacity factor for the first eluted peak (*k*1)	Nimodipine and impurities	[40]

Figure 8. Examples of AQbD applications.

Rafamantanana et al. [32] studied the HPLC-UV method to separate and quantify dicentrine in the alkaloidic extract of leaves Spirospermum penduliflorum Thouars (Menispermaceae). Therefore, the authors used full factorial design of 36 experimental conditions, varying the mobile phase of pH, the initial proportion of methanol and the gradient slope. The method provides accurate results and is suitable for routine analysis.

Shengyun Dai et al. [33] combined the design of experiments and design space methodology to optimize the HPLC separation Panax Notoginseng Saponins. Therefore, the temperature, the initial proportion of acetonitrile and the gradient slope using 17 experiments (Box- Behnken design) were varied. The resolution (Rs) and retention time were evaluated. The optimal condition obtained was validated, and was suitable for quantifying five compounds found, thus showing the importance of using DOE to develop the analytical methodology.

In Figure 8, other studies are shown using AQbD techniques to develop the analytical methodology.

According to Figure 8, AQbD is not used only for the improvement of the analytical method for quantification of the plant extracts but it is also used for water compounds analyses and final pharmaceutical products analyses as capsules, tablets and nanoparticles presents in medicaments.

Conclusion

Since the introduction of the US Food and Drug Administration, increasing importance has been given to Quality-by-Design (QbD) in the pharmaceutical industry. The main aim of QbD is to protect patients by maintaining quality in pharmaceutical products. Within this context, attention to quality should be given to develop the analytical methodology. Concerning the development of herbal medicines, one of the problems is developing an analytical method which can separate and quantify different compounds found in plant extracts.

Furthermore, the optimal method is obtained with a reduced number of experiments. When using an AQbD/DOE tool, it can (with a small number of experiments) optimize the analytical methodology, and study the influence of the individual effects and their interactions.

In complex samples, such as plant extracts using AQbD, as well as using DOE design helps to solve many problems. This is because the traditional method using one-factor-at-a-time does not take into consideration that the planning factors have a correlation, i.e., when change in response to the change in the factor level depends on the level of another factor. Therefore, the ideal method is obtained by carrying out many experiments. When using the AQbD/DOE tool, you can, with reduced number of experiments, the optimization of the analytical method, therefore, allows besides the study of individual factors, the analysis of the interactions between them.

Applying AQbD has been successful in terms of developing analytical methods and for robustness analysis of these methods.

However, there are few studies using herbal remedies. Thus, due to new tax arrangements for the herbal industry concerning quality and safety, AQbD has tended to increase. Since its application allows for the development of more efficient analytical methods which are more robust and resistant, it has survived the challenges of long-term use for the manufactures and quality control laboratories, thus reducing the probability of failure.

REFERENCES

[1] Carollo, Carlos A., and Daniel Pecoraro Demarque. 2011. "Análises de Produtos de Origem Natural por CLAE-RMN." *In Revisões em processos e técnicas avançadas de isolamento e determinação estrutural de ativos de plantas medicinais*, edited by Gustavo Henrique Bianco de Souza, João Carlos Palazzo de Mello and Norberto Peporine Lopes, 119-137. Ouro Preto: UFOP. ["Analysis of Products of Natural Origin by HPLC-NMR." In Advanced process reviews and techniques for insulation and structural determination of medicinal plant assets, edited by Gustavo Henrique Bianco de Souza, João Carlos Palazzo de Mello and Norberto Peporine Lopes, 119-137. Ouro Preto: UFOP].

[2] Peraman, Ramalingam, Kalva Bhadraya, and Yiragamreddy Padmanabha Reddy. 2015. "Analytical Quality by Design: a Tool for Regulatory Flexibility and Robust Analytics". *International Journal of Analytical Chemistry* 1-9. Accessed September 6, 2016. doi: 10.1155/2015/868727.

[3] Barros-Neto, Benício, Ieda S Scarminio and Roy Edward Bruns. 2010. *Como Fazer Experimentos: Pesquisa e Desenvolvimento na Ciência e na Indústria.* Porto Alegre: Bookman. [How to Do Experiments: Research and Development in Science and Industry. Porto Alegre: Bookman].

[4] Raman, N.V.V.S.S., Mallu, Useni Reddy, and Hanimi Reddy Bapatu. 2015. "Analytical quality by design approach to test method development and validation in drug substance manufacturing." *Journal of Chemistry* 1-9. Accessed September 6, 2016. doi: 10.1155/2015/435129.

[5] Neves, Célia F. C., Mônica M. A. M. Schvartzman and Elizabete Jordão. 2002. "Variables search technique applied to gas separation." *Química Nova,* 25:327-329.

[6] Schweitzer, Mark, Mathias Pohl, Melissa Hanna-Brown, Phil Nethercote, Phil Borman, Gordon Hansen, Kevin Smith, and Jaqueline Larew. 2010. "Implications

and opportunities of applying QbD principles to analytical measurements." *Pharmaceutical Technology* 34:52–59.

[7] Peixoto, Maria Paula G. 2005. "Obtenção do extrato seco de Syzygium cumini e avaliação da atividade hipoglicemiante." Ms diss., University of São Paulo. ["Preparation of dry extract of Syzygium cumini and evaluation of hypoglycemic activity." Ms diss., University of São Paulo].

[8] Torbeck, Lynn D. 2011. "OOS, OOT, OOC and OOSC." Pharmaceutical Technology, 35:46-47.

[9] Rozet, Eric, Ziemons, Eric M., Marini, R.D., Boulanger, B. and Philippe Hubert. 2012. "Quality by Design Compliant Analytical Method Validation." *Analytical Chemistry* 84:106–112. Accessed December 10, 2016. doi: 10.1021/ac202664s.

[10] Rozet, Eric, Pierre Lebrun, Benjamin Debrus, B. Boulanger, and Philippe Hubert. 2013. "Design Spaces for Analytical Methods." *Trends in Analytical Chemistry* 42:157-167. Accessed December 10, 2016. doi: 10.1016/j.trac.2012.09.007.

[11] Garg, Lovleen K., Vajrala S. Reddy, Shakil S. Sait, T. Krishnamurthy, Jafer Vali and A.Malleswara Reddy. 2013. "Quality by Design: Design of Experiments Approach Prior to the Validation of a Stability-Indicating HPLC Method for Montelukast." *Chromatographia* 76:1697–1706. Accessed December 10, 2016. doi: 10.1007/s10337-013-2509-4.

[12] Pereira, Sebastião César Assis. 2002. "Tratamento de incertezas em modelagem de bacias." PhD diss., Universidade Federal do Rio de Janeiro. ["Treatment of uncertainties in basin modeling." PhD diss., Universidade Federal do Rio de Janeiro].

[13] Borman, Phil J., Chatfield, Marion J., Nethercote, Phil, Thompson, Duncan, and Keith Truman. 2007. "The application of quality by design to analytical methods." *Pharmaceutical Technology* 31:142– 152.

[14] Elder, David P. and Phil Borman. 2013. "Improving an alytical method reliability across the entire product lifecycle using QbD approaches." *Pharmaceutical Outsourcing* 14:14–19.

[15] Davis, Bruce, Lundsberg, Line, and Graham Cook. 2008. "PQLI control strategy model and concepts." *Journal of Pharmaceutical Innovation* 3:95–104. Accessed December 10, 2016. doi: 10.1007/s12247-008-9035-1.

[16] Piriou, Johanne, Bernard Elissondo, Michel Hertschuh and Roland Ollivier. 2012. "Control Strategy as the keystone of the product life cycle, from product/process understanding to continuous process verification and improvement." *Pharmaceutical Engineering* 32:1–8.

[17] Scypinski, Stephen, Darryl Roberts, Mary Oates and Joseph Etse. 2002. "Pharmaceutical research and manufacturers association acceptable analytical practice for analytical method transfer." *Pharmaceutical Technology* 26:84–88.

[18] ICH Expert Working Group. 2005. "ICH Harmonized Tripartite Guideline, Validation of analytical procedures: Text and Methodology Q2 (R1)". Accessed December 14. http://www.ich.org/fileadmin/Public_Web_Site/ICH_Products/Guidelines/Quality/Q2_R1/Step4/Q2_R1__Guideline.pdf.

[19] Crotti, A. E. M., Carollo, C.A., Gobbo-Neto, L., Santos, M.D., Gates, P.J., and Norberto P. Lopes. 2006. "LC-Hyphenated techniques: uses in the structural elucidation of low-and high-molecular weight compounds." In *Modern Biotechnology in Medicinal Chemistry and Industry*, edited by Carlton A. Taft, 99-141. Bristol : Research Signpost.

[20] Exarchou, Vassiliki, Markus Godejohann, Teris A. van Beek, Ioannis P. Gerothanassis, and Jacques Vervoort. 2003. "LC-UV-Solid-Phase Extraction-NMR-MS Combined with a Cryogenic Flow Probe and Its Application to the Identification of Compounds Present in Greek Oregano." *Analytical Chemistry* 75(22):6288-6294. Accessed December 10, 2016. doi: 10.1021/ac0347819.

[21] Teixeira, Cristiane C. C., Tatiana P. F Cabral, João P. B Sousa, Simone P Teixeira, Jairo K.Bastos, and Luis A.P. Freitas. 2016. "Study of quality assurance for Poemus boldus M products by bothanic profiling, extracttion optimizaion, HPLC quantification and antioxidant assay." *Pharmacognosy Journal*, 8:254-272. Accessed December 10, 2016. doi: 10.5530/pj.2016.3.16.

[22] Collins, Carol H., Braga, Gilberto L., and Pierina S. Bonato. 2006. *Introdução a métodos cromatográficos.* Campinas: Editora da Unicamp. [Introduction to chromatographic methods. Campinas: Editora da Unicamp].

[23] Collins, Carol H. 2009. "Michael Tswett e o "nascimento" da Cromatografia." *Scientia Chromatographica* 1:7-20. Accessed August 28, 2016. http://www.scientiachromatographica.com/ files/v1n1/v1n1a1.pdf. ["Michael Tswett and the "birth" of Chromatography." *Scientia Chromatographica* 1:7-20. Accessed August 28, 2016. http://www.scientiachromatographica.com/ files/v1n1/v1n1a1.pdf].

[24] Lough, W.J., and I.W Wainer, 1995. *High Performance liquid chromatography: fundamental principles and practice.* London: Blackie Academic & Professional.

[25] Berger, Terry A. 2015. *Supercritical Fluid Chromatography.* USA: Agilent Technologies. http://hpst.cz/sites/default/files/attachments/5991-5509en.pdf (Berger 2015).

[26] Santos Neto, Álvaro J. 2009. "Problemas com o formato dos picos em cromatografia líquida, Parte 2." *Scientia Chromatographica* 1:55-61. ["Problems with the shape of the peaks in liquid chromatography, Parte 2. *Scientia Chromatographica* 1:55-61].

[27] Araujo, Rafael. R., Cristiane C. C. Teixeira and Luis A. P. Freitas. 2010. "The Preparation of Ternary Solid Dispersions of an Herbal Drug via Spray Drying of

Liquid Feed." *Drying Technology* 28:412-421. Accessed December 10, 2016. doi:10.1080/
07373931003648540.

[28] Teixeira, Cristiane C. C., Teixeira, Guilherme A., and Luis A. P. Freitas. 2011. "Spray Drying of Extracts from Red Yeast Fermentation Broth." *Drying Technology* 29:342-350. Accessed December 10, 2016. doi:10.1080 /07373937.2010.497235.

[29] Banga, J., and C.K.M. Tripathi. 2009. "Response surface methodology for optimization of medium components in submerged culture of *Aspergillus flavus* for enhanced heparinase production." *Letters in Applied Microbiology* 49:204–209. Accessed December 10, 2016. doi: 10.1111/j.1472-765X.2009.02640.x.

[30] Hamin Neto, Youssef A. A., Luis A. P. Freitas, and Hamilton Cabral. 2014. "Multivariate Analysis of the Stability of Spray-Dried *Eupenicillium javanicum* Peptidases." *Drying Technology* 32:614–621. Accessed December 10, 2016. doi:10.1080/07373937.
2013.853079.

[31] Beringhs, André O., Milene Dalmina, Tânia B. Creczynski-Pasa, and Diva Sonaglio. 2015. "Response Surface Methodology IV-Optimal design applied to the performance improvement of an RP-HPLC-UV method for the quantification of phenolic acids in *Cecropia glaziovii* products." *Revista Brasileira de Farmacognosia* 25:513-521. Accessed December 10, 2016. doi: 10.1016/ j.bjp.2015.05.007.

[32] Rafamantanana, Mamy H., Benjamin Debrus, Guy E.Raoelison, Eric Rozet, Pierre Lebrun, Suzanne Uverg-Ratsimamanga, Philippe Huber and Joelle Quetin-Leclercq. 2012. "Application of design of experiments and design space methodology for the HPLC-UV separation optimization of aporphine alkaloids from leaves of Spirospermum penduliflorum Thouars." *Journal of Pharmaceutical and Biomedical Analysis* 62:23–32. Accessed September 6, 2016. doi:10.1016/j.jpba.2011.12.028.

[33] Dai, Shengyun, Bing Xu, Gan Luo, Jianyu Li, Zhong Xue, Xinyuan Shi, and Yanjiang Qiao. 2015. "Application of Design of Experiment and Design Space (DOE-DS) Methodology for the HPLC Separation of Panax Notoginseng Saponins." *The Open Chemical Engineering Journal* 9:47-52.

[34] Kumar, Lalit, M. Sreenivasa Reddy, Renuka S. Managuli and Girish Pai K. 2015. "Full factorial design for optimization, development and validation of HPLC method to determine valsartan in nanoparticles." *Saudi Pharmaceutical Journal* 23:549-555. Accessed September 6, 2016. doi:10.1016/jsps.2015.02.001.

[35] Boussès, Christine, Ludivine Ferey, Elodie Vedrines and Karen Gaudin. 2015. "Using an innovative combination of quality-by-design and green analytical chemistry approaches for the development of a stability indicating UHPLC method

in pharmaceutical products." *Journal of Pharmaceutical and Biomedical Analysis* 115:114-122. Accessed September 8, 2016. doi: 10.1016/j.jpba.2015.07.003.

[36] Mittal, A., Imam, S.S., Parmar, S., Gilani, S.J., and M. Taleuzzaman. 2015. "Design of Experiment based Optimized RP-HPLC Method for Simultaneous Estimation of Amlodipine and Valsartan in Bulk and Tablet Formulations." *Austin Journal of Analytical and Pharmaceutical Chemistry* 2:1-6.

[37] Coscollà, Clara, Santiago Navarro-Olivares, Pedro Martí and Vicent Yusà. 2014. "Application of the experimental design of experiments (DoE) for the determination of organotin compounds in water samples using HS-SPME and GC-MS/MS." *Talanta* 119:544-552. Accessed September 8, 2016. doi: 10.1016/j.talanta.2013.11.052.

[38] Thummala, Veera R. R., Raja K. Seshadri, Satya S. J. M. Tharlapu, Mrutyunjaya R. Ivaturi, and Someswara R. Nittala. 2014. "Development and Validation of a UPLC Method by the QbD-Approach for the Estimation of Rabeprazole and Levosulpiride from Capsules." *Scientia Pharmaceutica* 82:307–326. Accessed December 10, 2016. doi: http://dx.doi.org/10.3797/scipharm.1310-17.

[39] Manranjan, Vayeda C., Devendra S. Yadav, Hitesh A. Jogia, and Praful L. Chauhan. 2013. "Design of Experiment (DOE) Utilization to Develop a Simple and Robust Reversed-Phase HPLC Technique for Related Substances' Estimation of Omeprazole Formulations." *Scientia Pharmaceutica* 81:1043–1056. Accessed December 10, 2016. doi: http://dx.doi.org/10.3797/scipharm.1306-06.

[40] Barmpalexis, Panagiotis, Feras I. Kanaze, and Emanouil Georgarakis. 2009. "Developing and optimizing a validated isocratic reversed-phase high-performance liquid chromatography separation of nimodipine and impurities in tablets using experimental design methodology." *Journal of Pharmaceutical and Biomedical Analysis* 49:1192-1202. Accessed September 8, 2016. doi: 10.1016/ j.jpba.2009.03.003.

In: Recent Developments in Phytomedicine Technology
Editors: L. A. Pedro de Freitas et al.
ISBN: 978-1-53611-977-0

Chapter 5

THE EXTRACTION OF BIOACTIVES FROM PLANTS

Rodrigo M. Martins, Luis Victor D. Freitas, Ana Carolina R. Montes and Luis Alexandre P. Freitas*

Faculdade de Ciências Farmacêuticas de Ribeirão Preto,
Universidade de São Paulo-USP, Brasil

ABSTRACT

One of the most important unit operations in the manufacture of phytomedicines is the extraction. Raw plant material is extracted to selectivelly obtain the main bioactives in higher concentrations, eliminating non wanted compounds. The extracts have higher load of bioactives, can be the final form of a phytomedicine or can be further dried for preparation of solid dosage forms. In this chapter main techniques for extraction of herbal medicines are presented and discussed, with highlight for the most recent microwave assisted, the ultrasound assisted and the supercritical fluid extraction, which now evolved from analytical applications to industrial scale. Also, the modern concepts of Green Extraction and use of GRAS solvents are discussed. As much as possible, examples of Quality by Design approach to herbal extraction are given.

Keywords: extraction equipment, factors, process optimization, recent techniques

INTRODUCTION

The extraction operation is probably the most important operation in the industrial processing of medicinal plants [1-4]. This is because if we consider that an important cost

---

* Corresponding Author Email:lapdfrei@fcfrp.usp.br.

in this industrial branch is the supply of vegetal raw material, their maximum exploitation as source of the bioactive is essential [4-27]. Of course, the essential character of other unit operations cannot be disregarded even because they also influence the extraction step. A classical example is the effect of plant raw material, like post-harvests drying and milling of leafs, roots or bark, which implies in powdered drug size distribution and the yields in extraction. As demonstrated in Chapter 3, all unit operations on phytomedicine manufacturing are tightly related and influence the whole process efficiency, e.g., yield and cost. The most common downstream and upstream operations for the extraction [1, 2] are shown in Figure 1. The drug raw material coming from agricultural site are stored in hoppers or silos (#1, Figure 1), the solvents are also stored in tanks that allow their mixtures in different proportions to vary polarity or pH (#2, #3, #4, Figure 1), a distillation column for solvent recovery and reuse (#5, Figure 1), the extraction is the main step in drug processing and the adequate choice of solvents and extraction equipment is essential to make the process feasible (#6, Figure 1), the extract can be filtered or centrifuged to separate the solid wastes (#7, #8, Figure 1), extracts are usually submitted to evaporation/drying to obtain standardized dried extract (#9, Figure 1), which are stored until packing (#10, Figure 1). Fine powder is collected in a filter (#11, Figure 1).

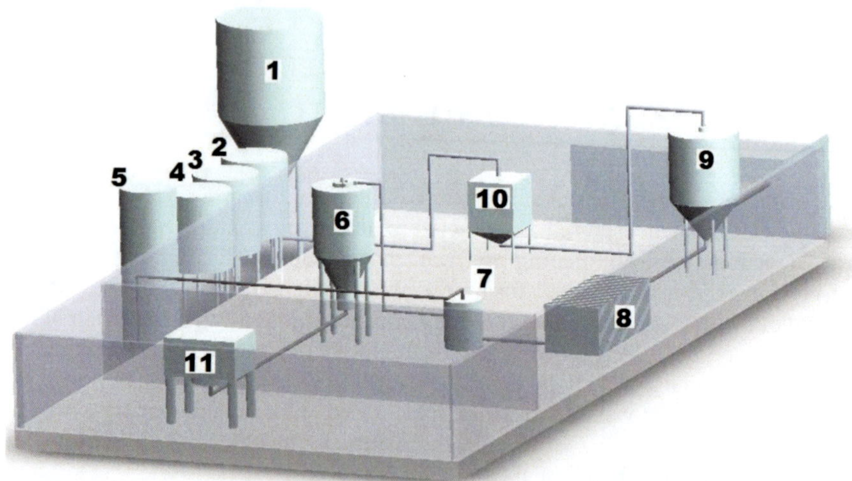

Figure 1. Plant for the production of standardized dried extracts of medicinal plants.

By solid/liquid extraction it is possible to selectively remove the chemical components having higher biological activity and therefore separate those from inert components of the plant material, such as cellulose [1-9]. Provided there is adequate choice of the solvents, extracting method [27-42] and operational conditions, final extract may be highly enriched with bioactives [42-87]. Further purification steps may result in the isolated phytochemicals, but for phytomedicines the extract may contain several other chemical compounds with synergistic activity.

The solid/liquid extraction or the extraction of compounds from a solid matrix is called leaching and involves the solubilization of a compound, which is usually called solute, from its mixture with an inert solid by using a specific solvent [10]. This transfer of a solute from a solid matrix to a solvent is a mass transfer operation, meaning the driving force for the transfer is the concentration difference or concentration gradient [10]. In the case of plant drug extraction the dried plant material is treated with a selected solvent to dissolve preferentially one or more compounds or bioactives of interest [11]. In the field of phytopharmaceutical technology, terms from Latin origin are commonly used and the solvent or mixture of solvents is called *menstrum* and the *menstrum* enriched with the extracted compounds is called *miscella* [1]. Also, it is important to look at the specificity of leaching vegetal material, which may be very different from other solid matrices. There are distinctive plant tissues with different basic life functions, including growth, reproduction, support, metabolism, circulation, and protection from the environment. Parenchyma cells, which are present in inner parts of leaves, stems, and roots, produce and store most of the compounds with pharmaceutical interest. The schematic diagram in Figure 2 depicts how the extraction from plant tissues can be described by two main mechanisms.

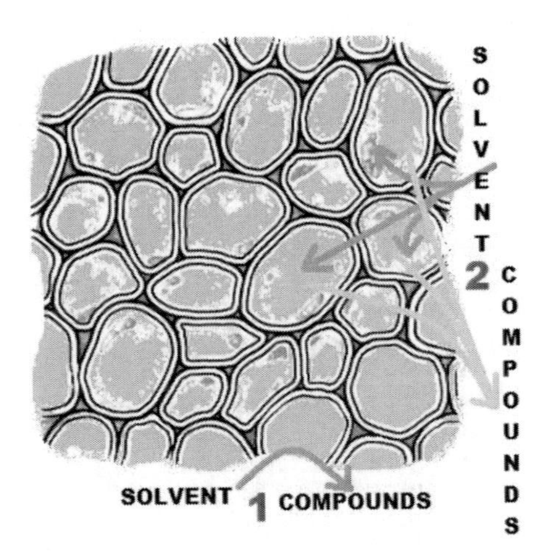

Figure 2. Mechanisms of extraction of compounds from a parenchyma tissue.

One of the mechanisms involves the washing or rising of the compounds from broken or damaged cells (#1, Figure 2). The other mechanism, which should be predominant, is the penetration of solvents through the tissue structure, including inter-cells and intra-cells pathways, followed by compounds solubilization and migration to outside of tissue (#2, Figure 2). The second mechanism is related to diffusion of both solvents in and compounds out of the tissue [1]. As said before, the driving force for the diffusive phenomenum is the concentration: a) diffusion of the solvent into the dried plant tissue due to concentration gradient until reaching the chemical equilibrium with environment; b) diffusion of solubilized compounds from inside the vegetal tissue to the extraction moiety. Both the phenomena follow the Fick´s First Law of Diffusion, given by Equation 1 for a binary mixture, and showing diffusive velocity relative to volume-average velocity [10].

$$J_A = -D_{AB}\frac{dc_A}{dx} \text{ and } J_B = -D_{BA}\frac{dc_B}{dx} \tag{1}$$

where: J_i = flux of entity i in mol per area x time; dc_i/dx = concentration gradient and D_{ij} = coefficient of diffusivity of i in j [1].

One must remember that driving force of diffusion is the concentration difference, which tends to move the compound in the direction from higher to lower concentrations as to equalize them, meaning the gradient will be decreased along time [10]. Specifically in solid/liquid extraction of plant compounds, the process can be described by three different stages [1]: a) diffusion of the solvent to plant tissues/cells and their consequent swelling; b) dissolution of compounds in the solvent and c) diffusion of solutes out of the tissues/cells. The swelling of tissues/cells plays an important role in the extraction, since it may increase the permeability of the cell walls and increase diffusion. Also, other important practical issue is that the limit to mass transfer is reached when the concentration in drug and solvent becomes equal in both phases, which is called *equilibrium*, thus ceasing the net transfer of compounds [10]. As a consequence, extraction process can be divided into two categories: a) exhaustive extraction and b) equilibrium extraction. The first category, exhaustive extraction, is often operated with continuous renewal of solvent during the extraction, i.e., when concentration gradient is very low, solvent is replaced by new fresh solvent [12]. However, many times in industrial practice, a reasonable production rate and solvent consumption indicate that equilibrium must be avoided and optimal manufacturing cost in plant extraction can be obtained before the equilibrium is reached [10, 12].

The solvents applied to phytomedicine technology have been widely discussed in other bibliographic materials on the subject [1]. The choice of solvent is mainly based on the characteristics of the compounds to be extracted, especially their solubility. However, in recent years, restrictions on various solvents have been imposed by regulatory agencies, drastically reducing the options for herbal medicines [13]. The solvents need to be non-toxic or easy to remove completely from the final product, preferably low cost and reusable after distillation, and also very importantly it must be selective in the extraction of the compounds with biological activity. All these characteristics needed for the solvents are inevitably linked to the cost of the extractive process. For example, if a solvent is restricted by legislation to very low concentration limits on the final product, the cost for its elimination is increased. Still, some solvents with flammable or toxic characteristics greatly increase the cost of insurance contracted for the industrial facility. The quantity or volume of solvent should also be considered, as well as, for example, the possibility of its recovery by distillation, which is also linked to cost issues. Among the solvents most used today, given the above considerations, are water and ethanol, as well as their mixtures in different proportions. Further there may be mentioned petroleum ether, n-hexane, dichloromethane, ethyl ether, methanol, acetone, methylacetone and ethyl acetate. However, as said before, the contemporary view for solvents choice should include also environmental and toxicity aspects, e.g., solvent should be preferably GREEN [12-14, 40-42] and GRAS [13]. GRAS is the American Food and Drug Administration, FDA, acronym for "generally recognized as safe" and designates chemicals considered by experts safe for human comsumption, and exempted from the usual Federal Food, Drug, and Cosmetic Act (FFDCA) food additive tolerance requirements. The list of GRAS solvents for pharmaceutical industry is given by ICH Q3C and FDA.

The characteristics of the plant material and chemicals of interest orientate the choice of the solvent system but also the extraction method. Among the drug characteristics there are the degree of comminution, swelling index, solvent uptake, solubility of bioactives and others. Concerning the extraction method, there are several technological options to carry out drug extraction. Some traditional laboratory-scale techniques of extraction are well known to the pharmacist such as soxhlet [3, 4, 7, 8], maceration [1, 2] percolation [1, 2], dynamic maceration [4, 11-14] and high pressure extraction [1], but today they compete with the latest techniques of turbolysis or supercritical fluid extraction, SFE [29-38], microwave assisted extractions MAE [39-64], ultrasound assisted extraction, UAE [65-87], and subcritical fluid extraction, SCE. However, the many factors influencing the selective extraction of chemical compounds from plant material may turn the development of this unit operation into a very meticulous task. One of the options to give high scientific value to this task is to adopt the ICH guidelines [15-18] and the quality by design, QbD, approaches [19-20] as shown in Chapter 3 of this book. Some of the factors that may influence the extraction of natural compounds are shown in the Ishikawa diagram [16] in Figure 3 [19-20]. It is possible to see that some of the factors are inherent to the environment, such as the installations (room) pressure, temperature and humidity, but the researcher must also remember the local regulations about plant/solvent toxicity, flammability, industrial hygiene, qualification of local workmanship and others. Plant material characteristics should be carefully controlled in post-harvest processing, like drug size distribution and moisture content, and other evaluated before the extraction development, like swelling index and solvent uptake. The solvent specifications should be in accordance to local rules, selectivity to the compounds of interest, suitability to the extraction method chosen, stability and possibility of recycling [13, 40-42]. Also, the solvent concentration, pH, polarity, volatility will influence the extraction yield and cost. The properties of the main chemical compounds, which are usually the bioactives, like their contents in the plant, polarity, pKa, and degradation under the effect of temperature, light, or ultrasound and microwave, should also be evaluated before extraction process development.

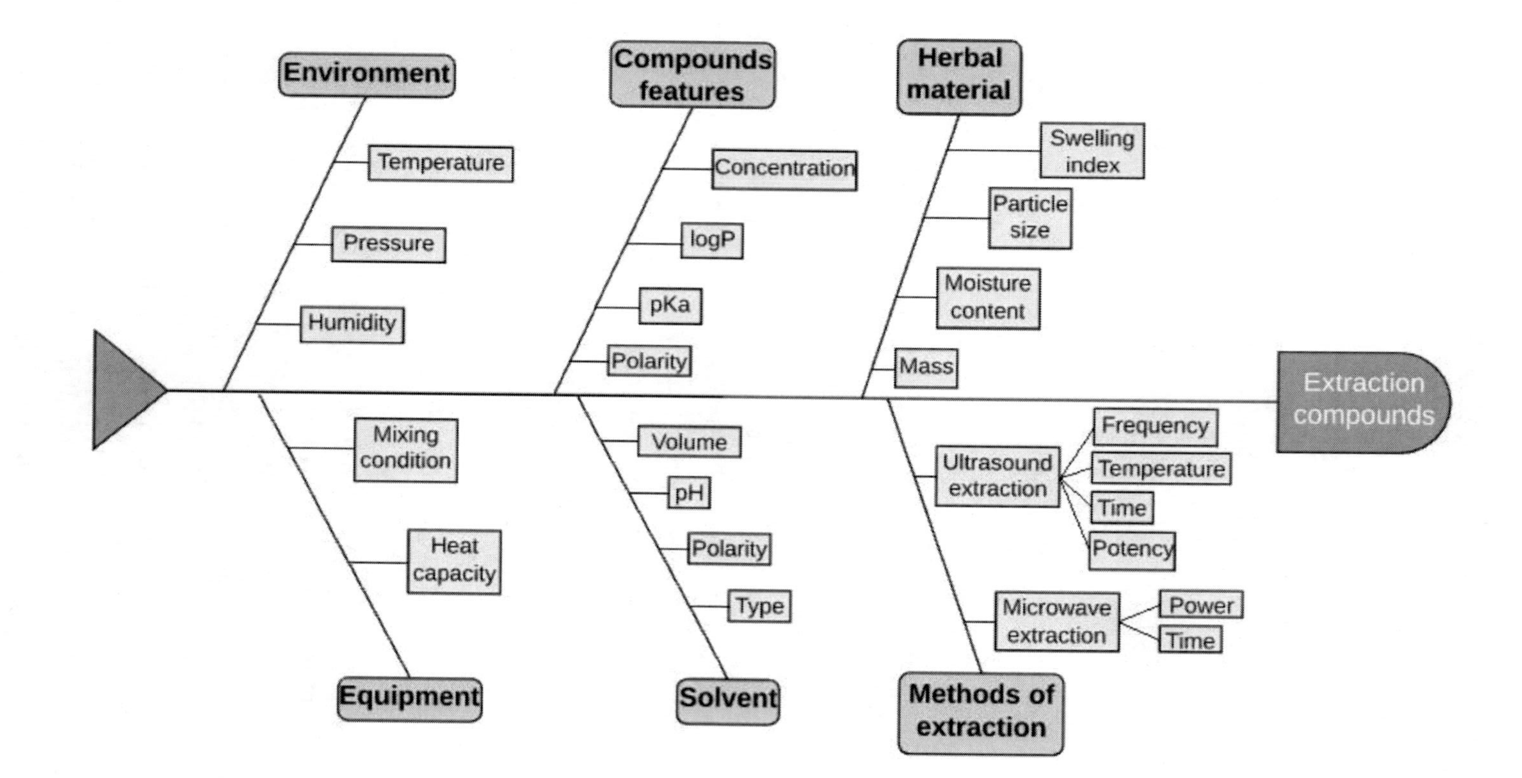

Figure 3. Ishikawa diagram showing some of the most important factors affecting the extraction of compounds from plant material.

Among the most used methods and equipment for extraction of bioactives from medicinal plant there are the exhaustive and the equilibrium methods. The main exhaustive and equilibrium methods are shown in Table 1. It must be clear that any of the equilibrium methods shown in Table 1 can be operated as an exhaustive extraction too, just by carrying out the extraction in several steps or stages, using always the same plant material (drug) but replacing solvent with amounts of fresh solvent in each stage.

The inconvenience of exhaustive extraction is the high consumption of solvent, but the advantage is the complete removal of the bioactives from the drug. However, in some extreme cases when the source of vegetal matter is scarce or very expensive, extracting all the bioactive may be the best manufacturing choice. As said before, a cost evaluation should answer which method is the most advantageous for a specific compound. The methods of extraction by Sohxlet, maceration, percolation, dynamic maceration, turbolysis, supercritical fluid, subcritical fluid, ultrasound and microwave will be discussed in detail in following topics.

Table 1. Typical exhaustive and equilibrium methods of bioactives extraction from plants

EXHAUSTIVE	EQUILIBRIUM
✓**Soxhlet**	✓**Maceration**
✓**Percolation**	•**Dynamic maceration**
✓Repercolation	•**Digestion**
✓Countercurrent extraction	•**Remaceration**
	✓**Turbolysis**
	✓**Supercritical Fluid**

Soxhlet

The Soxhlet is a well-known technique used over a century and invented by Franz von Soxhlet in 1879 whose initial proposal was a set up for lipids extraction from solid matrices [8]. Today Soxhlet technique is not limited to lipid extraction, but is widely accepted as laboratory scale technique for medicinal plants and is currently the main reference for performance comparison between extraction methods [1, 7]. This is certainly due to the Soxhlet apparatus configuration, which allows the exhaustive extraction of the bioactive compound and can be descrived as an intermittent process using constant solvent reflux [7, 8]. The device for Soxhlet extraction, also called Sochlet apparatus, is well known laboratory glassware with a settled design as shown in Figure 4, with four main sections: the solvent vapour reflux condenser; the percolation section, where the solvent permeates the drug bed; a filter section to avoid drug powder falling to the boiler; and the boiler section. The extraction occurs in the percolation section, where the drug powder is loosely packed and is permeated by condensed solvent from the reflux section, the powdered drug is hold by a filter, a thick filter paper for example, in the bottom of the section [7, 8]. The permeate accumulates in the chamber and the overflowing excess drops to the boiler section where solvent is evaporated to reflux condenser and bioactive compounds remain in the boiler. The compounds extracted accumulate in the boiler in a repeated cycle for long time, usually hours to allow the complete extraction of the compounds. The advantage of this system over other exhaustive methods such as percolation, is that much less solvent is used since within this process the solvent is distilled and reused simultaneously with extraction itself, and also obtaining a highly concentrated sample. After extraction is finished, the solvent can be removed by evaporation [1, 3].

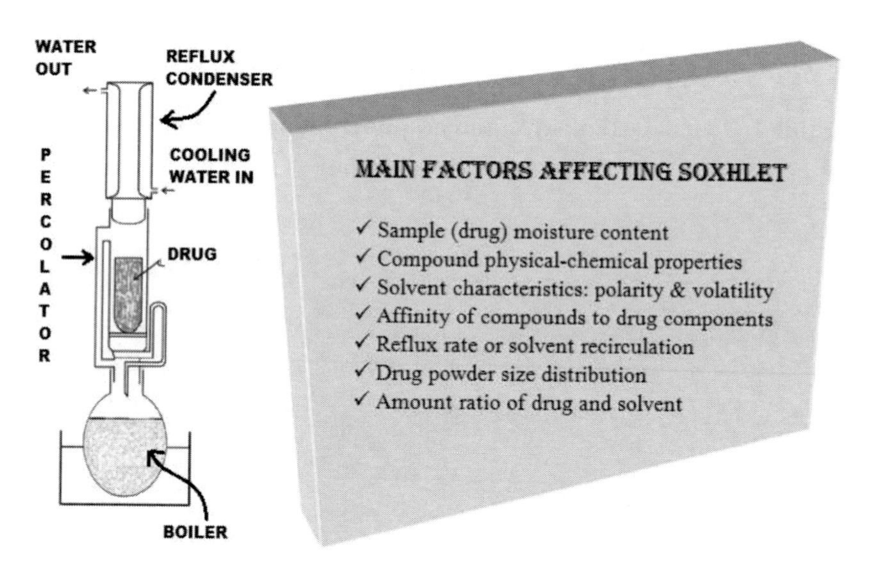

Figure 4. Schematic diagram of the Soxhlet apparatus.

The Soxhet method, however, is more applied at the laboratory level and is often used for analytical purposes and to determine the content of a substance in the plant material [7]. Being an exhaustive extraction method with low solvent consumption, Soxhlet is the favourite technique used for comparisons with other extractive methods [1-3, 7-8].

Among the main advantages of Soxhlet extraction there is the [3] the transfer equilibrium displacement by repeatedly bringing fresh solvent in contact with plant material; the relatively high temperature during process favouring extraction of compounds due to higher solubility; there is no need for filtration after leaching since it happens during the extraction; and finally, it is a simple and inexpensive method and apparatus. As said before, the Soxhet method is almost exclusively applied at the laboratory level, however the concepts involved in its configuration can be brought to industrial scale.

The main disadvantages of Soxhlet extraction are the non-selective extraction; laborious procedure; agitation to speed up the process is not possible; long delayed process; relatively large amount of solvent used; eventual use of dangerous and flammable solvents; and the potential of toxic emissions during extraction [1-7].

A suitable extraction solvent should be selected for the extraction of target compounds when using the Soxhlet extraction method. Different solvents yield different extracts and extract compositions. For example, the most commonly used solvent to extract vegetable oils is hexane. The boiling point is in the range of 63-69°C being an excellent solvent for extracting compounds with nonpolar characteristics. However, n-hexane, the main commercial hexane component, is listed as number 1 on the list of 189 hazardous air pollutants by the United States Environmental Protection Agency [1, 5, 6].

The use of alternative solvents such as isopropanol, ethanol, hydrocarbons, and even water, has increased due to safety and environmental issues, [13, 40-42]. However, alternative solvents often result in lower recovery, since there is a decrease in molecular affinity between solvent and solute. In addition, costs with alternative solvents can make the extractive process more expensive [7].

Percolation

The extraction is carried out by passing the extractive liquid through static layers of the plant material in the form of powder [1, 2, 4]. The material is placed in a container with a perforated screen at the bottom; the solvent is distributed at the top and permeates the powder layer driven by gravity. Figure 6 shows a schematic diagram of a percolator. The extraction chamber may have a cylindrical shape or, as shown in Figure 6a, conical or funnel shaped. An important measure is to distribute evenly the solvent on top of the drug bed, avoiding the creation of preferential pathways or channeling to the solvent. The usual low flow rate of solvent favors the distribution in the drug bed. The extraction by percolation can be described by two sequential phenomena, the first is the compounds wash-out and the second is the compounds diffusion to solvent. The wash-out occurs by solubilization of compounds from disintegrated cells of the drug plant and is rapidly finished as compared to diffusion. Literature proposes that wash out is completed after three parts of solvent has permeated one part of the drug powder, i.e., three volumes of solvent to one volume of drug [1]. However, one must remember that the solvent compromised with drug swelling can be very important in final micelle recovery and some drug can retain solvent amounts as high as three times their weight. So, pre-swelling is usual procedure before percolation. A part of this solvent can be recovered not by filtration but by permeate pressing [2]. The diffusion stage is long and requires large amount of fresh solvent to maintain the concentration gradient. The diffusion rate depends on the solvent feed rate, drug amount, solvent diffusion into drug cells and compounds diffusion into solvent and outside drug. The percolation method has the advantages of a low initial and operational cost, simplicity of operation and the possibility of extracting substances until the complete exhaustion of the vegetal drug. As disadvantages are the high solvent consumption and the long extraction time, which can be several days [1, 2].

Percolation is perhaps the most used method for plant drug extraction both in lab, pilot and industrial scale, due to its simplicity, low equipment cost and complete exhaustion of the drug. Operations are carried out at room temperature by simply controlling the solvent feed rate. The extraction by percolation can be widely improved in lab or industrial scale by using batteries of percolators. Figure 5b shows a common set up for percolators battery: solvent is stored in a tank, percolates drug in percolator 1, than is pumped to next percolators. After percolating the drug in percolator N, the solvent can be pumped back to percolator 1 and procedure is repeated. The assembly also allows removing the micella after each percolator, giving a great flexibility to operating conditions. There are not many factors to optimize extraction by percolation, however, solvent feed rate and degree of comminution of the drug play essential role in percolation efficiency. This is recognized by many Pharmacopoeias, such as United States, DAB, British and Brazilian Pharmacopoeia which specify the degree of comminution in the monographies of many plant drugs [1]. However, although coarse drug lead to low extraction rates, too fine drug is not recommended also because ultrafine powder may cause clogging of percolator. Other factors that may influence percolation efficiency were investigated before [1,2], and are listed in the literature [2]: selectivity of the solvent, contents of extractable compounds in drug, solubility of compounds in solvent, pre-swelling level and conditions, solvent feed flow rate, temperature, steeping time or time material is in percolator.

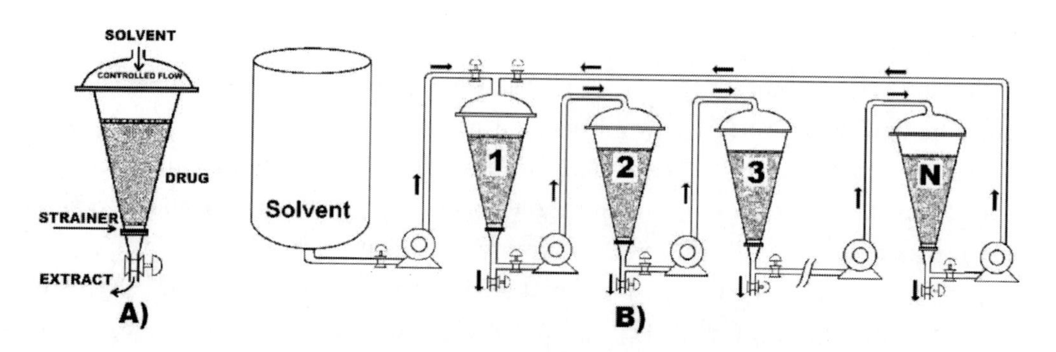

Figure 5. Percolation extraction: a) simple percolator; b) battery of N percolators.

Maceration

The extraction by maceration is done in a closed container where both the extractive liquid and the vegetal material are static, under occasional agitation without renewal of the extracting solvent. As there is no renewal of the extracting solvent, the extraction does not take place completely by virtue of a diffusional concentration gradient [1, 10] between the extracting solvent and the drug cells. However, in order for the diffusional equilibrium to be reached, the contact time of the plant material with the extractive liquid under these conditions becomes very long, typically many days or even weeks, which may compromise the chemical stability of some compounds. These may be important constituents for the extract biological activity and can undergo hydrolysis or other chemical degradation. Also, low concentrations of organic solvents in aqueous mixtures may even allow expressive microbiological contamination. At the end of the extraction the macerate is filtered and pressed [1, 2]. Maceration equipment are considered as low initial investment and operational cost since maceration can be performed in any sort of vessel, requiring no additional features such as mixing or agitation, heating source, instrumentation and others. Although maceration has low cost as an advantage, the long process times, low extraction efficiency, large space demand in the industrial plant can limit its application in many cases [1, 2].

To overcome these maceration limitations, many modifications of this method have been proposed, aiming at increasing maceration extractive capacity with some variations but maintaining the main advantage, which is actually the simplicity of the method. The most important methods derived from maceration are the digestion, the dynamic maceration and the remaceration [1].

DIGESTION

The digestion is characterized by heating the vessel containing extractive liquid and vegetal material to moderate temperatures, around 40 to 60°C and then allowing an increase of the extractive power and reduction of the extraction time [1]. However, digestion is still not capable of exhausting the drug and the increase in temperature may compromise the extractives composition by increasing the rate of their thermal degradation, which can be deleterious to highly thermal sensitive bioactives [2]. Digestion has intermediate equipment and operating costs, but allowed higher extraction efficiency, extraction time of the order of hours, as compared to maceration. The use high temperature usually diminishes the solvents consumption but increase the energy demand, so a cost evaluation is necessary to compare with maceration [1].

DYNAMIC MACERATION

The dynamic or kinetic maceration consists in the agitation of the extractive medium during the whole process, but there is no renewal of the extracting liquid [1, 2]. The agitation turns possible a more intimate contact between the drug particles and the solvent by reducing the boundary layer effect [10]. The mass transfer from a solid body to a liquid is limited by the concentration gradient formed around this solid. The liquid layers close to the solid surface becomes richer in the solute and its concentration decreases as it moves away from the surface of the solid [10]. This imposes a strong limitation to mass transfer in a static system because diffusion rates can be very low. When the liquid or solvent is forced to move around the solid, as in a stirred system, the liquid convection largely increases mass transfer due to turbulence. However, even under stirring there still remains a layer of static fluid, called *stagnant film*, which decreases in thickness as liquid velocity increases. So, under the light of the *film theory* [10], increasing stirring velocity may increase the rate of compounds extraction from the drug and that is the moto for dynamic maceration. The dynamic maceration is usually performed in conventional agitated tanks and can be performed with a variety of agitation impellers and other tank geometries [11-14]. The most common and most important geometric factors in the specification and study of an agited system are shown in Figure 6 [10]. All the details in tank geometry, represented by the proportions between the system dimensions Si, such as S1, the ratio of tank diameter, Dt, to agitator diameter, Da; or S2 the ratio between the impeller distance to tank bottom, E to the agitator diameter, Da; or the S6 which is the ratio of liquid height in the tank, H, to the agitator diameter, Da; play very important role in agitation efficiency. Other factors shown in Figure 6 are the impeller pitch, Θ, and height L; and the baffle thickness, J [10]. Also the type of impeller, such as marine propeller, straight-blade and the pitched blade propellers should be carefully evaluated in dynamic maceration studies.

Many dynamic maceration factors can be studied according to Quality by Design approach [15-20] and DOE [21], by first establishing the target quality product profile or QTPP, which is the rank of all product specifications and characteristics to reach the desired product therapeutical performance with minimum patient discomfort. Next step should be the preparation of an inventory of all critical quality attributes, CQAs of pharmaceutical product and the main critical process parameters, CPPs, for product quality [16] as shown in Chapter 3 of this book. The relationships between these stages of phytopharmaceutical development are illustrated in Figure 7 for a study of a plant material extraction by dynamic maceration, showing the application of DOE [21] for establishing the control space.

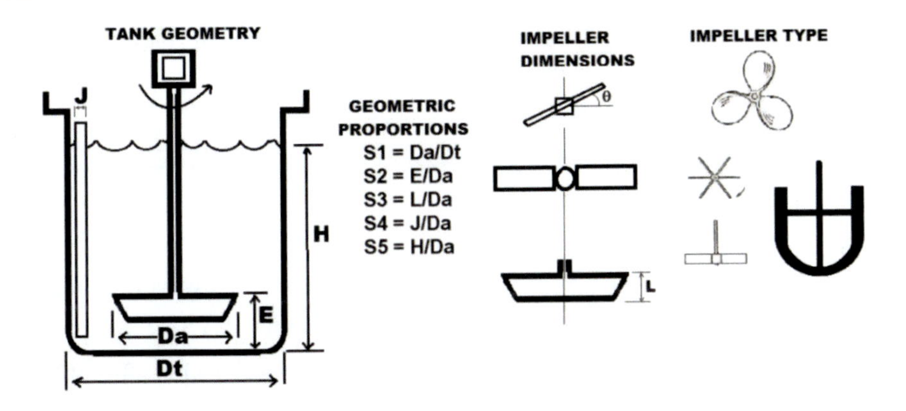

Figure 6. Tank and impeller geometries affecting dynamic maceration process.

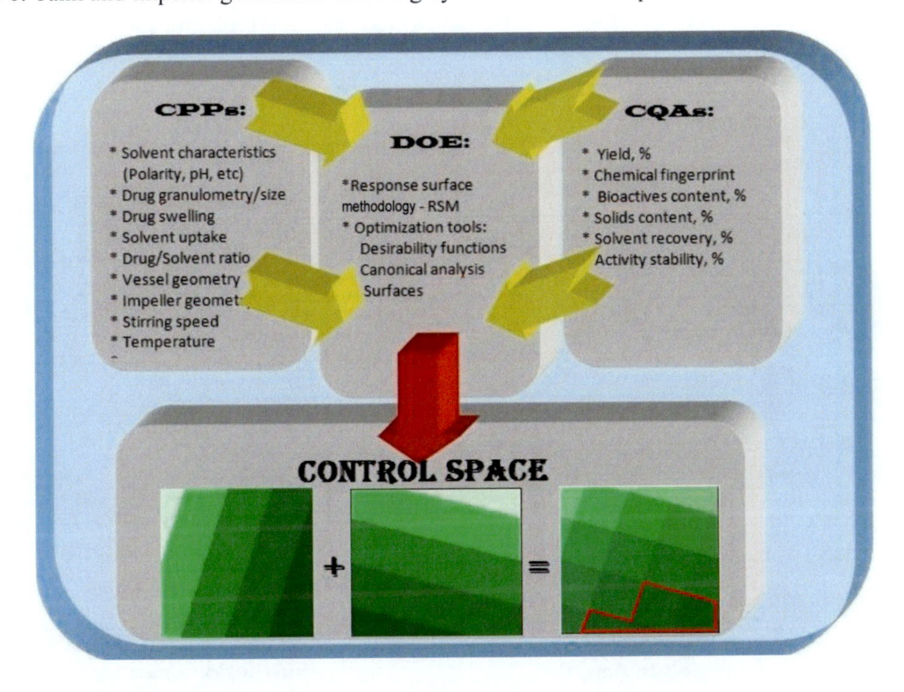

Figure 7. Illustration of QbD application to a dynamic maceration study.

As conclusion, dynamic maceration advantages include moderate equipment investment and operating costs, high extraction efficiency and short extraction times, in the order of hours [1, 9-14].

Re-Maceration

The process is the same as in conventional maceration, but the extracting liquid is replaced after the system reaches diffusion equilibrium. This process is repeated until the extractive capacity is exhausted. The process times are in the order of days but have high extraction efficiency since it is an exhaustive process, and demands for large spaces in the industrial plant. Also there is the need to use high volumes of solvents, increasing operational cost [1, 2]. Sequential dynamic maceration stages with fresh solvent, or re-maceration, were used to exhaustively extract stevioside and rebaudioside A from *Stevia rebaudiana* leafs [13]. The exhaustion of the main glycosides from drug was attained after 18 hours and 4 stages which were clearly shown by the asymptotic trend in the curves of glycosides content in *micella*, as shown in Figure 8. However, it is interesting to note that the authors compared the yields of glycosides reached in 18 hours re-maceration to an optimized conventional (one step) dynamic maceration and concluded that their yields were comparable. This result testifies the effective performance of a dynamic maceration method optimized by QbD approach, achieving high yields in much shorter times and low solvent consumption than exhaustive methods, such as re-maceration.

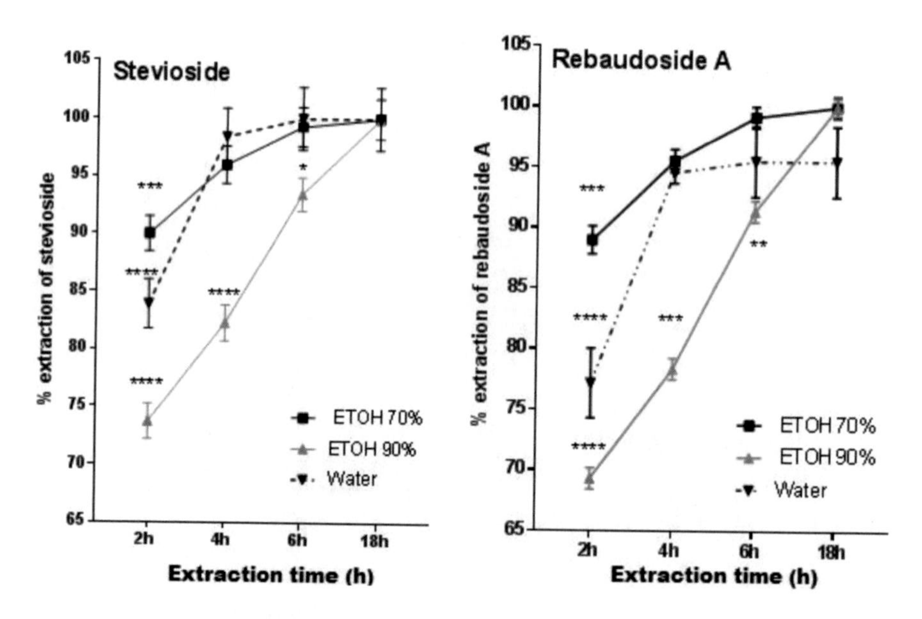

Figure 8. Re-maceration of *S. rebaudiana* leafs for stevioside and rebaudioside A extraction. Cumulative percent extracted in each step. Solvents water, ethanol 70% and ethanol 90%. *$p < 0.05$. (From ref. [13]. With permission, Rev. Bras. Farmacogn., Elsevier©).

Turbo Extraction

The turbo extraction, also called turbolysis or vortical extraction differs from dynamic maceration by the type of agitator and the rotational speed of the device [1]. In turbo extraction, the agitation is done by a high shear mixer, which is most like a colloidal mill than an agitator. Usually, the high shear mixer has two parts: one is the stator and other is the rotor that turns in a very high velocity, much above the typically applied in conventional agitation. The small gap between stator and rotor, together with the high rotation speed causes a very strong shear in the suspension, and causing the powder comminution. The assembly of a high shear mixer and its positioning in a tank are shown in Figure 9.

Initially indicated for lab scale, such as extraction for analytical purposes, the high shear mixers are available today for large capacity applications. A typical lab scale high shear apparatus can be used in rotation speeds up to 27,000 rpm, with a consumption of 0.3kW per liter. Pilot and industrial scale high shear mixers for 30-50L at 3,000 rpm up to 5,000-20,000L at 1,000 rpm have power consumptions from 1.1 to 110 kW, respectively, and are available from many equipment suppliers. One of the advantages of turbolysis is the short extraction times, low solvent consumption, high efficiency of extraction and moderate equipment investment and operational cost [1].

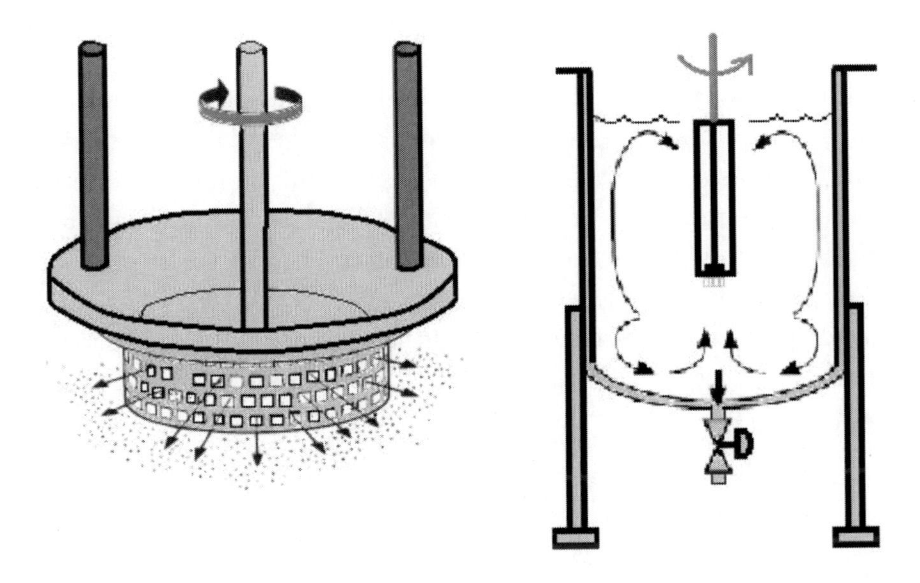

Figure 9. High shear mixer and positioning in the extraction tank.

Counter Current and Other Moving Bed Extractors

In moving bed extractors, the drug and solvent are also mixed in a continuous movement, but in this class of extractors the movement is not caused by a stirrer, as in dynamic maceration, but by some other mechanical principle. There is a great diversity of equipment assemblies for handling and mixing the drug/solvent mixture. Most of these equipment or assemblies were brought in from other industrial processes, such as the Hildebrandt or the Bollman extractors [1, 10], which were originally designed for the chemical and mining industries and are also called counter current extractors. In counter current extractors, drug is mechanically transported in one direction while the extracting solvent flows in the opposite direction. Figure 10 shows the Hildebrandt 10a, and the

Bolllman, 10b, extractors. The Hildebrandt extractor consists of a U-shaped screw conveyor that transports the drug in the opposite direction of the solvent flow. The Bollman extractor, shown in Figure 10b, has a principle similar to the Hildebrandt, but buckets elevator is used instead of screw conveyors. The bottom of each bucket is perforated and allows solvent flow by gravity. As shown in Figure, Hildebrandt extractor usually operates with partial bypass of solvent. The main advantages of the counter current extractors is that fresh solvent is fed at the same side of drug exit, allowing higher concentration gradients through the extractor and also they can be operated in continuous mode, while most of other extractors in phytomedicines manufacturing operate in batch or discontinuous mode.

Other moving bed equipments, which do not operate in counter current mode, are shown in Figure 11. The most used equipment are the screw or ribbon conveyor, shown in Figure 10a, the bin mixer in 10b and the Nauta mixer, shown in Figure 10c. The moving bed equipments for drug extraction shown in Figure 10 are commonly indicated for drug that cannot be handled in a tank with conventional agitation, or dynamic maceration. In these cases, agitated tanks are not efficient in drug/solvent movement and more drastic options should be applied, such as the case of bin mixer, where the whole bin is mechanically rotated by a motor. One example of the efficient drug/solvent movement patterns provided by such equipment is shown in Figure 10d, demonstrating the flow of drug/solvent in a Nauta extractor. As can be seen in 10d, Nauta screw rotates to bring the drug upwards, the screw also circulate around vessel axis close to the wall, giving a spiral movement to the drug and when the drug reaches the top of the screw it moves downward in the center of the vessel.

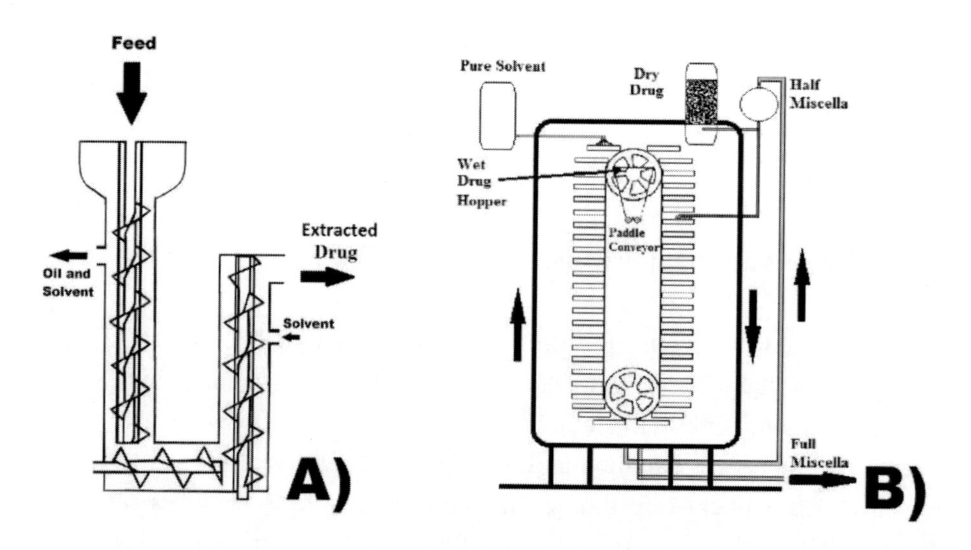

Figure 10. Counter current extractors used in phytomedicines manufacturing: A) Hildebrandt and B) Bollman extractors.

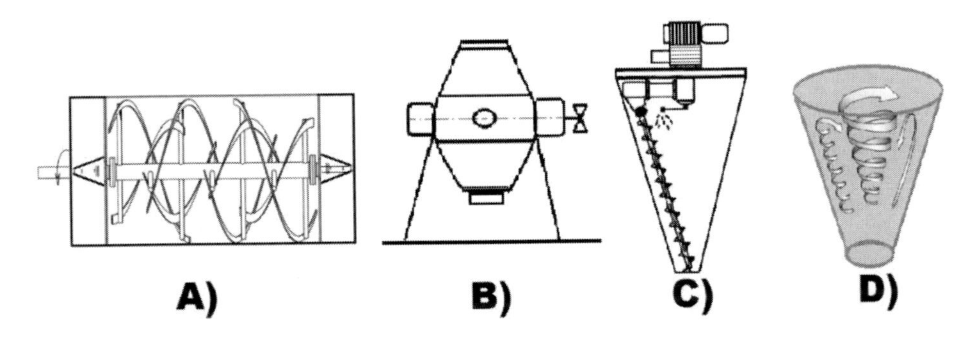

Figure 11. Moving bed extractors: a) the ribbon mixer, b) bin mixer and c) Nauta mixer.

Supercritical Fluid Extraction

Extraction of compounds from natural sources is the most widely studied application of supercritical fluids (SFEs). SFE has immediate advantages over traditional extraction techniques, being a flexible process due to the possibility of continuous modulation of the solvent, allowing the use of less polluting organic solvents and eliminating the solvent used after the extraction process [4-6, 22-41].

Each fluid is characterized by a critical point, which is defined in terms of its critical temperature and pressure. The fluids cannot be liquefied above the critical temperature regardless of the pressure applied, but may reach a density close to a liquid state. Supercritical fluid is any substance that is in conditions of pressure and temperature higher than its critical parameters [24].

The physical properties of a supercritical fluid are intermediate between typical gases and liquids, as shown in Figure 12a. SFEs have low viscosity as gases, high density as liquids and intermediate diffusivity between gases and liquids. As the density of a supercritical fluid is 100 to 1000 times greater than that of a gas, the molecular interactions are strong, allowing to decrease [24, 30] its intermolecular distances, which promotes greater solvation capacity for various chemical substances. The extraction of the substances by this process is facilitated due to the similarity between the viscosity of the supercritical fluids and that of the gases, and because its diffusion coefficient is greater than that of liquids [36-38]. In addition to density and viscosity, other properties such as diffusivity, heat capacity and thermal conductivity make SFEs suitable for extraction processes. High density values of SFEs contribute to greater solubilization of compounds, while lower viscosities allow penetration into solids causing SFE to flow with less friction. The manipulation of the temperature and pressure above the critical points can affect the properties of SFEs increasing their capacity to extract certain molecules of vegetal raw materials [27].

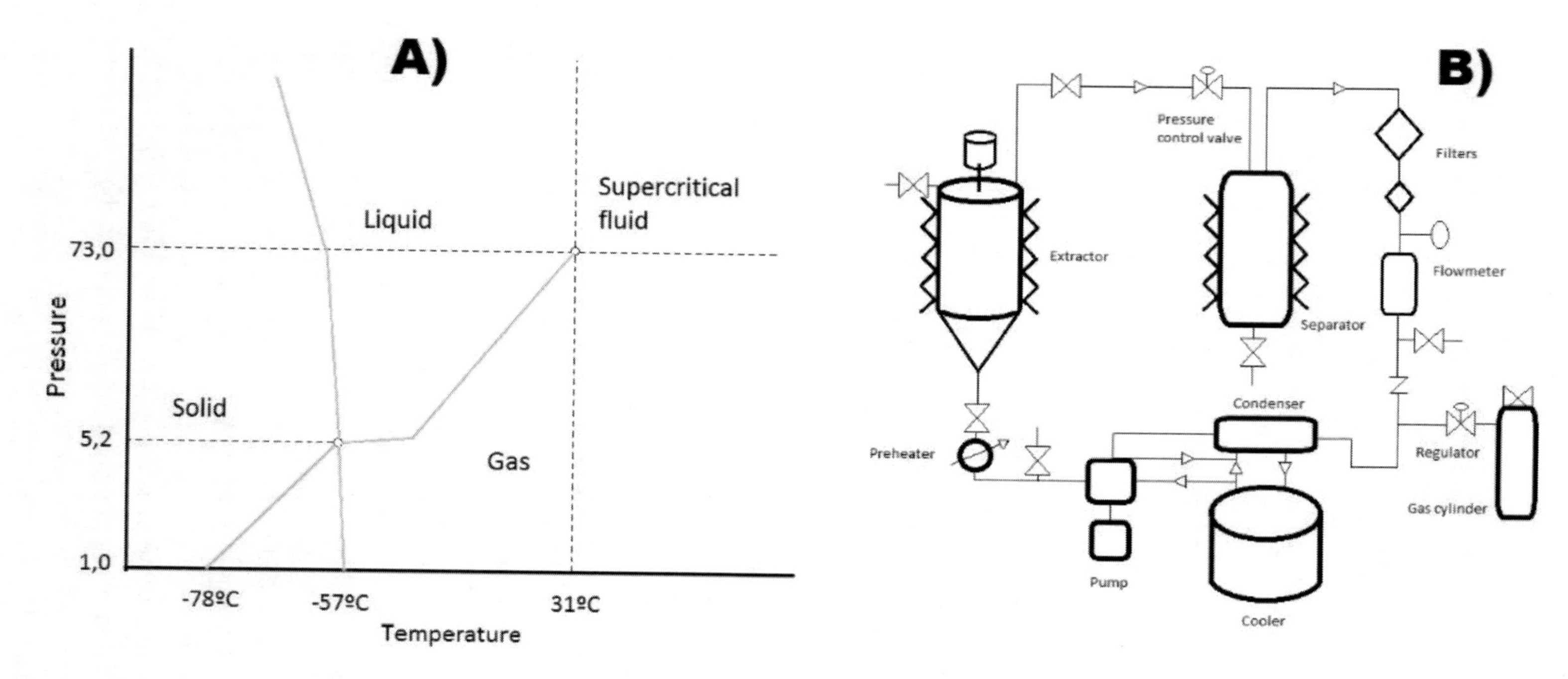

Figure 12. Supercritical fluid extraction for drugs. a) phase diagram showing supercritical condition. b) supercritical fluid extraction set up.

Supercritical CO_2 is the most used solvent for the extraction of compounds of vegetal origin, since it favors the extraction of thermo sensitive materials. In addition, CO_2 allows a high level of recovery [26]. It is easily separated from the solute, non-toxic, does not cause environmental problems, and is non-flammable and low cost. It is the solvent indicated for the extraction of a great range of natural substrates. Its extraction selectivity can be adjusted for each substrate by changing the temperature and pressure within the supercritical region. From an economic point of view, working with low pressures and low temperatures, is of great interest to reduce the cost in the extraction [22]. Table 2 shows other solvents that are used in the SFE extraction processes.

SFE extraction has several advantages compared to conventional extraction methods. Firstly, SFE can penetrate the pores of solid materials more efficiently than techniques that use liquid solvents, allowing faster mass transfer in less time. Second, SFE is continuously pumped through the plant material and can provide complete extraction and the solvation power of the fluid can be manipulated by changes in pressure / temperature and addition of co-solvent promoting high selectivity. The most relevant advantage of the art is the easy separation between the solvent and the extracted material, which does not require subsequent steps of filtration and concentration. The effect of extraction equipment, as shown in Figure 12b, is that the temperature and pressure are usually higher than the room temperature and pressure [29-38]. Table 3 shows some SFE extraction studies performed on plant materials.

The extraction of compounds from solid substrates by SFE has been performed on a commercial scale for more than two decades and in recent years. Large-scale processes are found in the food industry such as decaffeination of coffee beans or black tea leaves and extraction of bitter (alpha-acids) hop flavor. Small-scale processes include the extraction and concentration of essential oils, oil-resins from high-value compounds of herbs and spices, and the removal of pesticides from plant material [29-38].

Table 2. Main SFE solvents, with their respective temperatures and critical pressures

Solvents	Tc (°C)	Pc (MPa)
Ethylene	9.4	5.04
Carbon dioxide	31.1	7.38
Ethane	32.3	4.87
Nitrous oxide	36.6	7.26
Propane	96.8	4.25
n-Hexane	234.5	3.01
Acetone	235.1	4.70
Methanol	239.6	8.09
Ethanol	240.9	6.14
Ethyl Acetate	250.2	3.83
Water	374.1	22.06

Tc – critical temperature, Pc - crítical pressure.

Table 3. Studies involving SFE in the extraction of compounds from plants

Drug	Product	Traditional Process	Reference
Turmeric	curcumin	maceration	[23]
S paludosum	bioactives	maceration	[22]
Chamomile	oil	hydrodestillation	[25]
Copaifera l	afzelin	organic solvent	[26]
Origanum	oil	hydrodestillation	[31]
fish oil	fatty acids	organic solvent	[37]
coffee beans	caffeine	organic solvent	[34]
Rice bran	oil	organic solvent	[30]
Citrus	naringinin	organic solvent	[33]

Briefly, SFE extraction presents high efficiency and extraction selectivity. The extraction times can vary from minutes to several hours. The SFE method has the disadvantage of high equipment and operational costs, making the option for SFE reserved for specific materials demanding high selectivity in extraction due to post-extractive expensive purification. SFE also has high energy demand and requires skilled workmanship.

Microwave

Microwaves are non-ionizing electromagnetic waves of frequency between 0.3-300 GHz and are therefore located between X-rays and infrared in the electromagnetic spectrum, which can penetrate certain materials and interact with polar molecules such as water producing and releasing heat [39-64]. The MAE technique allows very quick extraction of bioactive from vegetable sources.

The microwave extraction is carried out in a microwave environment, which causes the vibration of molecules with magnetic dipole causing stirring and heating at the molecular level [44-49]. The extraction provides a rapid release of energy to the total volume of solvent and solid plant material with subsequent heating of all the material (solvent and solute) with optimum efficiency and homogeneity. This is because water inside the plant matrix absorbs microwave energy, causing cellular disruption by internal overheating, facilitating the extraction of chemicals from the matrix, and consequently improving its recovery [50-59]. In addition, the presence of dissolved ions increases the penetration of the solvent within the matrix and thus facilitates the release of the chemical constituents. The effect of microwave energy is thus strongly dependent on the dielectric susceptibility of both the solvent and the plant matrix depending directly on both [60]. Better recoveries can be obtained by moistening the samples with a substance having a relatively high dielectric constant, such as water.

Other factors may influence the recovery of chemical constituents, such as particle size and distribution, solubility of extracts of interest, interaction between solvent and plant matrix and temperature [60].

The particle size and size distribution of the plant material to be extracted usually has a significant influence on the efficiency of the microwave extraction. The size of the vegetable matrix particles used are generally in the range of 100 μm to 2 mm [62]. Very fine powders favor the extraction because the limiting step of the extraction is often the diffusion of chemicals from the plant matrix. The diffusion is favored by an increase in the surface area of the powder providing a more effective contact between the matrix of the plant and the solvent [63].

Generally, the solvent chosen should have a high dielectric constant and strongly absorb the microwave energy. The most commonly used solvents that present these characteristics are ethanol, methanol and water [63]. Table 4 shows the main solvents used for the extraction and their respective dielectric constants. Non-polar solvents with low dielectric constant such as hexane and toluene generally do not have adequate characteristics to be used in microwave extraction. The selectivity and the ability of the solvent to interact with microwaves can be modulated using solvent mixtures. One of the most used blends is hexane-acetone [60]. A small amount of water (e.g., 10%) may also be added in non-polar solvents such as hexane, xylene, toluene, improving the rate of heating [60].

Table 4. Main solvents used for microwave extraction and their respective dieletric constants and dipole momment

Solvent	Dielectric Constant (20°C)	Dipole Moment (25°C)
Hexane	1.89	< 0.1
Toluene	2.04	0.36
Dichloromethane	8.9	1.14
Acetone	20.7	2.69
Ethanol	24.3	1.69
Methanol	32.6	2.87
Water	78.5	1.87

Adapted from [60].

During extraction, the volume of solvent should be sufficient to ensure that the plant matrix is fully immersed. A higher amount of solvent volume in the vegetable matrix may lead to an increase in recovery. However, large amounts of solvent can produce low recoveries due to an inadequate stirring of the solvent during the extraction process.

Temperature is another important factor that contributes to recovery performance. High temperatures result in greater extraction efficiency. However, for the extraction of thermolabile compounds, high temperatures can cause the degradation of certain constituents. In this case, the power chosen during microwave extraction has to be adjusted correctly to avoid very high temperatures leading to a possible degradation of the solute [59].

There are two types of microwave systems available commercially: microwave extraction with closed system under pressure and controlled temperature and microwave at atmospheric pressure. These systems may or may not be aided by mechanical agitation [58-64].

The main advantages that make microwave extraction a potential technique for solid-liquid extraction of plant metabolites are the reduced extraction time and amount of solvents; increased extraction yield and results comparable to other modern extraction techniques, such as SFE. As a disadvantage one may cite the need for additional filtration or centrifugation to remove the solid residue. In addition, MAE efficiency may be very low when both compounds of interest and the solvents are non-polar, or when they are volatile [64-67].

In summary, the MAE generally presents high efficiency with extraction time in the order of minutes. MAE has very high equipment and operating costs and the application is restricted to solvents with dipole moment, such as water or mixtures thereof. MAE requires highly specialized labor and is an alternative to conventional techniques involving heating and long extraction times [39-64].

Ultrassound

Ultrasound assisted extraction, UAE, is another technique used to accelerate extractive processes. UAE is usually performed using ultrasonic probes or ultrasonic baths which may or may not be assisted by mechanical agitation. Mechanical agitation becomes an important auxiliary in MAE because it reduces the temperature surge produced by ultrasonic energy and allows handling larger amounts of drug in the vessel [68].

The extraction is done with the application of ultrasonic frequency vibrations through, for example, the "sonicator" probe or "horn", that causes cavitation and accelerates the extraction. But what is cavitation? Cavitation is one of the phenomena responsible for the acceleration of solid-liquid extraction. This is the generation of "cavities" inside the liquid, due to sudden and localized gradients of pressure [64-87]. When the fluid is moved very quickly, as in turbulent processes, the displacement of portions of the fluid generates a sudden and local drop in pressure. If the local pressure reaches values lower than the vapor pressure of the solvent at that temperature, it will vaporize and form bubbles. When the bubbles become in contact with higher pressure waves they are "imploded," generating highly energetic shock waves and micro-jets, responsible for high mechanical tensions and elevation of the temperature. These waves and micro wells end up causing a greater interaction between the solid and liquid phases, reducing the resistance to mass transfer that originates from the *stagnant layer*, or *film resistance* [10], between the phases. In addition to extraction, ultrasound has been widely used in the preparation of emulsions, disruption of cells and heterogeneous chemical reactions [73-79].

In addition to selecting the appropriate ultrasonic type configuration, it is very important to optimize different operating parameters such as extraction time, process temperature and most importantly the type of solvent. The choice of the most suitable solvent for extracting the components of interest from the sample matrix is a key step in the development of any extraction method. The solvent type, amount and concentration of solvent and solute solvent ratio have significant effect on extraction efficiency, since the efficiency of the extraction by ultrasound depends on the ability of the solvent to absorb and transmit the energy of the ultrasound [72].

The solvent polarity is another important feature that influences the extraction efficiency. Water is the most appropriate solvent due to its ecologically correct and low cost nature. However, depending on the characteristics of the plant material components, water is not able to extract them completely. Therefore, organic solvents such as ethanol, methanol, n-butanol, isopropanol, hexane, acetone, acetonitrile, ethyl acetate, dichloromethane, ether, etc. are most commonly used. The use of water miscible solvents in different proportions such as ethanol and methanol are generally chosen by combining the extractive properties of the solvents composing the blend. Alkalinized ether and sometimes inorganic solutions such as KOH, NaOH may also be used [70-79].

Another set of important factors in the extraction by ultrasound is that the parameters of the extraction process must be properly optimized. The most important are frequency and ultrasound power. For the complete removal of the compounds from the extracts located in the innermost parts of the plant material sufficient ultrasonic energy must be provided. The scientific literature has reported that in general the combination of frequencies from 20-100 kHz together with power from 100-800 W result in good yields. It has been observed that the ultrasonic frequency of 20 kHz is effective in the maximum extraction of compounds from drugs. In the case of low frequencies, for example, 20 kHz, the physical effects of ultrasound dominantly promote cavitation [73-87].

The use of ultrasound for laboratory scale extraction is already widespread, and is a well-studied technique to optimize analytical methods. The sonicator probes for laboratory scale work at very high amplitudes and power densities, but are not capable of transmitting significant power to liquids because their tips are small, which restricts the zone or volumes where cavitation actually occurs. In this way, these probes are not suitable for industrial scale because they are effective for only a small portion or volume of the liquid in their surroundings. However, they are recommended for data collection and extractive process information and can then be used for scale-up studies [92].

Its application on an industrial scale is still incipient and many researchers believe it is not feasible on larger scales. However, this does not correspond to the reality and manufacturers of these instruments have recently launched ultrasound horns for scales of hundreds of kilograms. In addition, some scientific work confirms the potential for transposition of scale using transducer-assisted ultrasound. The use of ultrasonic reactors with a working capacity of 700-850 L of solvent in the extraction of plant-derived compounds was reported [33]. According to the authors, the design of a large-scale industrial reactor must achieve a uniform distribution of the cavitational activity above the threshold necessary for the sufficient intensification of the extraction operation, which would be possible with the use of transducers to obtain a higher cavitational yield [33].

Regarding ultrasound adaptations to make its industrial application viable, manufacturers have developed variants of sonicator horns whose main advantage is the coverage of a greater volume of cavitation within the liquid with a single rod. The challenge is, therefore, to establish the shapes of the horns capable of producing the ultrasonic energy in larger volumes of liquids while operating in large amplitudes [93].

In short, ultrasound is a high-efficiency extraction technique that can be performed within a few minutes. However, the cost of the equipments are today very high, but with a trend of price reduction. Energy consumed is also high and skilled laborship is desirable. In some cases ultrasound can be effectively combined with other techniques to increase extraction yields, such as SFE and dynamic maceration. This is the case of vacuum distillation for the extraction of flavoring compounds, due to the increased concentration of oxygenated compounds [85].

REFERENCES

[1] List, P. H., Schmidt, P. C. *Phytopharmaceutical Technology*. CRC Press, Boca Raton, Fl, USA, 374 p., 1984.

[2] Wijesekera, R.O.B. *The Medicinal Plant Industry*. CRC Press, Boca Raton, Fl, USA. 2000.

[3] Luque de Castro, M.D.; Garcia-Ayuso, L.E. Soxhlet extraction of solid materials: an outdated technique with a promising innovative future. *Analytica Chimica Acta* 369 1-10, 1998.

[4] Wang, L.; Weller, C. L. Recent Advances in Extraction of Nutraceuticals from Plants. *Trends in Food Science & Technology*. 17: 300-312, 2006.

[5] Sahena, F.; Zaidul, I. S. M.; Jinap, S.; Karim, A.A.; Abbas, K. A.; Norulaini, N. A. N.; Omar, A. K. M. Application of supercritical CO_2 in lipid extraction – A review. *Journal of Food Engineering*, 95: 240–253, 2009.

[6] Mamidipally, P. K.; & Liu, S. X. First approach on rice bran oil extraction using limonene. *European Journal of Lipid Science and Technology,* 106: 122–125, 2004.

[7] Zarnowski, R.; Suzuki, Y. Expedient Soxhlet extraction of resorcinolic lipids from wheat grains. *Journal of Food Composition and Analysis,* 17: 649–664, 2004.

[8] Herzfeld: Franz von Soxhlet †. In: Die Deutsche Zuckerindustrie Jg. 51, 1926, S. 501-502.

[9] Li, H., Pordesimo, L.; Weiss, J. High intensity ultrasound assisted extraction of oil from soybeans. *Food Research International*, 37: 731–738, 2004.

[10] McCabe, W.; Smithm, J.; Harriott, P. *Unit Operations of Chemical Engineering*. 7th edition, McGraw Hill, London, 2004.

[11] Tacon, L. A.; Freitas, L. A. P. Box-Behken design to study the bergenin content and antioxidant activity of Endopleura uchi (L) Bark extracts obtained by dynamic maceration. *Rev Bras Farmacogn*, 23(1): 67-71, 2013.

[12] Costa-Machado, A. R. M.; Freitas, L. A. P. Dynamic maceration of Copaiba langsdorffii leaves: a technological study using fractional factorial design. *Rev Bras Farmacogn.* 23(1): 79-85, 2013.

[13] Mello, P. M.; Thorat, B. N.; Lanchote, A.; Freitas, L. A. P. Green extraction of glycosides from Stevia rebaudiana (Bert) with low solvent consumption. *Res Effic Technol*, 2(4): 247-253, 2016.

[14] Paulucci, V. P.; Couto, R. O.; Teixeira, C. C. C.; Freitas, L. A. P. Optimization of the extraction of curcumin from Curcuma longa rhizomes. *Rev Bras Farmacogn,* 23(1): 94-100, 2013.

[15] Q7-ICH, International Conference on Harmonization of Technical Requirements for Registration of Pharmaceuticals for Human Use. Q7 Good Manufacturing Practice. ICH Expert Working Group, 2009. http://www.ich.org/products/guidelines /quality/article/quality-guidelines.html.

[16] Q8-R2-ICH, International Conference on Harmonization of Technical Requirements for Registration of Pharmaceuticals for Human Use. Q8(R2) *Pharmaceutical Development*. ICH Expert Working Group, 2009.

[17] Q9-ICH, International Conference on Harmonization of Technical Requirements for Registration of Pharmaceuticals for Human Use. Q9 Pharmaceutical Quality Risk Management. ICH Expert Working Group, 2009. http://www.ich.org/products /guidelines/quality/article/quality-guidelines.html.

[18] Q10-ICH, International Conference on Harmonization of Technical Requirements for Registration of Pharmaceuticals for Human Use. Q10 Pharmaceutical Quality System. ICH Expert Working Group, 2009. http://www.ich.org/products/guidelines /quality/article/quality-guidelines.html.

[19] Xu, B.; Shi, X.; Qiao, Y.; Wu, Z.; Lin, Z. Establishment of design space for production process of Chinese traditional medicine preparation. *China Journal of Chinese Materia Medica*. 38(6): 924-929, 2013.

[20] Yan, B.; Li, Y.; Guo, Z.; Qu, H. Quality by Design for Herbal Drugs: a Feedforward Control Strategy and an Approach to Define the Acceptable Ranges of Critical Quality Attributes. *Phytochem. Anal.* 2014, 25, 59–65.

[21] Box, G. E.; Hunter, J. S.; Hunter, W. G. *Statistics for experimenters: Design, innovation and discovery*. 2nd Edition. John Wiley & Sons Inc, 2005.

[22] Siqueira, S.; Falcão-Silva, V. S. Agra, M. F.; Dariva, C.; Siqueira-Júnior, J. P. Fonseca, M. J. V. Biological activities of Solanum paludosum Moric. extracts obtained by maceration and supercritical fluid extraction. *The Journal of Supercritical Fluids*, 58: 391–397, 2011.

[23] Wakte PS, Sachin BS, Patil AA, Mohato DM, Band TH, Shinde DB 2011. Optimization of microwave, ultra-sonic and supercritical carbon dioxide assisted extraction techniques for curcumin from Curcuma longa. Separation and Purification Technology 79: 50-55.

[24] Brunner, G., Gas Extraction. An Introduction to Fundamentals of Supercritical Fluids and the Application to Separation Processes. Springer, New York, NY, 1994.

[25] Reverchon, E.; Senatore, F. Supercritical Carbon Dioxide Extraction of Chamomile Essential Oil and Its Analysis by Gas Chromatography-Mass Spectrometry. *J. Agric. food Chem.* 42: 154-158, 1994.

[26] Costa, A. R. M.; Freitas, L. A. P.; Mendiola, J.; Ibanez, E. Copaifera langsdorffii supercritical fluid extraction: chemical and functional characterization by LC/MS and in vitro assays. *J Supercritical Fluids.* 100: 86-96, 2015.

[27] Andras, C. D., Simandi, B., Orsi, F., Lambrou, C., Missopolinou-Tatala, D., Panayiotou, C., et al. Supercritical carbon dioxide extraction of okra (Hibiscus esculentus L) seeds. *Journal of the Science of Food and Agriculture*, 85: 1415–1419, 2005.

[28] Bruni, R.; Guerrini, A.; Scalia, S.; Romagnoli, C.; & Sacchetti, G. Rapid techniques for the extraction of vitamin E isomers from Amaranthus caudatus seeds: Ultrasonic and supercritical fluid extraction. *Phytochemical Analysis*, 13: 257–261, 2002.

[29] Dobbs, J. M.; Wong, J. M.; Lahiere, R. J.; Johnston, K. P. Modification of supercritical fluid phase behaviour using polar co-solvents. *Industrial & Engineering Chemistry Research*, 26: 56–65, 1987.

[30] Dunford, N. T., Teel, J. A., King, J. W. A continuous counter current supercritical fluid deacidification process for phytosterol ester fortification in rice bran oil. *Food Research International* 36: 175–181, 2003.

[31] Ertugrul, S.; Aeskenazi, O.; Akman, U.; Hortaçsu, O. Distributions of origanum oil components in oil and sub:super critical carbon dioxide phases, in: Proceedings of the Fourth International Symposium on Supercritical Fluids, B: 417–4201, 997.

[32] Fattori, M., Bulley, N. R., Meisen, A. Carbon dioxide extraction of canola seed:oil solubility and effect of seed treatment. *Journal of the American Oil Chemists Society* 65: 968–974, 1988.

[33] Giannuzzo, A. N.; Boggetti, H. J.; Nazareno, M. A.; Mishima, H. T. Supercritical fluid extraction of naringin from the peel of citrus paradise. *Phytochemical Analysis*, 14: 221–223, 2003.

[34] Peker, H.; Srinivasan, M. P.; Smith, J. M.; McCoy, B. J. Caffeine extraction rates from coffee beans with supercritical carbon dioxide. *AIChE Journal,* 38: 761–770, 1992.

[35] Richter, M.; Sovova, H. The solubility of two monoterpenes carbon dioxide. *Fluid Phase Equilibria,* 85 285-300, 1993.

[36] Sass-Kiss, A.; Simandi, B.; Gao, Y.; Boross, F.; Vamos-Falusi, Z. Study on the pilot-scale extraction of onion oleoresin using supercritical CO_2. *Journal of the Science of Food and Agriculture*, 76: 320–326, 1998.

[37] Staby, A. Mollerup J. Separation of constituents of fish oil using supercritical fluids: a review of experimental solubility, extraction, and chromatographic data. *Fluid Phase Equilibria*, 91: 349-386, 1993.

[38] Vinatoru, M. Mass transfer enhancement in supercritical fluids extraction by means of power ultrasound, *Ultrason. Sonochem*. 8: 303–313, 2001.

[39] Mandal, V.; Mohan, Y.; Hemalatha, S.; Microwave Assisted Extraction – An Innovative and Promising Extraction Tool for Medicinal Plant Research. *Pharmacognosy Reviews*, 1: 7-18, 2007.

[40] C. Capello, U. Fischer, K. Hungerbuhler, What is a green solvent? A comprehensive framework for the environmental assessment of solvents, *Green Chem*., 9(2007) 927-934.

[41] F. Chemat, N. Rombaut, A. S. Fabiano-Tixier, J. T. Pierson, A. Bily, Green extraction: from concepts to research, education and economical opportunities, In: *Green Extraction of Natural Products: Theory and Practice*, 1st edition, Eds F Chemat & S Struhe, Wiley-VCH Verlag GmbH & Co, Berlin, 2015, pp 1-36.

[42] F. Chemat, M. A. Vian, G. Cravotto, Green extraction of natural products: concept and principles, *Int J Mol Sci*., 13(2012) 8615-8627.

[43] Kaufmann, B., & Christen, P. Recent extraction techniques for natural products: Microwave-assisted extraction and pressurized solvent extraction. *Phytochemical Analysis*, 13: 105–113, 2002.

[44] Mandal V, Mohan Y, Hemalatha S 2008. Microwave assisted extraction of curcumin by sample–solvent dual heating mechanism using Taguchi L9 orthogonal design. *Journal of Pharmaceutical and Biomedical Analysis* 46: 322-327.

[45] Brachet, A., Christen, P.; Veuthey, J.L. Focused microwave-assisted extraction of cocaine and benzoylecgonine from coca leaves. *Phytochemical Analysis,* 13, 162–169, 2002.

[46] Pan, Y.; He, C.; Wang, H.; Ji, X.; Wang, K.; Liu, P. Antioxidant activity of microwave-assisted extract of Buddleia officinalis and its major active component. *Food Chemistry, 121*: 497-502, 2010.

[47] Talebi, M.; Ghassempour, A.; Talebpour, Z.; Rassouli, A.; Dolatyari, L. Optimization of the Extraction of Paclitaxel from Taxus baccata L. by the Use of Microwave Energy. *J. Sep. Sci.,* 27: 1130-1136, 2004.

[48] Chen, Z.; Zhang, L.; Chen, G. Microwave-assisted extraction followed by capillary electrophoresis-amperometric detection for the determination of antioxidant constituents in Folium Eriobotryae. *Journal of Chromatography A*, 1193: 178-181, 2008.

[49] Da Porto, C., Decorti, D. Ultrasound-assisted extraction coupled with under vacuum distillation of flavour compounds from spearmint (carvone-rich) plants: comparison with conventional hydrodistillation, *Ultrason. Sonochem.* 16: 795–799, 2009.

[50] Dabiri, M.; Salimi, S.; Ghassempour, A.; Rassouli, A.; Talebi, M. Optimization of Microwave-Assisted Extraction for Alizarin and Purpurin in Rubiaceae Plants and its Comparison with Conventional Extraction Methods. *J. Sep. Sci.,* 28: 387-396, 2005.

[51] Deng, J.; Xiao, X.; Tong, X.; Li, G. Preparation of bergenin from Ardisia crenata sims and Rodgersia sambucifolia hemsl based on microwave-assisted extraction/high-speed counter-current chromatography. *Separation and Purification Technology*, 74: 155-159, 2010.

[52] Farhat, A.; Fabiano-Tixier, A.S.; Maataoui, M.E.; Maingonnat, J. F.; Romdhane, M.; Chemat, F. Microwave steam diffusion for extraction of essential oil from orange peel: kinetic data, extract's global yield and mechanism. *Food Chemistry,* 125: 255-261, 2011.

[53] Flamini, G.; Tebano, M.; Cioni, P.L.; Ceccarini, L.; Ricci, A.S.; Longo, I. Comparison between the conventional method of extraction of essential oil of Laurus nobilis L. and a novel method which uses microwaves applied in situ, without resorting to na oven. *Journal of Chromatography* A, 1143: 36-40, 2007.

[54] Font, N.; Hernandez, F.; Hogendoorn, E.A.; Baumann, R.A.; Van Zoonen, P. Microwave-assisted solvent extraction and reversed-phase liquid chromatography–UV detection for screening soils for sulfonylurea herbicides. *Journal of Chromatography A*, 798: 179–186, 1998.

[55] Inglett, G. E.; Rose, D. J.; Chen, D.; Stevenson, D. G.; Biswas, A. Phenolic content and antioxidant activity of extracts from whole buckwheat (Fagopyrum esculentum Meoench) with or without microwave irradiation. *Food Chemistry,* 119: 1216-1219, 2010.

[56] Kaufmann, B.; Christen, P.; & Veuthey, J.L. Parameters affecting microwave-assisted extraction of with anolides. *Phytochemical Analysis,* 12: 327–331, 2001.

[57] Kwon, J. H.; Belanger, J. M. R.; Jocelyn Pare, J. R.; Yaylayan, V. A. Application of microwave-assisted process (MAP TM) to the fast extraction of Ginseng saponins. *Food Research International*, 36: 491–498, 2003.

[58] Sharma, A.; Verma, S. C.; Saxena, N.; Chadda, N.; Singh, N. P.; Sinha, A. K. Microwaver- and Ultrasound Extraction of Vanillin and its Quantification by High-Performance Liquid Chromatography in *Vanilla planifolia*. *J. Sep. Sci.,* 29: 613-619, 2006.

[59] Song, J.; Li, D.; Liu, C.; Zhang, Y. Optimized microwave assisted extraction of total phenolics (TP) from Ipomoea batatas leaves and its antioxidant activity. *Innovative Food Science and Emerging Technologies*, 12: 282-287, 2011.

[60] Spar Eskilsson, S.; Bjorklund, E. Analytical-scale microwave-assisted extraction. *Journal of Chromatography* A, 902: 227–250, 2000.

[61] Szentmihalyi, K. Vinkler, P. Lakatose, B. Iles, V.I. M. Then, Rose hip (Rosa canina L.) oil obtained from waste hip seeds by different extraction methods, *Bioresour. Technol*. 82: 195–201, 2002.

[62] Wang, H.; Chen, L.; Xu, Y.; Zeng, Q.; Zhang, X.; Zhao, Q.; et al. Dynamic microwave-assisted extraction coupled on-line with clean-up for determination of caffeine in tea. *LWT-Food Science and Technology,* 44: 1490-1495, 2011.

[63] Zhanga, H-F.; Yang, X-H.; Wang, Y.; Microwave assisted extraction of secondary metabolites from plants: Current status and future directions. *Trends in Food Science & Technology*, 22: 672-688, 2011.

[64] Zheng, X.; Wang, X.; Lan, Y.; Shi, J.; Xue, S. J.; Liu, C. Application of response surface methodology to optimize microwave-assisted extraction of silymarin from milk thistle seeds. *Separation and Purification Technology,* 70: 34-40, 2009.

[65] Costa FSO, Araújo Júnior CA, Silva EJ, Bara MTF, Lima EM, Valadares MC, Marreto RN 2011. Impact of ultrasound-assisted extraction on quality and photostability of the Pothomorphe umbellata extracts. *Ultrasonics Sonochemistry* 18: 1002-1007.

[66] Chemat, S.; Lagha, A.; AitAmar, H.; Bartels, P. V.; Chemat, F. Comparison of conventional and ultrasound-assisted extraction of carvone and limonene from caraway seeds. *Flavour and Fragrance Journal,* 19: 188–195, 2004.

[67] Gu, X.; Cai, J.; Zhu, X.; Su, Q. Dynamic Ultrasound-Assited Extraction of Polyphenols in Tobacco. J. Sep. Sci., 28: 2477-2481, 2005.

[68] Mason, T. J.; Paniwnyk, L.; Lorimer, J. P. The uses of Ultrasound in Food Technology. *Ultrasonics and Sonochemistry,* 3: S253-S260, 1996.

[69] Patist, A.; Bates, D. Ultrasonic Innovations in the Food Industry: From the Laboratory to Commercial Production. *Innovative Food Science & Emerging Technol.,* 9:147-154, 2008.

[70] Ebringerova, A. Hromadkova, Z. An overview on the application of ultrasound in extraction, separation and purification of plant polysaccharides, *Cent. Eur. J. Chem.* 8: 243–257, 2010.

[71] Adje, F.; Lozano, Y. F.; Lozano, P. Adima, A.; Chemat, F.; Gaydou, E.M. Optimization of anthocyanin, flavonol and phenolic acid extractions from Delonix

regia tree flowers using ultrasound-assisted water extraction, *Ind. Crops Prod.* 32: 439–444, 2010.

[72] Albu, S., Joyce, E., Paniwnyk, L., Lorimer, J. P., & Mason, T. J. Potential for the use of ultrasound in the extraction of antioxidants from Rosmarinus officinalis for the food and pharmaceutical industry. *Ultrasonics Sonochemistry*, 11: 261-265, 2004.

[73] Alupului, A.; Calinescu, I.; Lavric, V. Ultrasonic vs Microwave Extraction Intensification of Active Principles from Medicinal Plants. AIDIC Conference Series 09:1-8, 2009. DOI: 10.3303/ACOS0909001.

[74] Barbero, G. F.; Liazid, A.; Palma, M.; Barroso, C.G. Ultrasound-assisted extraction of capsaicinoids from peppers, *Talanta* 75: 1332–1337, 2008.

[75] Barbero, G. F.; Liazid, A.; Palma, M.; Barroso, C.G. Ultrasound-assisted extraction of capsaicinoids from peppers, *Talanta* 75: 1332–1337, 2008.

[76] Ghafoor, K.; Choi, Y. H.; Jeon, J. Y.; Jo, I. H. Optimization ofultrasound-assisted extraction of phenolic compounds, antioxidants and anthocyanins from grape (Vitis vinifera) seeds. *Journal of Agricultural and Food Chemistry*, 57: 4988-4994, 2009.

[77] Hromádková, Z.; Ebringerová, A.; Valachovic, P. Comparison of Classical and Ultrasound-Assisted Extraction of Polysaccharides from *Salvia officinalis* L. *Ultrasonics Sonochemistry,* 5: 163-168, 1999.

[78] Jadhav, D.; Rekha, B. N. Gogate, P. R. Rathod, V. K. Extraction of vanillin from vanilla pods: a comparison study of conventional soxhlet and ultrasound assisted extraction, *J. Food Eng*: 93 421–426, 2009.

[79] Japon-Lujan, R.; Luque-Rodríguez, J. M.; Luque de Castro, M. D. Dynamic ultrasound-assisted extraction of oleuropein and related biophenols from olive leaves. *Journal of Chromatography A,* 1108: 76-82, 2006.

[80] Jerman, T.; Trebse, P.; Vodopivec, B. M. Ultrasound-assisted solid liquid extraction (USLE) of olive fruit (Olea europaea) phenolic compounds, *Food Chem:* 123 175–182, 2010.

[81] Piyasena, P.; Mohareb, E.; McKellar, R.C. Inactivation of Microbes using Ultrasound: A Review. *International J. of Food Microbiology*, 87: 207-216, 2003.

[82] Santos Jr., D.; Krug, F. J.; Pereira, M. G.; Korn, M. Currents on Ultrasound-Assisted Extraction for Sample Preparation and Spectroscopic Analytes Determination. *Applied Spectroscopy Reviews,* 41: 305-321, 2006.

[83] Shirsath, S. R.; Sonawane, S. H.; Gogate, P. R. Intensification of extraction of natural products using ultrasonic irradiations-A review of current status. *Chemical Engineering and Processing*, 53: 10-23, 2013.

[84] Sivakumar, V.; Verma, V. R.; Rao, P. G.; Swaminathan, G. Studies on the use of power ultrasound in solid–liquid myrobalan extraction process, *J. Clean. Prod.* 15: 1813–1818, 2007.

[85] Soria, A. C. Villamiel, M. Effect of ultrasoundon the technological properties andbioactivity of food: a review. *Trends in Food Science & Technology,* 21: 323-331, 2010.

[86] Thongson, C.; Davidson, P. M.; Mahakarnchanakul, W.; & Weiss, J. Antimicrobial activity of ultrasound-assisted solvent-extracted spices. *Letters in Applied Microbiology*, 39: 401-406, 2004.

[87] Valachovic, P.; Pechova, A.; Mason, T. J. Towards the Industrial Production of Medicinal Ticntures by Ultrasound Assisted Extraction. *Ultrasonics and Sonochemistry*, 8: 111-117, 2001.

[88] Wu, J.; Lin, L.; Chau, F. Ultrasound assisted extraction of ginseng saponins from ginseng roots and cultured ginseng cells, *Ultrason. Sonochem*. 8: 347–352, 2001.

In: Recent Developments in Phytomedicine Technology ISBN: 978-1-53611-977-0
Editors: L. A. Pedro de Freitas et al.

Chapter 6

RECENT DEVELOPMENTS IN DRYING EXTRACTS

Rayssa Aparecida S. P. Reis, Ana Rita M. Costa, Luciana A. Tacon, Cristiane C. C. Teixeira, and Luis Alexandre P. Freitas*

Faculdade de Ciências Farmacêuticas de Ribeirão Preto,
Universidade de São Paulo-USP, Brasil

ABSTRACT

Drying processes are some of the most commonly used techniques in industries, especially in the pharmaceutical industry. They are some of the most used unit operations due to their many advantages related to solid dosage forms, such as increased stability and the fact that they are easy to transport and store. Furthermore, they are versatile techniques as they can be used for products of synthetic and biological origin. The aim of this chapter is to present the theoretical foundations involved in drying processes, as well as the most used technologies in processing plant extracts for phytotherapy. In addition, scientific papers will be presented that use these techniques to develop these pharmaceutical products.

Keywords: drying, excipients, fluid bed dryer, freeze dryer, phytomedicines, spray dryer, vegetal extracts

* Corresponding Author Email: lapdfrei@fcfrp.usp.br.

INTRODUCTION

Using herbs as complementary or isolated therapy has always been part of the world´s history. In recent years, due to worldwide phytopharmaceutical market trends, industrial manufacturing of herbal medicines has grown considerably [1].

Herbal medicinal products - or phytomedicines are standardized herbal preparations exclusively containing one or more plants in the form of a liquid, solid (powdered extract) or viscous preparations [1, 2, 3]. In addition, according to the World Health Organization (WHO), these medicines have active ingredients, such as parts of plant materials in a crude or processed state, containing secondary constituents, i.e., solvents, diluents or preservatives. Usually, the active principles responsible for their pharmacological action are unknown [1, 4].

Although the regulation and legislation quality of marketed herbal medicines changes from country to country, validated and standardized analytical methodologies are required for the production of reliable products. Thus, the WHO has established some guidelines to ensure the quality, safety and efficacy of the products [2, 5, 6]. Different phytomedicines are commercially available from a comminuted plant material, extracts, tinctures, oils or resins, resulting in liquid or solid pharmaceutical preparations [1, 2, 7]. In this context, compared to theliquid forms, powdered extracts show advantages such as better physical and microbiological stability and easier standardization of the solid dosage form [7, 8].

Concerning industrial manufacturing of phytomedicines, dry extracts are the main raw material used to produce solid dosage forms, often as tablets or capsules. Usually, these powders are highly hygroscopic and are highly sensitive to atmospheric moisture. Consequently, the particle interactions contribute to poor flow and compactability properties. Furthermore, their hygroscopic nature and chemical complexity favors degradation reactions, such as oxidations and hydrolyses. Therefore, to overcome these limitations, suitable excipients can be incorporated into the liquid extracts and be co-dried.

Therefore, the powder obtained containing a high content of dry herbal extracts is appropriate for other pharmacotechnical processes, such as direct compression or wet granulation [9, 10, 11]. Thus, factors such as the properties of the crude herb, the extraction method and the type of excipient can affect the physical characteristics of the powder extract, and therefore it is useful to previously investigate the behavior of selected excipient carriers of dry extracts [12]. The "Review on Pharmaceutical Excipients" by PAWAR et al. (2015) divides up the excipients, commonly used in the pharmaceutical industry, according to different categories, such as origin, and function. It also introduces new pharmaceutical excipients [13]. In the same way, other reviews and guides from The International Pharmaceutical Excipients Council provide essential information for choosing the most suitable excipients for a particular pharmaceutical formulation [14, 15].

In this chapter, the different drying techniques for obtaining powdered vegetable extracts will be described. It should be emphasized that selecting the most appropriate methodology depends on the characteristics related to the chemical complexity of botanicals, as well as the desirable pharmacotechnical properties [16].

FUNDAMENTAL ASPECTS: DRYING PHARMACEUTICAL PRODUCTS

Drying is among the most usual *processes in* industrial operations and has a significant impact on the properties of the final product. In this process, moisture (often water) is thermally removed to yield a solid [17] and the heated gas causes the conversion of this moisture from the liquid to the vapor state in a mass and heat transfer phenomenon [18,19,20]. This complex process can lead to numerous physical changes in the material, such as: shrinkage, puffing, crystallization, glass transition, solubility changes, bioavailability, color, taste, odor, etc. Moreover, depending on the purpose of the product, these changes can be desirable or undesirable [18,20].

The reasons for removing moisture from a product are diverse and mainly include:

- Preservation and storage: Products with lower humidity have greater physical chemical and microbiological stability;
- Powdered products are easy-to-handle and transport: powdered material often occupies a smaller volume, which often ends up being a great advantage as it decreases the physical space for storage and transportation.

In the pharmaceutical industry, drying is used in synthetic and biological products for oral, ocular and even transdermal applications [21, 22, 23]. Therefore, *these* products were made in various different forms: tablets, capsules, suspensions, solutions, nanometric particle size, enzymes, proteins, etc. Due to the high added value of these products, selecting the most appropriate drying method should take into account aspects such as: the physical properties of the wet material, its thermal sensitivity, drying kinetics and equilibrium properties, as well as the final characteristics of the product and the economic and energy costs [20]. Due to the significant impact on the characteristics of the final pharmaceutical product, if inadequate drying conditions are used, it may lead to irreversible damage in terms of product quality and, hence, cause *financial losses* [18,24].

During the drying process, the heat exchange between the drying gas and the wet product should be sufficient for the moisture to vaporize and then diffuse through the material, being subsequently transported by the drying gas stream. Thus, in any drying operation, heat and mass transfer between the drying agent and the wet product is a common process and, therefore, extremely important in terms of understanding the drying steps.

Understanding this operation requires an explanation of some important terms, which will be presented in the context of water, but can be applied to various other solvents, such as ethanol (a solvent commonly used in the production of plant extracts). Therefore, in the following topics, some fundamental aspects of the drying *phenomenon will be explained.*

Moisture Content

Moisture content (MC) is a measure the total amount of solvents contained in the solid and is an important parameter to be evaluated because the MC influences the properties of a pharmaceutical formulation. Mathematically, MC can be expressed as:

$$MC = \frac{\text{Weight of moisture in sample}}{\text{Weight of dry sample}} \times 100$$

During drying, the MC of wet feedstock granules *continually decays* until they reach the equilibrium moisture content with the drying air.

Dry Bulb and Wet Bulb Temperature

During the drying process, the absolute humidity and relative humidity values are extremely important in terms of controlling the final humidity of the dried product. Both measurements (absolute humidity and relative humidity) are difficult to determine directly. Thus, by using a hygrometer, the moisture content of a material can be obtained.

A psychrometer consists of two thermometers, one that is kept moist with distilled water and one that is dry. In the wet bulb thermometer, the temperature decreases due to the heat removed to evaporate the water, until it is stationary. It is expected that the evaporation in the wet bulb is higher due to the drying air and therefore, the greater the cooling is in this thermometer. It should be mentioned that the dry bulb temperature is measured using a standard thermometer. The relative humidity is obtained from tables that relate the observed temperatures in the dry bulb and wet bulb. *A larger difference between* the *wet* and *dry bulbs* of the psychrometer *means* that the *relative humidity* is *lower*. The smaller difference means higher relative humidity. If the temperature observed in both thermometers is identical, the air is saturated and therefore no evaporation will occur [25, 26, 27].

Dew Point Temperature

The dew point is the temperature at which air becomes saturated with water vapor and, thus, water begins to condense [28, 29, 30].

Vapor Pressure

Vapor pressure or equilibrium vapor pressure is a measure of a liquid´s evaporation rate. It is defined as the pressure of the vapor over a condensed phase (liquid or solid) at a given temperature in a closed system.

The vapor pressure of any substance increases non-linearly with the temperature. Thus, higher temperatures allow for higher amounts of vapor gas in the system, while lower temperatures allow for smaller amounts [28, 29, 30].

Relative Humidity (%RH)

The relative humidity is expressed as the ratio of partial pressure of water vapor to the saturated vapor pressure of water at a particular temperature in an air-water mixture.

Thus, relative humidity is indicative of how close the air is to saturation, rather than indicating the actual amount of water vapor in the air.

The following equation expresses this relation [28, 29]:

$$\% \text{RH} = \frac{\text{Partial pressure of water vapor}}{\text{Saturated vapor pressure of water}}$$

*at a particular temperature.

Bound and Unbound Moisture

Moisture in a solid can exist as either *bound moisture* or *unbound moisture.*

Bound moisture is defined as being chemically bound to the microstructure of the solid, i.e., it is located internally in the structure of the material. Moreover, the vapor pressure at a given temperature is lower than that observed for the pure solvent. Thus, the energy used to evaporate it is more than that used to remove unbound moisture and, therefore, it is not removed easily by physical drying processes.

Unbound moisture is defined as the moisture content in the solid which exerts an equillibrium vapour pressure equal to the saturated vapor pressure of the pure solvent. This type of moisture can be easily removed from a wet solid. Therefore, in a non-hygroscopic material, all the liquid is unbound, while in a hygroscopic material, the liquid in excess of the equilibrium moisture content is the unbound moisture. The free moisture of a solid is the moisture content in excess of the equilibrium moisture content. Thus, the free moisture is the same as the unbound moisture, under saturation conditions [31, 32].

Water Activity

Water Activity (Aw) is a qualitative measure that represents the availability of water to favor microbial growth and chemical reactions. Aw is obtained by the ratio of the water vapor pressure in the product (Ps) to the vapor pressure of the pure water (Po), at a constant temperature [2, 5].

$$\mathbf{Aw} = \frac{\mathbf{Ps}}{\mathbf{Po}}$$

Ps = Partial water vapor pressure above the sample
Po = Vapor pressure of pure water at the same temperature

High levels of moisture and water activity in pharmaceutical and foods products are associated with deterioration and loss of stability. Some materials have high free moisture content, which results in high values of Aw. Consequently, they are more likely to undergo microbial growth and chemical and biochemical reactions [20].

Additionally, at a constant temperature, the water activity is related to the equilibrium relative humidity present in the atmosphere [33]:

$$\mathbf{Aw} = \frac{\text{Relative moisture}}{100}$$

Drying Mechanism

During drying there are two phases: the *constant rate drying* period and the falling rate drying period occur concomitantly with heat and mass transfer mechanisms [35, 36].

In the first phase, the surface moisture contained in the wet feedstock granules is removed by diffusion from the surface by stationary air film, which is in contact with it. This process occurs at a constant rate of drying, depending mainly on the temperature and humidity at which the drying air is transmitted to the material. Thus, the maximum drying rate is limited by the heat transfer between the drying air and the wet solid. If the drying process continues, the critical moisture content will be reached.

In the second phase, the falling rate drying period starts when the drying rate begins to drop. During *this phase*, the moisture inside the wet feedstock granules diffuses to the surface of the particle and is removed. Then, as result, a concentration gradient between the inside and outside of the particle is formed.

The duration and speed at which the drying occurs are determined mainly by the ability of the drying air to absorb and carry away the moisture. Both properties can be controlled by air temperature and air flow rate. Thus, the higher the temperature of the drying air, the greater its vapor holding capacity [18, 19, 37, 38].

Excessive removal of moisture can lead to irreversible changes in the product, leading to economic loss. Therefore, different ways are used to determine the drying end point. One of these techniques is to collect small samples of the product at different stages of the drying process. Then, a drying curve is established, relating the moisture content of the sample and the drying time. When the product temperature starts going up, the drying finishes at specific and desired product-moisture content. Other techniques with physico-chemical fundamentals include Karl Fischer titration and Loss-on Drying (LOD) moisture analyzers, which are routinely used [38].

Equilibrium Moisture Content and Sorption Isotherms

During a drying process, the rate of drying is limited by two processes: heat and mass transfer. Owing to the fact that drying is a process of thermal nature, heat transfer has a fundamental role in the drying operation. The main heat transfer mechanisms are convection, conduction, radiation and dielectric or microwave heating [36] and will be discussed later in the section on "Classification of Drying Operations."

The moisture flow from the region of higher vapor pressure to that of lower pressure occurs until the moisture content of the solid is in equilibrium with the humidity of the air. At this point, which is called equilibrium moisture content of a solid; the solid neither gains nor loses moisture. Thus, the residual moisture of a dry solid cannot be less than the equilibrium moisture content, corresponding to the humidity of the inlet gas [18, 19, 34, 36]. The equilibrium moisture value remains unchanged if the humidity and temperature of the environment also remain unchanged and it depends on factors such as: the physicochemical properties of the solid to be dried, the way in which the water is held by the material, the processing conditions, the temperature, pressure, relative humidity and flow rate of the drying agent. From this information, equilibrium moisture curves or equilibrium isotherms are traced and provide information of fundamental importance to the drying process modeling, as well as the development of packages that preserve and maintain the quality of the product [17, 34, 39].

There is a relationship between moisture content of a material and relative humidity for a given temperature. Therefore, the equilibrium moisture content can be plotted as a function of relative humidity and these graphical representations are generally called equilibrium isotherms. An equilibrium isotherm obtained when the dry material is exposed to increasing humidity is called the adsorption isotherm. On the other hand, desorption isotherm can be traced when the wet material is exposed to decreasing values of moisture. Due to many types of interactions, such as colligative, surface effects and capillary between water and the solid components, the moisture sorption isotherm is unique for each product and specific temperature. The difference between the adsorption and desorption curves is called *hysteresis* [18, 20,3 4, 39].

As shown in Figure 1, a *sorption isotherm* comprises three regions (A, B, C) which are distinguished by the amount of moisture in the system and the different water binding mechanisms on the solid matrix. In *region A*, the water is strongly bound in monolayer, which are high-energy polar sites and its enthalpy of vaporization is higher than that of pure water. In this region, there is no distinction between adsorption and desorption isotherms. They are usually non-free and are not available for chemical or biochemical reactions. *Region B* delimits a region where additional layers of water settle into smaller capillaries forming a multilayer system. In this region, the water molecules are bound less firmly than in region A, and thus are available as a solvent for low-molecular-weight solutes and for some biochemical reactions. This region shows the transition from the bound to the free type of water.

Region C comprises Aw values greater than 0.7 and, thus, the water approaches the condensed condition on the surface of the solid and is available for reactions as a solvent [18, 19, 40].

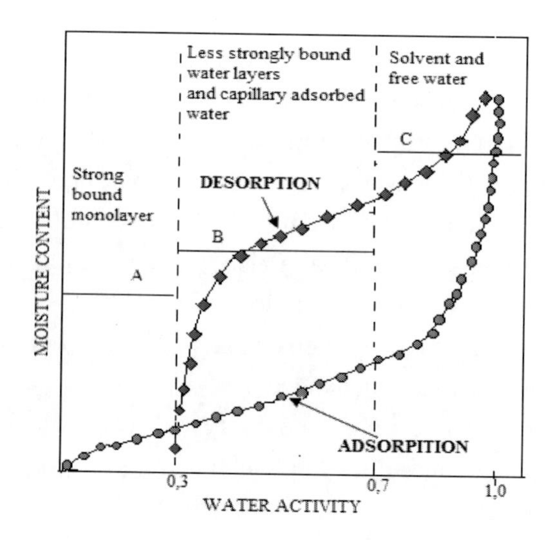

Figure 1. General type of sorption isotherm and hysteresis phenomenon.

The information provided through the sorption isotherm is essential in the drying process and also for storing the product as it can obtain the minimum and maximum equilibrium moisture values that a solid is subjected to after drying at a constant temperature. The process to construct a sorption isotherm consists of collecting the Aws and the moisture values of a solid, using gravimetric techniques and moisture analyzers [34, 41].

Many scientific *publications* present empirical and theoretical models with the purpose of adjusting the experimental results obtained in the sorption isotherms. In 1940, Brunauer et al. classified isotherms into 5 different types, in which the Langmuir's adsorption isotherm is the most important theoretical model and is based on the forces acting on the monomolecular layer of the solid. BET (Brunauer, Emmett and Teller) and GAB (Guggenhein-Anderson-deBoer) isotherms are extensions of Langmuir's adsorption isotherm. These models, commonly used, describe sigmoidal shapes of the isotherms and support the multi molecular layers [43, 44]. Additionally, Limousin et al. (2007) reported on details of various experimental methods for acquiring an isotherm of sorption. In 1978, Iglesias and Chirife described some of the mathematical relationships used to prepare isotherms. All these scientific publications contributed in some way to establishing different empirical or mechanistic models and give details of various experimental methods to acquire sorption isotherm [42].

BEHAVIOR OF SOLIDS DURING THE DRYING PROCESS

During the processing of pharmaceutical solid dosage forms, various factors may lead to increased moisture in the product obtained. Moisture comes from various sources such as manufacturing processes, bulk drug, inactive excipient and environmental conditions, among others. Moreover, the water can interact in different ways with the solid and it has a great impact on the physical and chemical properties of the final product. As a result, it can influence the stability of the product, its flow properties and also some industrial processes such as tablet compaction and wet granulation. Therefore, it can influence the product stability, powder flow properties and some industrial processes such as tablet compaction and wet granulation [45].

It should be mentioned that the physical-chemical properties of a pharmaceutical active ingredient is important information in the drug *development* process. Probably, the structural organization of atoms and molecules of the solid is one of the most essential properties during drying. Its importance is due to the fact that during the drying process, the product is subjected to conditions that can be modified giving rise to materials with different physical and chemical characteristics [46, 47].

The structural organization of a solid may be of the crystalline type or amorphous type. For a crystalline drug, the most common forms found are polymorphs and solvates

[46, 48]. In crystalline materials, the internal structures are arranged homogeneously and uniformly in three dimension spaces. A drug is defined as a polymorph when it can exist in the solid state with two different crystal structures. In the solvated crystalline forms, the water molecules are connected by capillarity; they are present between the interstitial spaces of the particles and are removable using little energy expenditure. Therefore, the equilibrium moisture content is close to zero. Commonly the materials in this category are inorganic and, consequently their physical chemical properties are not very affected by the heating. This category includes products commonly used as excipients in the pharmaceutical industry, such as zinc oxide, calcium sulfate and magnesium oxide [33].

On the other hand, the absence of a crystallization pattern characterizes so-called non-crystalline or amorphous solids. These materials do not have a well-defined molecular organization and due to this, the diffusion of the solvent molecules occurs at a slower rate through the interstitial spaces of the solid and consequently, this solid has high equilibrium moisture content. Therefore, amorphous solids are more difficult to dry [33, 49].
In the pharmaceutical industry, amorphous solid dosage forms are quite desirable because of their physical and chemical stability; higher solubility, higher dissolution rate and sometimes better compression characteristics than the corresponding crystals. The following can be found in this category: casein, aluminum hydroxide, yeast, proteins, peptides and some sugars and polymers [47].

Various papers have been *presented* about the moisture sorption isotherms of crystalline and amorphous forms of some pharmaceutical excipients. Based on this data, important information can be found concerning the interaction of these compounds with the moisture [18].

CLASSIFICATION OF DRYING OPERATIONS

Drying operations can be classified in several ways. Typically the classification criteria are: temperature, pressure, working regime and mechanisms of heat supply [34, 51]. Concerning the temperature during the drying operation, it can change according to the characteristics of the desired material and may be lower or higher than the boiling temperature of the *moisture content* in the *solid*. During drying by vaporization, the temperature is greater than the boiling point of the solvent. On the other hand, during lyophilization, drying takes place through the phenomenon of sublimation. In this condition, the low pressures used in the system allow the frozen water, present in the material structure, to pass directly from the solid phase to the vapor phase without being unfrozen. Lyophilization is a drying methodology widely used in the pharmaceutical industry and its main advantage is the suitability to thermo sensitive products [35, 42].

Regarding the production system used, the types of industrial dryers available on the market can operate under two modes of operation: batch/mix or continuous mode. The first type is ideal for pilot-scale production regimes, where the product volume is small and production cycles are short. In the second type, feeding the equipment and unloading the dried material is done continuously, one example is producing excipients [34, 51].

Handling solids during drying may occur in the presence or absence of agitation of the material to be dried. Moreover, the drying beds can be classified as static bed dryers and fluidized bed dryers.

Heat transfer mechanisms, convection, conduction and dielectric (or radiation) phenomena are a criterion for the classification of dryers in direct and indirect types [53]. In the first type, the heat transferred and subsequent vaporization of the moisture contained in the solid occurs through a convection phenomenon between a heated gas and the wet material. In this type, the vaporizing liquid is carried away by the drying medium. Dryers using this mechanism are called adiabatic or direct dryers [17]. On the other hand, indirect or non-adiabatic dryers perform heat transfer through conduction. In this type, the temperature gradient is formed as a result of the contact between the solid and the heated gas, which comes from the heated metal wall of the dryer or from a source of radiation [31, 51, 54].

Approximately 85% of industrial dryers are convective type, applying hot air directly to the wet material. This model of dryer has much higher thermal efficiencies compared to indirectly heated dryers. However, convection drying is not always accepted because it can contaminate the product, thus in such cases, indirect heating must be used [33, 34, 54, 55].

SELECTING DRYING EQUIPMENT

Choosing the ideal industrial dryer is not a simple task and although there are different guidelines for selecting a dryer, it should be recognized that the standards presented are probably not suitable for all the pharmaceutical products [13]. The choice of drying equipment should be made in order to minimize these possible changes in the dry product [34, 51] taking into account factors such as the physical properties of the pharmaceutical active (thermo-sensitivity, friability, flammability, total moisture, drying kinetics), properties of the mixture between the drying agent and moisture, drying kinetics of the material and also the capacity of the equipment to produce the product with the required quality and requirements [34, 56]. In addition, the dryer must also operate reliably, safely, and economically [18, 19, 51, 53].

Some examples of the most used dryers in the phytopharmaceutical industry are described in the next section.

Drying Equipment

Fluidized Bed Dryer

In 1942, the fluidization technique first appeared in the petrochemical industry on a large scale due to the catalytic petrochemical cracking process known as Fluidized Catalytic Cracking (FCC). Since then, fluidization has spread to various other sectors of the chemical, food and pharmaceutical industries. Its success story is mainly due to its versatility and it can be applied to different processes such as drying, coating, granulation and mixing solids [57].

One of the reasons for the wide acceptance of fluidized beds in the pharmaceutical industry is that there are numerous variations of this equipment for laboratory and industrial use, which allows the use of different particle flow regimes of varying sizes, shapes and densities [57].

In a fluidization system, solid particles are freely suspended in an upward stream of gas. The velocity of the air flow used in the process should be greater than the sedimentation velocity of the particles and less than the velocity for pneumatic transport. At this rate, the particles are in continuous motion and all surfaces are exposed to the drying air. The air passes through the particles of the product causing them to move in a perpendicular direction. As a result, the particles of the solid acquire a flow regime which resembles boiling. In this situation, the solid mixture and air stream behave as a liquid and the system is said to be fluidizing. The process ends when the desired humidity is reached [33, 58].

At low speeds, the displacement of the fluid is insufficient to move the particles and the regime is called a fixed bed. As the fluid velocity increases the bed begin to expand to the condition where the drag exerted by the fluid on the particles equals the weight thereof, cancelling out the compressive forces between adjacent particles. In this condition, the regime is said to be incipient fluidization or minimum fluidization [57]. The minimum fluidization is a characteristic of the particle, depending on its size, shape and specific mass and therefore is not affected by the characteristics of the equipment and its determination is very important.

There are different kinds of fluidization regime and the particles behave as the fluid flow increases. Some examples of fluidization regimes are:

- Bubbling (it has a formation of preferential channels, such as bubbles, movement of the most vigorous solid),
- Slugging (piston) (Bubbles begin to coalesce and grow, movement of the particles in pistons),
- Turbulent (still higher flows, very vigorous and agitated movement, very fast flow);

- Pneumatic Transport (the flow is so high that the transport of the particles occurs, leaving the bed) [59].

  Figure 2 shows an illustration of the fluidizations regimes.

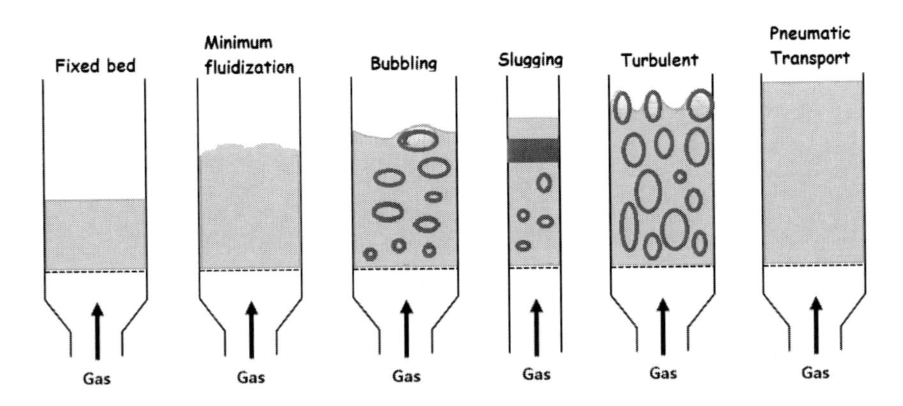

Figure 2. Illustration of fluidization regimes.

In the solid-liquid flow regime, drying occurs through a combined heat and mass transfer mechanism. Moreover, the high degree of contact between the two phases promotes a high heat transfer, allowing this technique to have greater thermal efficiency in relation to other drying processes. For example, the fluid bed dryer has been shown to be thermally efficient two to six times over a tray dryer [33, 34]. Other advantages relate to the wide versatility of the dryer, such as: the ability to work with wide feed ranges from a few grams to tons per hour, coating, mixing, granulating, pelleting and drying and the instrumentation and process control are user-friendly. These characteristics enable the fluidized bed to be used in sequential operations of drug production [33]. The limitations in the fluidization process include friability or large particle products [58, 60].

Figure 3 presents some main variants for the pharmaceutical industry: fluidized beds of the bottom spray type, top spray or tangential spray. In Figure 3.a, the first bed is called the "WURSTER chamber." In this model, the atomizer nozzle is positioned directly into the bed of the product and is useful in terms of coating and granulation processes. In Figure 3.b, the TOP SPRAY type bed is useful in terms of granulation and coating processes. The apparatus consists of a conical chamber with a cylindrical top, where an atomizer nozzle and a filter with automatic discharge/ cleaning. In Figure 3.c, the TANGENTIAL SPRAY bed can be observed. In this model, the nozzle that is located tangentially to the wall of the chamber atomizes the solution over the solids being moved through the air flow from the bottom region of the bed.

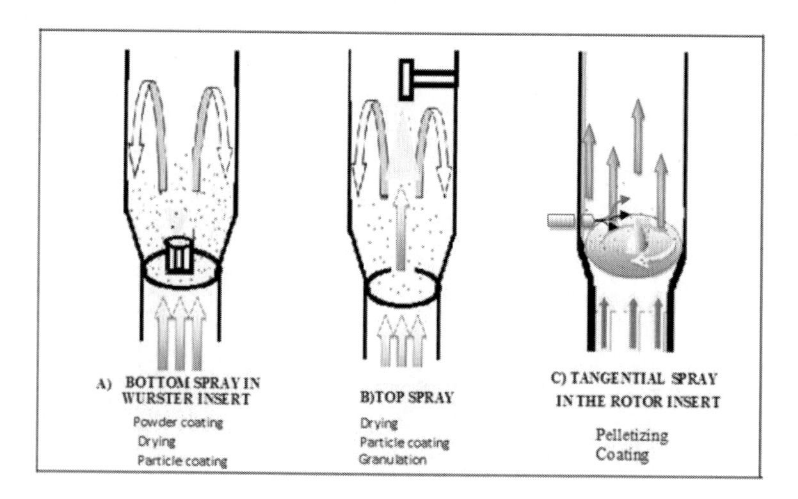

Figure 3. Fluidized Bed System used in Pharmaceutical Industry.

The fluidization regime in a spouted bed is characterized by the formation of three regions with different gas-solid flows. These regions are described below and can be seen in Figure 4:

a) the central or spouted region, where the particles are dragged by the stream of air passing at high ascending velocity;
b) the annular region around the central region where air passes at low velocity - about 30% of the total air passes through this region - and the particles have a downward movement under gravity until they re-enter the gushing region
c) fountain, where the particles that were spilt fall back into the annular region.

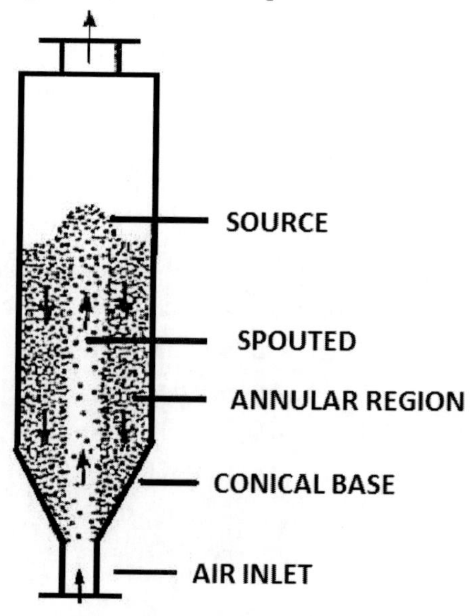

Figure 4. Regions of the spouted bed.

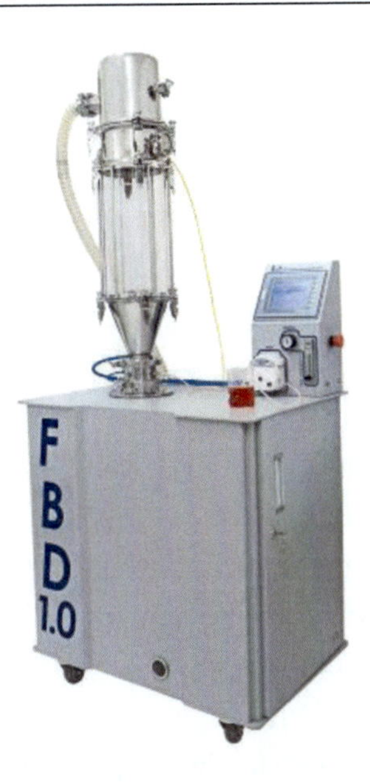

Figure 5. Fluid bed dryer. Laboratory scale, MODEL FBD 1.0- Courtesy: Labmaq do Brasil Ltd.

A variation of the fluidized bed widely used in the pharmaceutical industry is the spouted bed. The main distinction is related to the size of the particles used as the fluidization. Particles larger than 1 millimeter, when fluidized tend to develop undesirable regimes such as slugging and channeling [61]. Thus, the spouted bed is recommended for larger particles and difficult-to-fluidize products [59, 62] and is a low cost drying equipment option that can be used in coating, granulation, drying paste, solutions and suspensions (dry fruit pulp, animal blood, fungi and plant extracts) [61, 64, 65]. There are fluid bed equipments for several scales of powder manipulation, from few grams at lab scale, Figure 5, to several tons in industrial scale. An example of lab scale fluidized bed dryer can be seen in Figure 5, showing the FBD 1.0 (from *Labmaq do Brasil Ltd., Brazil*) for 1 kg load of solids.

Marreto, Freire and Freitas (2006) conducted a study to evaluate drying plant extracts and microcapsules in spouted beds. The authors compared the morphology of indomethacin microcapsules obtained from a spray dryer and a spouted bed. The microcapsules obtained in the spouted bed showed a tendency to retain the drug in their matrix, however according to the authors, the reasons for this behavior are not clear [64]. Also, by monitoring the major chemical markers of Guarana and Annato extracts the authors concluded that the operational conditions used in spouted bed drying provide good preservation of active principles and adequate moisture content in dry powders. Particularly, the Annatto drying process has shown to be competitive when compared to commercial methods.

Freeze Drying

Many products from the pharmaceutical industry, such as proteins, microorganisms, pharmaceuticals, tissues & plasma lose their viability in the liquid state or deteriorate easily if subjected to drying at high temperatures, oxygen or atmospheric pressure. In this context, considering products with these characteristics, the freeze drying/lyophilization technique is an excellent method for preserving a wide range of heat-sensitive materials [19, 33].

The technique uses the sublimation process to remove ice or other frozen solvents and the desorption process to remove bound water molecules from a substance [66]. During the whole process, the temperature of the product must be low enough to avoid changes in the dried product´s appearance and characteristics. The process consists of three steps: pre-freezing, sublimation drying and secondary drying.

Pre-freezing is an essential step because an inadequate time and temperature of freezing can result in undesirable characteristics of the lyophilized material, such as ice crystals and large pores [51].Usually, in the pharmaceutical industry, the temperatures range from -10ºC to -40ºC [33].

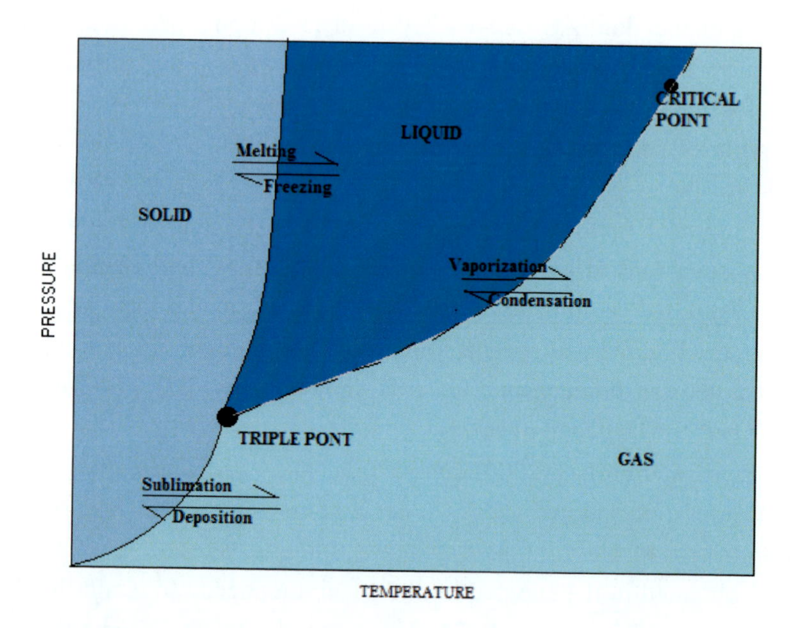

Figure 6. Pressure-temperature diagram for water, showing the conditions for various phases.

During sublimation, the frozen material changes from the solid state directly to a vapor, without first going through its liquid phase [67]. During this endothermic stage, the water present in the structure of the solid is removed by providing heat which may be by conduction or radiation. To prevent melting ice and consequently physical-chemical and structural damage of the material, the temperature of the ice should be below the melting temperature of the solvent in the absolute operating pressure [34]. At the final stage, called secondary drying desorption of all the frozen moisture takes place that is bound to the structure of the material, then all the frozen solvents will pass directly to the gaseous state. This transition occurs below the triple point at 25°C and 60°C, and the system must be under a reduced pressure [67].The phenomenon described above is shown in Figure 6. Moreover, Figure 7 presents the parts of hypothetical *freeze drying*.

In the pharmaceutical industry, the applicability of the freeze drying technique extends to products of biological origin such as blood, plasma, antibiotics, hormones, bacterial cultures, vaccines. Furthermore, freeze-drying is widely used in the food industry to preserve food. [36, 67, 68, 69].

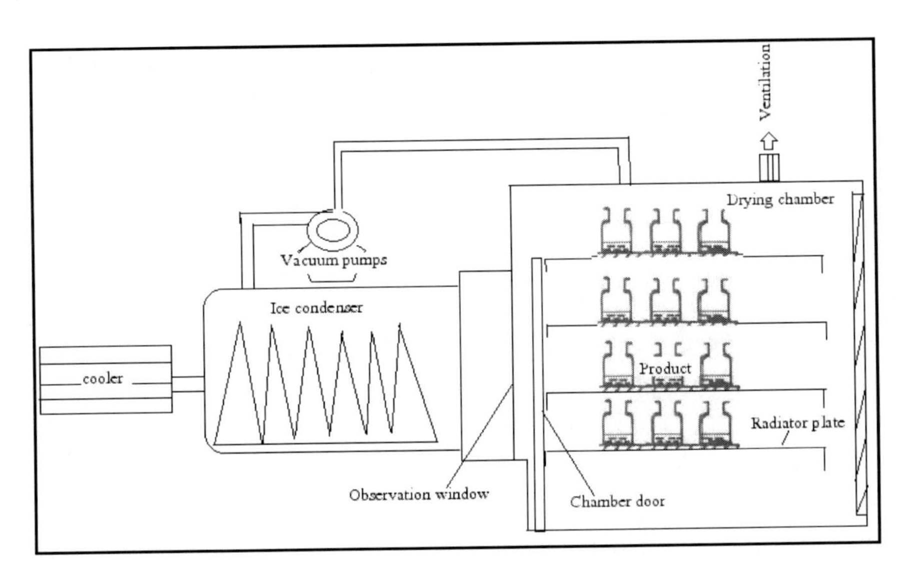

Figure 7. Schematic freeze drying.

Spray Drying

The spray drying technique is one of the most versatile for processing powdered products. It began in the mid-18th century with an atomization and heating process for drying eggs. Soon after, approximately in 1920, it spread to industries in the form of milk and soap powder. Afterwards, it was used in the food, chemical, electronics, and pharmaceutical and biopharmaceutical industries [24, 70]. This technique differs from other types of drying processes because it converts solutions, suspensions and pastes into dry matter in a few seconds [18, 33, 71].

In the pharmaceutical industry, it is widely used to produce raw drugs, excipients or microparticles and can be applied to a wide range of materials, including heat-sensitive, water-soluble and water-insoluble drugs [72-74]. This is a useful method to obtain spherical particles that have a small size and a narrow distribution. The advantages of the method include the fact that the drying process is completed in one step and that the residence time of particles inside the dryer does not exceed 30 seconds. It is also suitable for drying thermo sensitive materials such as plant extracts [2, 9, 16, 75], microorganisms [76], proteins, etc. [33, 55, 73, 78, 79], pilot or industrial scales (easy scale-up) [18]. In addition to the modulation of the physical-chemical properties of the material, such as moisture content, density, flow ability, morphology and particle size, it can be achieved by modifying the operational variables such as air inlet temperature, feed flow rate and drying air used in the spray dryer *[24, 80, 81]*. In addition, the spray drying technique is used to obtain liposomal systems and also nanoparticles for novel pulmonary drug delivery formulations [82], as well as producing microparticles and microcapsules for cosmetic and therapeutic purposes [74, 83, 84].

The effect of spray drying on the physical chemical properties of carbamazepine, indomethacin, piroxicam, and nifedipine was studied by Martins et al. (2012). These compounds have high permeability and low solubility and due to this they are attractive targets for research aiming to increase solubility and dissolution rates (85).

The experimental results demonstrate a correlation between the decrease in particle size and increase in the dissolution rate of the spray dried drugs, while the relative crystallinity, solubility and density of the four compounds were minimally affected by spray drying.

Thus, the data demonstrate that a decrease in drug article size induced by spray drying can enhance drug dissolution. Moreover, the authors point out that spray drying technique may lead to other physicochemical changes in active pharmaceutical ingredients, however they were unable to correlate these changes and the increase in drug dissolution [86].

Mendonça et al. (2015) evaluated the antioxidant and antigenotoxic effects of curcumim solid dispersion microparticles produced by the spray drying technique. Curcumin is the main active component derived from the rhizome of Curcuma longa (Curcuma longa L.) and although it has many therapeutic properties, low concentration is detected when it is administered orally. Thus, the formulation of solid dispersion microparticles is a key strategy for improving the solubility and bioavailability of this poorly water soluble compound.

In this study, the antioxidant and antigenotoxic effects of the solid dispersions were compared to those of the unmodified curcumin and it was concluded that the therapeutic effects remain in both products and the water soluble increases in curcumin solid dispersion microparticles [87]. Table 1 show some spray dryer studies performed on medicinal plant extracts.

The operating mechanism is based on the atomization of the sample into small diameter droplets and subsequent dispersion into a stream of heated air. When the drop comes in contact with the flow of heated gas, its temperature rapidly increases and is slightly higher than the wet bulb temperature of the drying gas. The solvent contained in the sample evaporates rapidly before the dry solid reaches the wall of the drying chamber and then the dried particle is charged by the air stream to a reservoir system [33, 58].

Table 1. Studies involving spray dry studies performed on plant materials

Drug	Product	Objective	Reference
Tanacetum parthenium	Bioactives	Enteric coated tablets	88
Eugenia dysenterica	Bioactives	Spray-dried extracts	89
Syzygium cumini	Bioacives	Spray-dried extracts	90
Turmeric	Curcumin	Solid dispersion	91-93
Green coffee oil	Oil	Microencapsulation	94

Figure 8 shows the atomization and formation of dry particles. In this heat transfer and mass process, after removing the solvent, a thin solid film forms on the surface of the particle. In later stages, the rest of the moisture should evaporate and, for this to happen, the solvent should diffuse to the surface of the droplet. Energetically, the solvent diffusion rate through the droplet is inversely proportional to the heat transfer and, therefore, the accumulation of heat causes the liquid within the droplet to evaporate and raise its internal pressure. As a result, the droplet swells and its surface diameter decreases, causing an increase in the diffusion rate of the internally located solvent. However, if the drop is not elastic and permeable, the elevation of the internal pressure will lead to the rupture of the droplet and the formation of small dry solid fragments [33, 54, 96, 97, 103]. An interesting review on spray drying in the pharmaceutical industry was written by Jain M.S. et.al. (2011) and Vehring (2007).

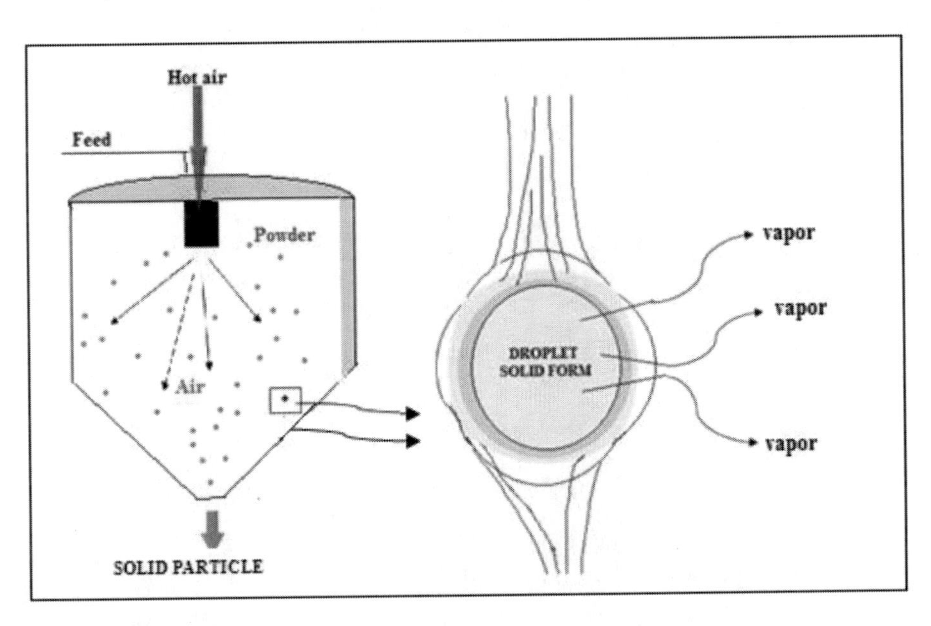

Figure 8. Atomization and formation of solid particle.

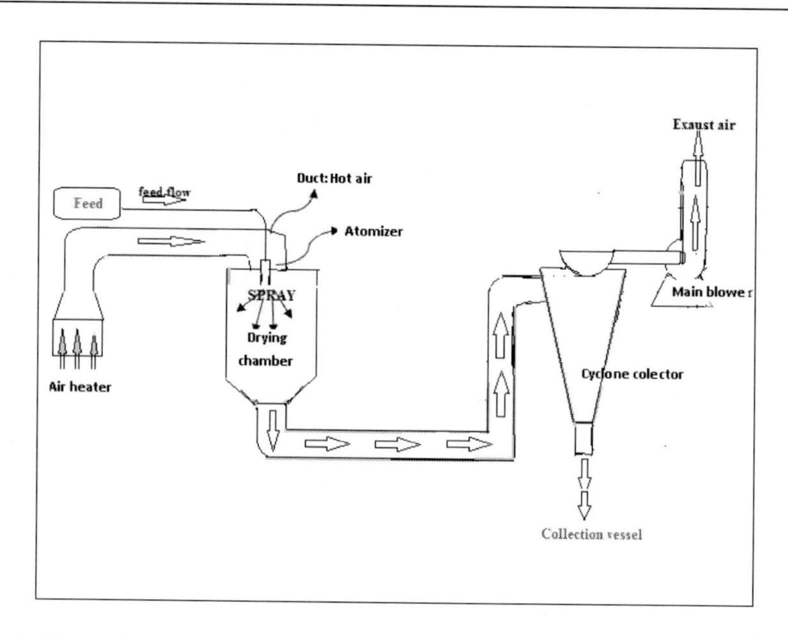

Figure 9. Typical Spray drying system flowsheet.

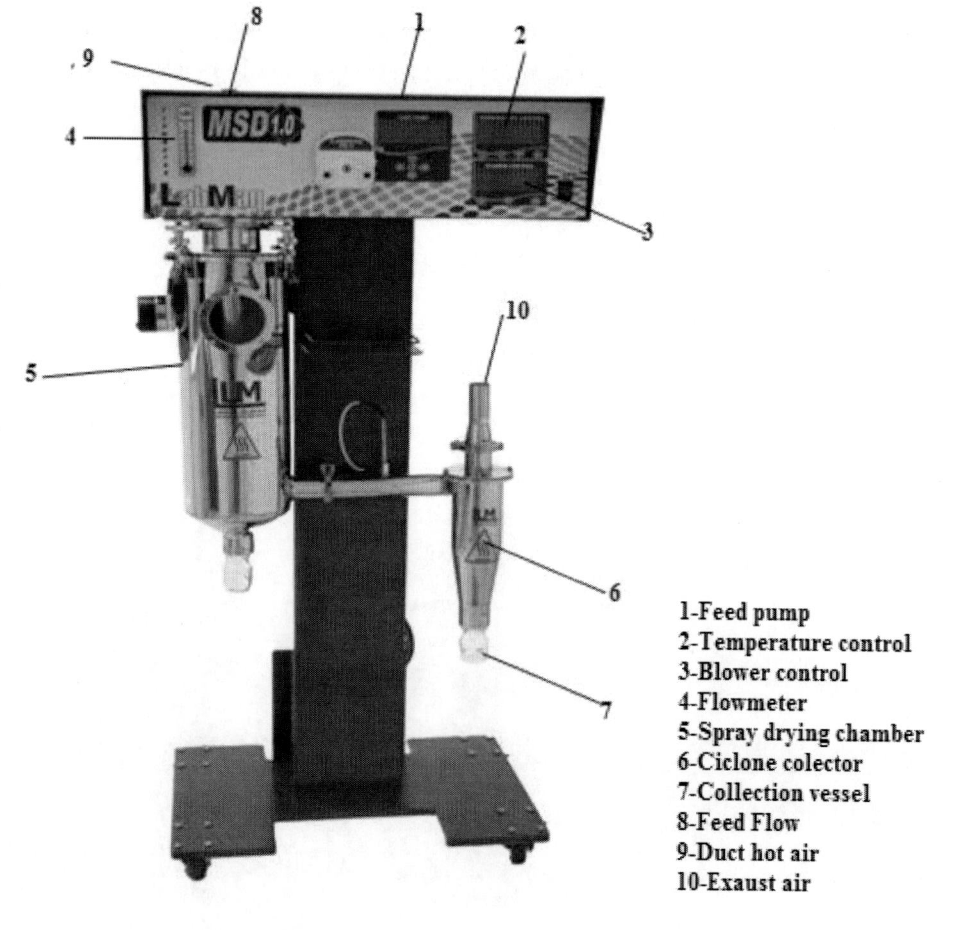

Figure 10. Spray Dryer - Model: MSDi 1.0 - Courtesy LABMAQ do Brasil.

All types of spray drying comprise the basic components of a feed delivery system, atomizer, drying chamber, solid-gas separator, heated air supply and product collection system [54], as shown in Figure 9. Figure 10 shows a spray dryer, MSD 1.0 model from LABMAQ DO BRASIL.

Some operating variables such as the atomizing nozzle, feed and flow rate and temperature can be altered, by spray drying to adjust and modify some morphological properties, such as particle size, surface and shape of the powder. These changes have a *direct influence* on *physical* and *chemical properties* of the pharmaceutical powder [19, 33, 51, 96].

Guimarães et al. (2015) evaluated the most important factors to control during the spray drying of D-mannitol in order to obtain particles of spray-dried mannitol with a high value of circularity. To select the best spray-drying operational parameters, the multivariate experimental design was used. The authors concluded that the drying outlet temperature, ethanol and the concentration of the feed solution (mannitol solution) are the operational parameters that contribute to the surface and size variation of spray dried manitol particles [98].

Using drying additives is a very important tool in spray drying as they can cause an increase in the glass transition temperature, and therefore, the material can be dried under conditions where adequate evaporation of the solvent occurs without adhesion of the product [70, 99]. There is a wide range of additives that can be used to improve drying yield, reducing losses by adhesion to the walls of the equipment. Some of these additives are still responsible for modifying dry powder properties such as stability, controlled release of actives [72, 100-102].

Below is a summary of the main additives and their functions used in the drying process

- Colloidal silicon dioxide: antiadhesive, decreases density and hygroscopicity
- Modified starches: antiadhesive, physical barrier, diluent, antiadhesive
- Maltodextrins, Physical barrier, diluent
- Cellulose derivatives (CMC, Ethylcellulose, HPMC): modified release, physical barrier.
- Gelatins, physical barrier, diluent
- Goma Arabica: physical barrier for volatiles.
- Sugars (Sorbitol, malitol, mannitol): antiadhesive, diluent
- Acrylate derivatives modified release functions (pharmaceutical coating).

In the section, “Excipients for dried medicinal extracts,” a case study proposed by Mello Costa (2016) will be presented. This study present a framework to define optimal excipient for a plant extract, using the drying of Copaifera langsdorffii extracts in a spray dryer as an example.

Figure 11, obtained by scanning electron microscopy, shows the morphology of a spherical powder particle, obtained using the spray drying technique.

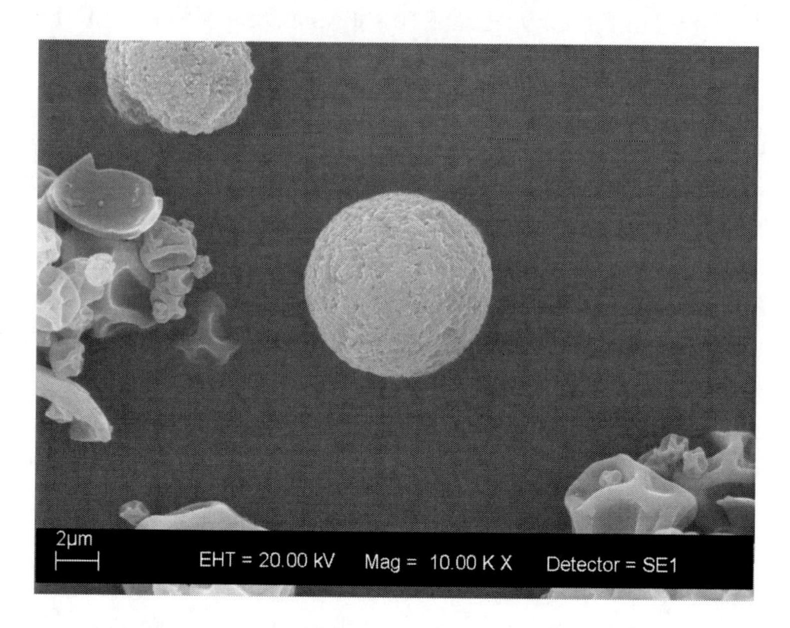

Figure 11. Photomicrography of the powder increasing by 10,000 x. Powder of the Endopleura uchi extract with starch and aerosil® (Source: Tacon, 2012 [103]).

Spray Congealing

Spray congealing is a drying technique also known as spray chilling or spray cooling [104]. It has been widely studied in the pharmaceutical field, as well as in the food industry [105-108]. It is used in these areas due to the fact that this technique allows the formation of controlled release microparticles, a mixture of active substances that are not soluble in water, which have low stability, high reactivity in aqueous medium, improved solubility and reduced hygroscopicity [107]. This technique is a variation of a spray dryer, whereby instead of aqueous solutions, the vehicle used as a carrier is lipid materials. By melting this matrix and its components, it is transported to an atomizing nozzle and, as the spray dryer, after atomization, a droplet is transformed into millions of droplets that will result in microparticles. The solidification and consequently formation of these microparticles occurs through contact with cold air (generally below 25°C and above 1°C). Generally, the higher the melting point of the lipid matrix, the cooler the drying air needs to be [105]. An illustration of this technique can be seen in Figure 12.

Depending on the model of the equipment, the particles can be collected in two locations: in the drying chamber (large particles) and in the cyclone (small diameter particles).

It is a low-cost technique that does not require organic solvents, it does not work at high temperatures and it is fast.

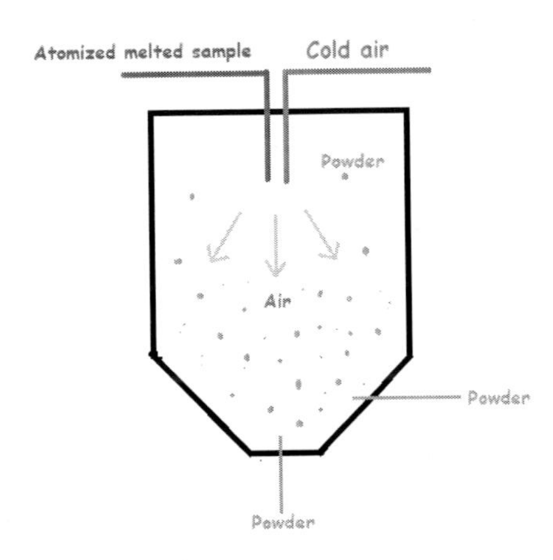

Figure 12. Schematic spray congealing technique.

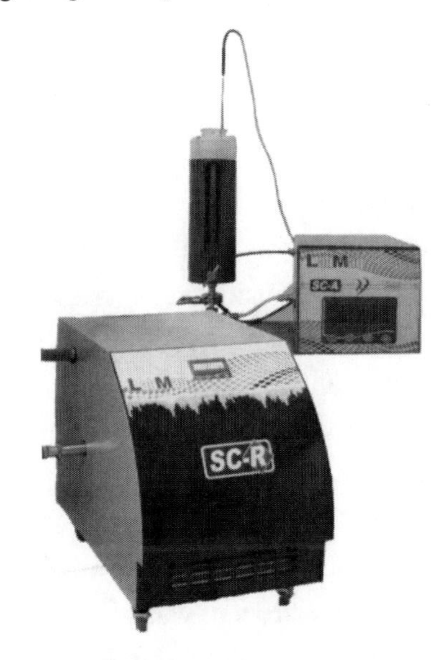

Figure 13. Equipment for the spray congealing technique in lab scale. Courtesy Labmaq do Brasil Ltd, Brazil.

There are various materials that are studied and used as lipid matrices. Some of these examples are: beeswax, castor oil, almond oil, polyethylene glycols, Gelucire®, Poloxamer®, palm oil, cocoa butter, among others [106-109]. The lipid matrix should be carefully chosen based on the substance to be loaded. In some cases, a mixture of them is needed for best results. A study by Martins et al. (2012) evaluated the solid dispersions of carbamazepine using congealing spray.Using a three-factor, three-level Box-Behnken design, they evaluated the effects of the operating conditions of congealing spray on the carbamazepine solubility. The experimental results indicated spherical microparticles and changes in the crystalline state of the drug. As a result, there was an increase in the solubility and dissolution rate of spray-dried carbamazepine compared to the raw drug [110]. Despite the advantages of this technique, there are still very few studies concerning drying extracts. A study conducted by Passerin et al. (2012) obtained promising results with the increase of the bioavailability of S*ilybum Marianum* bioactives through the association of mechanochemical activation and spray congealing [116]. Figure 13 shows the accessories used for the spray congealing technique.

Spray Freeze Dryer and Fluid Bed Atmospheric Spray Freeze Drying

These are new techniques that are being studied and evaluated in the pharmaceutical and food areas for pharmaceuticals, nanocomposites, food, bioproducts and others. These techniques have characteristics of both the spray drying process and the freeze-drying process. Furthermore, phytomedicines require exceptional chemical and physical stability, as well as low microbial growth, which in turn can be best achieved by their dried powder. In addition to more stability, powdered vegetable extracts allow for the preparation of tablets and capsules.Drying heat sensitive substances, such as natural and biotechnological products, has been of the utmost importance for biotechnologists, chemists and engineers.

Freeze-drying can produce high quality powder and preserved characteristics for thermo-sensitive products, however it is an expensive and time consuming technique. Spray drying is a very fast technique, with high productivity, however it is not used for thermo-sensitive products [111-115]. Considering these recent techniques, the samples are dried at low temperatures (<-5°C). Thus, they can be used for thermally sensitive samples, such as proteins, microorganisms, peptides and plant compounds. In addition, the samples are atomized, which allows for the formation of spherical particles of small diameters and with good flow [111-114].

The samples are atomized and form small droplets, and as in the spray dryer, they come in contact with cold air, causing the particles to freeze, and then they are subjected to the drying process to remove the frozen water that is formed together with the particles. There are numerous variables to be controlled: air temperature, cold air flow, sample concentration, feed rate, drying time, among others. This may interfere to a lesser or greater extent with characteristics such as porosity, solubility and average particle diameter of the final product [112].

Despite the complexity and various parameters, it has advantages compared to the other techniques as it joins together aspects from various techniques. It can be used for products that need to be dried at low temperatures and it has a spherical shape and a good flow [111]. Figure 14 shows an illustration of the fluidized bed atmospheric spray freeze drying technique.

Some of the additives used in spray freeze drying and fluid bed atmospheric spray freeze drying techniques can be used to decrease hygroscopicity, increase solubility, protect the active, control the release of drugs and also as a diluent. Some examples are: mannitol, trehalose, maltodextrins, cellulose derivatives and PVP. [111].

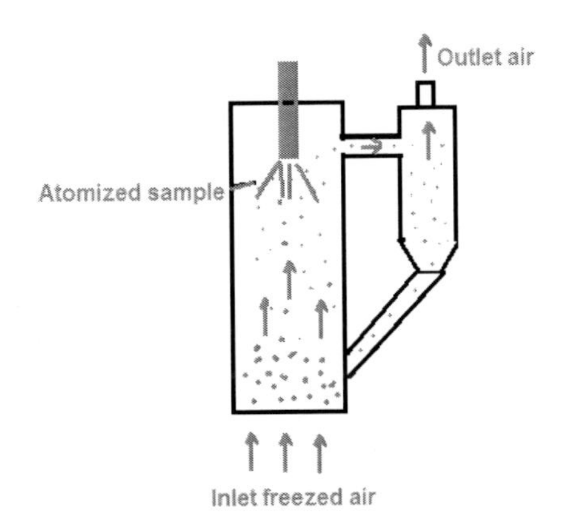

Figure 14. Fluidized bed atmospheric spray freeze drying technique.

Perfecting this process will bring numerous benefits to processing plant and biotechnology products for very specialized applications, such as phytomedicines and biopharmaceuticals. Table 2 shows some spray freeze and atmospheric freeze drying studies performed on plant materials. Figure 15 shows an example of an atmospheric spray freeze dryer.

Other advantages of using excipients in the spray drying process are to increase the dissolution rate, helping in manufacturing processes such as tableting or capsule filling [127, 128], taste masking for oral forms [126], overcoming common problems or limitations during drying heat-sensitive materials [129, 130], such as chemical degradation reactions and loss of biological activity [125, 131].

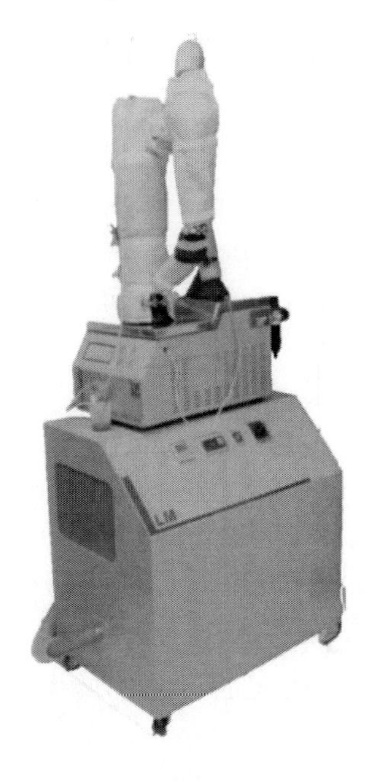

Figure 15. Fluidized bed atmospheric spray freeze dryer – Courtesy: Labmaq do Brasil.

Excipients for Dried Medicinal Extracts

The possibility of adding excipients to liquid plant extracts to produce intermediates for solid phytopharmaceutical forms is one of the factors responsible for the interest in the spray drying and other techniques [122]. Excipients may help to supply adequate physical properties for the powders since they provide specific characteristics such as a decrease in powder hygroscopicity, improvement in flowability and packing, etc. [123-125]. High capacity for compression and packing are also important processing parameters [127].

Table 2. Studies involving spray freeze and atmospheric freeze drying of compounds from plants

Drug	Product	Process	Reference
Coffee	volatile compounds	atmospheric freeze drying	[117]
Rabbiteye blueberry	bioactives	freeze-drying	[118]
Apium graveolens	bioacives	freeze drying	[119]
Averrhoa bilimbi	bioacives	freeze drying	[119]
Centella asiatica	bioacives	freeze drying	[119]
Mentha arvensis	bioacives	freeze drying	[119]
Psidium guajava	bioacives	freeze drying	[119]
Sauropus androgynous	bioacives	freeze drying	[119]
Solanum nigrum	bioacives	freeze drying	[119]
Polygonum minus	bioacives	freeze drying	[119]
Olea europaea	bioacives	freeze drying	[120]

In the previous sections, some excipients were described which can be used in drying. In this section, a study will be presented by Mello Costa (2016). In this study, a critical analysis of eight different excipients was performed for medicinal plant dried extracts and the chemical-chemical properties of the powders were compared. The plant researched as a case study, *Copaifera langsdorffii*, is a new and important plant which can supposedly treat kidney stones. The excipients were: maltodextrin, colloidal silicon dioxide, corn starch, D-mannitol, lactose monohydrated, sorbitol, microcrystalline cellulose and modified corn starch. Physical analyses were performed to evaluate flowing and packing of the dried extracts, as well as chemical analyses to evaluate the degradation of their constituents.

Moisture content values (*Mc*) for the *C. langsdorffii* dried extracts ranged from 4 to 6% (wet basis). Moisture sorption values (*Ms*) ranged from 6 to 17% w/w for the colloidal silicon dioxide and sorbitol, respectively. All dried extracts became darker after analysing the moisture sorption except for the colloidal silicon dioxide one. The process yield (*Py*) ranged from 12.8% w/w for the *C. langsdorffii* dried without any excipient to 60.9% w/w for the *C. langsdorffii* dried extract containing colloidal silicon dioxide (Table 3 and Figure 16).

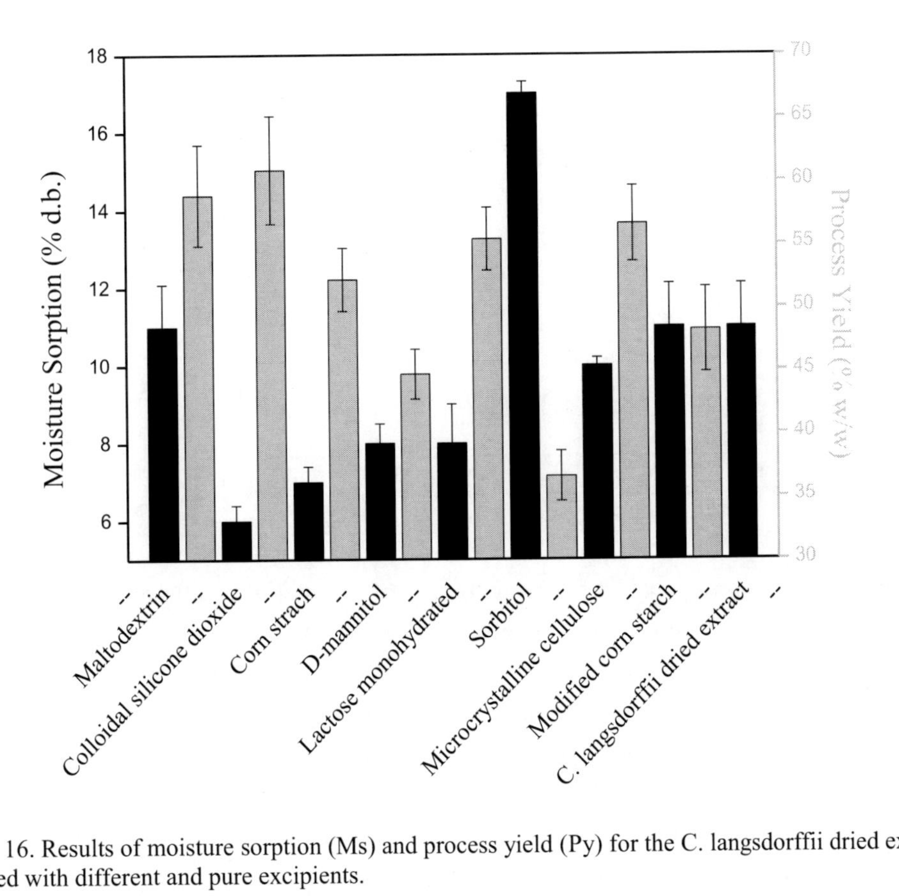

Figure 16. Results of moisture sorption (Ms) and process yield (Py) for the C. langsdorffii dried extracts obtained with different and pure excipients.

The moisture content (*Mc*), as discussed earlier in this chapter, is an important property of dried extracts and it is an indicator of the efficiency of the drying process. Powder packing, flowability, bulk density, particle agglomeration and even the color tonality of the powder are all affected by moisture content. Moreover, this parameter is extremely important in the development of various pharmaceutical forms, because it shows a major effect on the chemical and microbiological stability, as well as the physical properties of the product, especially regarding the flow properties and the particle size distribution. According to the literature, pharmaceutical powders, for example, spray-dried extracts, moisture content values within the range of 3 to 7% (w/w) are considered acceptable [122, 123]. The moisture content values (*Mc*) obtained for the *C. langsdorffii* dried extracts containing different excipients were adequate regarding the spray drying parameters used.

Table 3. Results of bulk density (ρb), tapped density (ρt), Carr index (Ic), Hausner ratio (Hr) and angle of repose (θ) for the *C. langsdorffii* dried extracts obtained with different and pure excipients

C. langsdorffii dried extract with	P_b (g/cm^3)	ρ_t (g/cm^3)	Ic	Hr	θ (°)
Maltodextrin	0.156 ± 0.007	0.237 ± 0.010	34.3 ± 1.3	1.52 ± 0.03	28 ± 1
Colloidal silicon dioxide	0.256 ± 0.017[a]	0.377 ± 0.022[a]	32.1 ± 1.1	1.47 ± 0.03	25 ± 3
Corn strach	0.198 ± 0.007	0.298 ± 0.015	33.7 ± 1.8	1.51 ± 0.04	28 ± 1
D-mannitol	0.277 ± 0.018[a]	0.380 ± 0.020[a]	27.3 ± 1.3[a]	1.38 ± 0.03[a]	22 ± 1[a]
Lactose monohydrated	0.133 ± 0.006	0.205 ± 0.012	35.0 ± 1.1	1.54 ± 0.03	31 ± 1
Sorbitol	0.202 ± 0.011	0.315 ± 0.012	35.8 ± 1.1	1.56 ± 0.03	27 ± 1
Microcrystalline cellulose	0.207 ± 0.005	0.339 ± 0.004	39.0 ± 0.7	1.56 ± 0.02	30 ± 2
Modified corn starch	0.167 ± 0.002	0.262 ± 0.012	36.0 ± 2.6	1.64 ± 0.06	30 ± 0
---	0.156 ± 0.007	0.156 ± 0.006	34.0 ± 1.5	1.57 ± 0.03	29 ± 1

The moisture sorption (*Ms*) is the tendency of a material to attract and retain water molecules from the environment by absorbing and adsorbing and it may change its physical state increasing its volume or becoming sticky. Hence, the obtained dried extracts were kept well-covered when not in use [134]. As expected, the *C. langsdorffii* dried extract containing sorbitol was the one that most absorbed water in a 75.3% RH chamber during 72h and the colloidal silicon dioxide was the one which most protected the *C. langsdorffii* dried extract. In fact, the latter was the only one which avoided a huge difference in the physico-chemical properties of the dried extracts in these conditions. Thus, the importance of keeping the dried extracts in airtight packaging is clear.

Bulk and tapped densities are defined as the mass of particles that occupies a unit volume of a container. Therefore, high values of bulk and tapped densities mean that a gram of the powder occupies small volumes helping transport vehicles and storage vessels [135]. Table 3 shows the bulk and tapped densities of the *C. langsdorffii* dried extract.

The *C. langsdorffii* dried extract dried with mannitol, sorbitol, microcrystalline cellulose and colloidal silicon dioxide presented bulk and tapped densities above 0.200 and 0.300 g/cm^3 and could be considered the fourth best density results of the studied dried extracts. Perhaps, other powder features could favor high densities such as:

1) *Span*. Mannitol, sorbitol and microcrystalline cellulose provided wider size distribution for the dried extract observed by a *span* greater than 2.0, which allowed the fine particles to settle and fill the voids.
2) *Shape*. The mannitol, sorbitol and colloidal silicon dioxide presented round shape particles that have also helped pack powder.
3) *Particle mean size*. The size distribution of the dried extract containing colloidal silicon dioxide was narrow. The mean particle size of the spherical shape helps to obtain high densities

The other excipient did not provide high densities for the dried extracts, possibly because the other powder features were not favorable, for example, low particle size distribution (*span*), non-delineable particle agglomerates, irregular shapes and the chemical interaction.

Abdullah & Geldart [138] observed that for powders containing a mixture of fine and large particles, the maximum tapped densities are achieved with 60 to 80% of larger particles which closely matches the 35% of fine particles in mixtures predicted by them before. The particle size ratio of large to fine particle about 10:1, or higher, is also related to maximum tapped densities as the porosity of bulk powders is filled with fine particles increasing the tapped density.

Powders must present good flow in order to help manufacturing processes, such as tableting or capsule filling without any difficulty. This parameter is essential to obtain the uniform target dosage of the active [122].

As the Carr index (*Ic*) and the Hausner ratio (*Hc*) present good correlation for the flowability [31], they were determined from the bulk and tapped densities. Values below 15 for the *Ic* are excellent, 15 to 25 are average and *Ic* values above 25 mean poor flowability. The *Hr* values between 1.00 and 1.18 indicate good or even excellent, whereas values from 1.18 to 1.34 indicate average and above 1.34 poor flowability [137].

In Table 2, the *C. langsdorffii* dried extract containing mannitol presented the lowest *Ic* (27.3 ± 1.3) and *Hr* (1.4 ± 0.03). The other studied excipients were not able to provide such a good flowability for the *C. langsdorffii* dried extracts presenting *Ic* values above 30 and *Hr* above 1.5 and is statistically significant ($P = 0.05$). Therefore, mannitol was the excipient that provided the best flowability to the *C. langsdorffii* dried extract.

The angle of repose was also determined and has been widely used to characterize the powder flow and is related to the interparticle friction or resistance to movement among the particles. Angle of repose values below 30° represent excellent flow property, from 30° to 50° passable flow and above 50°, the flow is rarely acceptable for manufacturing purposes. [23] The angle of repose for the *C. langsdorffii* dried extract with mannitol (22° ± 1) presented the lowest significant value as shown in Table 3.

The mannitol was the excipient that indicated the best flowability to the *C. langsdorffii* dried extract. Possibly, factors such as its round and non-spherical shape and its wide particle size distribution (span) could have helped its flowability. It is also important to consider the molecule interaction between the extract constituents and excipient that was coincidently ideal.

The colloidal silicon dioxide, microcrystalline cellulose and sorbitol demonstrated good powder packing but did not present good results of the Carr index (*Ic*), Hausner ratio (*Hr*) and angle of repose (θ). Possible explanations to these cases are:

1) *Particle mean size.* Flowability increases to almost all powders when the particle size increases. Microcrystalline cellulose and sorbitol dried extracts presented the lowest values of the particle mean size (d_{50}), 206 and 208 μm, respectively, which could promote more cohesiveness. The mannitol resulted in a particle mean size of 212 μm, but good flowability, whereas the colloidal silicon dioxide provided a particle mean size of 339 μm, but poor flowability. This was coherent because an increase in the particle size of powder mixture is always accompanied by a decrease in cohesiveness. Abdullah & Geldart [138] observed the same trend for the angles of repose for both spherical and angular materials where the angle of repose gradually decreases as the mean size increases, indicating that both types of powder, whatever their shapes, change from cohesive to free-flowing and the mean size increases.
2) *Span.* The microcrystalline cellulose and sorbitol provided better packing only after taps in spite of having presented wide size distribution. This is likely due to the cohesive and fluffy powder properties.
3) *Molecular interaction.* The colloidal silicon dioxide dried extract could have provided a kind of molecular interaction with the extract constituents making the dried extract cohesive which was a more significant disadvantage than the advantages, such as the large particle mean size and round shape morphology. On the other hand, good molecular interaction of mannitol with the chemical constituents of the dry extract is responsible for the powder flowability. *Moisture sorption.* Sorbitol was another excipient which provided good powder packing, but poor flowability probably because of its moisture sorption that is a well-known feature.

The other dried extracts that did not present good flowability properties could have been influenced by several other factors, such as moisture sorption (*Ms*) in the case of maltodextrin, cohesiveness as a common feature of corn starch, as well as an effect of some kind of molecular interaction.

The powder packing and flowability depend on the particle mean size, the particle size distribution, the particle shape and the morphology among several other aspects. Hence, the particle mean size (d_{50}) and the particle size distribution (*span*) were determined by a series of sieves, as well as the morphology of the particles which was observed by electronic scanning microscopy of the dried extracts.

The d_{50} of the dried extracts varied from 206 to 365 μm, as shown in Figure 17A. They could also be classified as the particle size of approximately 200 μm and above 300 μm, as well as the *span* above or below 2 (Figure 17B). The *C. langsdorffii* dried extracts that presented finer particles and higher polidispersivity were the ones containing microcrystalline cellulose (d_{50}= 206 ± 31μm, *span* = 2.92), sorbitol (d_{50}= 208 ± 20μm, *span* = 2.57) and mannitol (d_{50}= 212 ± 0μm, *span* = 2.47).

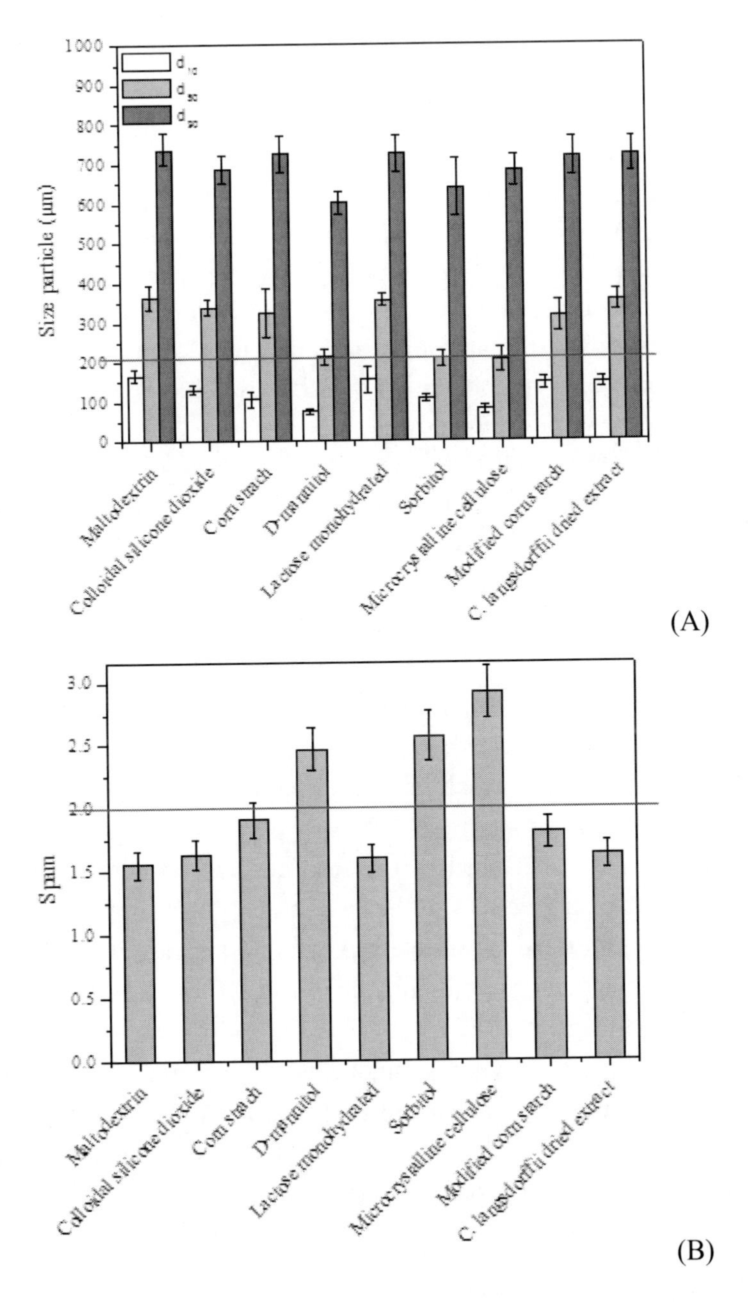

Figure 17. (A) Results of particle sizes (d50, d10 and d90). The horizontal line indicates the border value of 200 μm to d50. (B) Results of span for the C. langsdorffii dried extracts obtained from different excipients and as pure excipient.

The morphology in the micrographics (Figure 18) of the *C. langsdorffii* dried extracts with corn starch, lactose and microcrystalline cellulose presented particles as agglomerates and are unable to observe the particle delineation. The *C. langsdorffii* dried extract with maltodextrin and without any excipient also revealed agglomerates, however the particles are delineated. Moreover, the beginning and end of each one can be observed. The *C. langsdorffii* dried extract with colloidal silicon dioxide, mannitol and modified corn starch presented disperse particles and, as a result, it was easier to observe few-particle agglomerates and each particle seemed to be well delineated. It is likely that the sorbitol provided non-agglomerated particles as agglomerate was not observed on the micrographics. The *C. langsdorffii* dried extracts with colloidal silicon dioxide, sorbitol and modified corn starch presented a round shape while the one with mannitol showed irregular shape particles; some round and others sharp. The *C. langsdorffii* dried extract with sorbitol revealed a pear shape, which was smooth and not agglomerated.

The particle mean size from 206 to 365 μm was expected since the spray dryer provides a particle size in the range of 50 to 200 μm or larger depending on the spray drying parameters especially the nozzle orifice diameter [155-157]. This larger particle size can be explained by the agglomeration of particles and it is a usual feature of spray dried powders due to the electrostatic power.

Couto et al. (2013) [89] studied the spray drying process of the *Eugenia dysenterica* DC extract using maltodextrin, mannitol and colloidal silicon dioxide as excipients. The mean particle size of the dried extracts ranged from 370 to 1226 μm obtained by a pneumatic (two-fluid) spray nozzle with an inlet orifice of 1.5mm diameter and determined by the cumulative size distribution using a series of sieves.

It is generally accepted that the larger the particles, the better the flow. Particles larger than 250 μm are usually free-flowing. As the particle size decreases below 100 μm, powders become cohesive and flow problems are likely to occur. Powders having a particle size less than 10 μm are usually extremely cohesive and resist flow under gravity [139, 140].

Particle size is usually increased as the feed concentration or viscosity increases. Masters [24] reports that surface tension has a minimal effect on particle size, although other authors report an increase in particle size with an increase in feed surface tension and density, as well as with concentration and viscosity. If the feed rate is increased, the particle size will increase again [141].

It is known that the spray drying technique can lead to particles presenting several different characteristics as its parameters are guided and controlled [141]. The spray dried particle size can be guided by various parameters in the process. As all the parameters of the *C. langsdorffii* drying process were kept constant, it can be observed that the average particle size depends only on the excipient characteristic. The difference between properties of the *C. langsdorffii* dried extracts given by the excipients can be explained by the intrinsic excipient features.

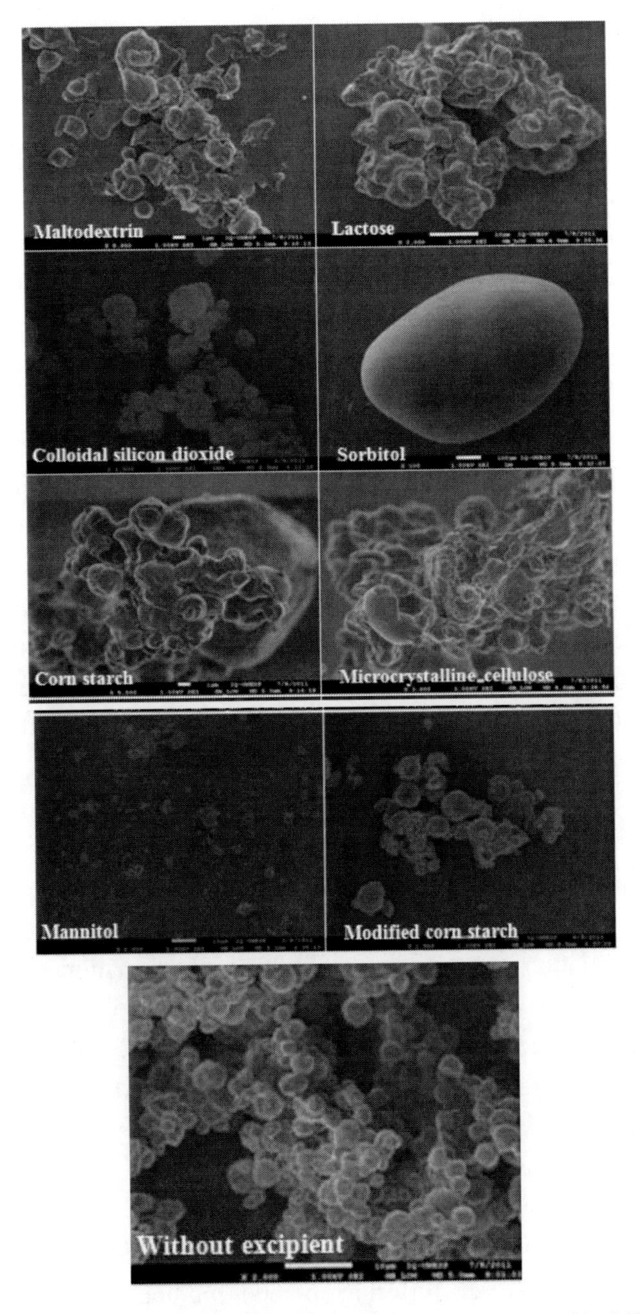

Figure 18. Micrographies of the SEM for the C. langsdorffii dried extracts with different and without excipients.

Some of the *C. langsdorffii* dried extracts, such as those containing corn starch, lactose and microcrystalline cellulose, had agglomerated particles and were unable to detect the particle design.

One explanation is that these particles have agglomerated before drying avoiding single particle formation. It is likely that these particles act as a non-porous barrier that hinders mass transfer. In fact, plastic materials present this behavior bringing about particle distortion as they promote vapor pressure delivery during drying allowing the particle to inflate following a particle break and hole formation. This kind of particle is inevitably hollow [142, 143].

The *C. langsdorffii* dried extracts with maltodextrin and without any excipient also presented agglomerates, however the particles are delineated and the beginning and end of each one can be observed.

Meanwhile, the *C. langsdorffii* dried extract with maltodextrin, colloidal silicon dioxide, mannitol, modified corn starch and without any excipient also presented a sort of agglomerates, however the particles are delineated and the beginning and end of each one can be observed. Thus, the agglomerates could be formed after completely drying each particle.

The *C. langsdorffii* dried extract quantification is illustrated in Figure 19. The theoretical content for total flavonoids, quercitrin and afzelin was around 34.0, 27.7 and 8.3 mg/g, respectively because the dried extracts containing the excipient presented a proportion of 3:1 *C. langsdorffii* dried matter to the mass of excipient. The dried extract without any excipient resulted in theoretical contents of 45.2 mg/g of total flavonoids and 36.8 mg/g of quercitrin and 10.9 mg/g of afzelin contents. These values are higher than the dried extracts containing excipient because the dried extract without any excipient was a hundred percent of *C. langsdorffii* dried matter.

The modified corn starch provided the most similar practical content for the total flavonoids (33.8 mg/g) and the quercitrin (27.5 mg/g) and afzelin (8.3 mg/g) contents. The microcrystalline cellulose provided the lowest practical contents of the whole analysis: 27.3 mg/g for the total flavonoids, 21.8 mg/g for quercetin and 6.6 mg/g for afzelin and the degradation was approximately 20%. The remaining dried extracts, even the dried extract without any excipient, presented less than 11.5% degradation.

The microcrystalline cellulose presented the lowest values of flavonoids, quercitrin and afzelin contents. The results were lower than the dried extract without any excipient meaning the microcrystalline cellulose was either unable to protect or increase the degradation more than if there was no excipient.

On the other hand, both kind of starches and maltodextrin provided contents near the theoretical values. This fact is very interesting as cellulose and starch are glucose polysaccharide molecules, which differing in their binding. The starch presents α-D-glucose linkages while cellulose presents β-D-glucose linkages. Perhaps this different inter glucose linkage influenced the protection of the chemical constituents provided by the excipient [145].

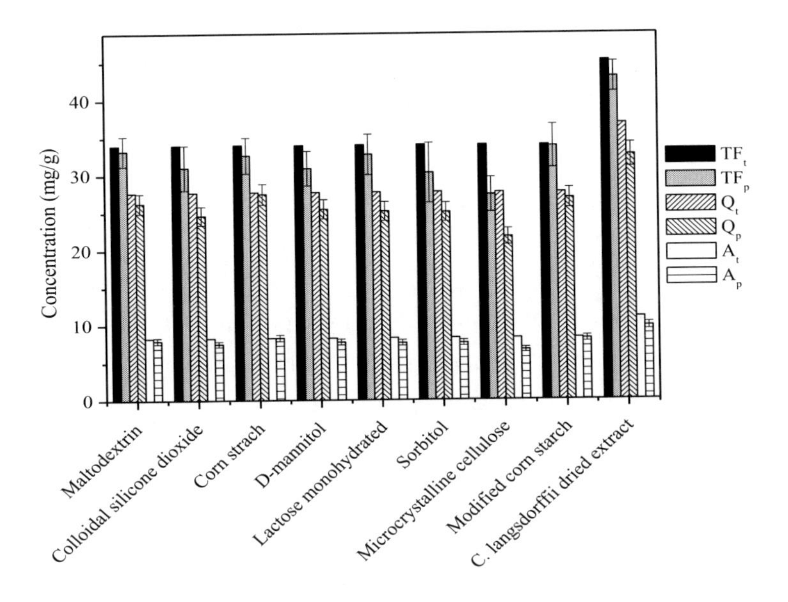

Figure 19. Results of the chemical constituent quantification from the C. langsdorffii obtained from the different excipients.

EVALUATING THE PEARSON AND SPEARMAN CORRELATIONS AMONG THE DRIED EXTRACTS CHARACTERISTICS

In order to evaluate if there was any correlation between the characteristics of the dried extracts, such as moisture sorption, process yield, bulk density, tapped density, Carr index, Hausner ratio and angle of repose, the Pearson and Spearman correlation coefficients were calculated. The Spearman correlation is a non-parametric test, therefore it does not assume normal distribution for the data. It is applied to measure any association between two variables which can be linear or not [146].

The Pearson correlation measures the strength between the association of two variables. If the association is monotonic (both variables decrease or increase) and linear, when the value of the coefficient is closer to one in the module, the greater its association [146].

It can be observed by analysing the Pearson and Spearman correlation coefficients the variables have a correlation when their values are approximately 1 in module. If their values are zero, it means the variables do not present a correlation. Not necessarily both correlation coefficients provide similar values. As written above, this is because the Spearman correlation considers any kind of correlation, linear or not, whereas the Pearson correlation coefficient is near 1 only when there is a linear correlation between the variables. This case can be observed in the coefficients between the *Py* and the *Ic* where the Pearson correlation coefficient was 0.080 and the Spearman´s was 0.533 (Table 4) [146].

Generally, for both correlation coefficients the positive signal indicates monotonicity which means a direct proportion between the variables. On the other hand, a negative signal indicates an inverse effect in the variables, which means while one of the variable increases the other decreases. This case was observed for the *Py* and *Ms* (Pearson coefficient -0.454 and Spearman coefficient -0.600) and it is justified due to the rapid absorption of water by the material, which tends to adhere in the spray drying chamber, resulting in a low yield.

The Spearman coefficient also provided good correlation (values between 0.533 to 0.833) for powder flowability indexes (*Ic*, *Hr* and θ) and *Ms,* as well as for *Py*. Therefore, powders which present good flowability characteristics do not usually stick to the equipment walls because of non-absorption of water and can flow better making it easy to be collected in the spray dryer cyclone.

Table 4. Results for the Pearson (above) and Spearman (below) correlation among the variables for the dried extracts obtained from each excipient

Variable	*Ms (% d.b.)*	*Py (% w/w)*	ρ_b (g/cm^3)	ρ_t (g/cm^3)	*Ic*	*Hr*	θ (°)
Ms *(% d.b.)*		-0.454 -0.600	-0.281 0.633	-0.215 -0.483	0.419 0.533	0.490 0.833	0.188 0.533
Py *(% w/w)*	-0.454 -0.600		0.183 0.133	0.475 -0.317	0.080 0.533	-0.216 0.833	-0.216 0.533
ρ_b (g/cm^3)	-0.281 0.633	0.183 0.133		0.913 0.950	-0.591 0.533	-0.732 0.833	-0.871 0.533
ρ_t (g/cm^3)	-0.215 -0.483	0.475 -0.317	0.913 0.950		-0.319 -0.283	-0.566 0.833	-0.677 0.533
Ic	0.419 0.533	0.080 0.533	-0.591 0.533	-0.319 -0.283		0.840 0.800	0.851 0.533
Hr	0.490 0.833	-0.216 0.833	-0.732 0.833	-0.566 0.833	0.840 0.800		0.853 0.733
θ (°)	0.188 0.533	-0.216 0.533	-0.871 0.533	-0.677 0.533	0.851 0.533	0.853 0.733	

The coefficient values correlating bulk and tapped densities (ρ_b and ρ_t) were very high (0.913 and 0.950) indicating a strong and monotonic correlation. This result is satisfactory as similar values of ρ_b and ρ_t indicate that the powder presents a good flow which was generally confirmed by the high correlation coefficients (>0.5) of the densities and the flowability indexes.

Decision-Making

In order to choose the excipient that provided the best overall characteristics for the *C. langsdorffii* dried extract, a decision-making technique by criteria and weight was performed [147]. In this decision-making technique, the criteria of quality for the dried extracts was identified and a weight of importance was rated for each criteria. Considering this, the impact of different characteristics on the dried extract quality was estimated by rating the parameters: process yield, moisture (including moisture sorption and content), powder packing (including bulk and tapped densities), powder flowability (including Carr index, Haussner ratio and angle of repose) and the quantification of the constituents. The criteria and set weight given for the parameters are presented in Table 5 and discussed below. At the end, the rates for each dried extract were scored and summed. The dried extract with the best characteristics was the one which scored the highest number.

For the process yield, the weight was set at 1 and the minimum value was 50% due to the fact that the process yield values of bench scale equipment are commonly observed with values lower than 50% [122, 148], which was observed in the results of the dried extracts throughout this work.

Powders are able to adsorb/absorb water from the environment. However, moisture sorption can be successfully controlled and avoided by good package and proper storing conditions. Thus, the weight of the moisture sorption was set at 1 and its value was defined as a maximum of 8% of mass gain.

It is interesting that the tapped density of powders presents high values because, by doing this, the powders occupy a tiny space favoring their storage. Regarding the tapped density, the value of 0.350 g/cm^3 and weight 1 were set. Therefore, the dried extracts with values higher than 0.350 g/cm^3 scored 1, but the ones below 1 scored zero.

The Carr index refers to the flowability of the powder and low values provide good flowability characteristics. For this reason, a weight of 2 for the Carr index was provided for the dried extracts that presented values below 30.

The lower the angle of repose the better the flowability of a powder. In the literature, angle of repose values below 25° are considered good flow parameters. Since the flowability is considered an important characteristic for several unit operations such as compression and packing, it received a weight of 2. Consequently, angle of repose values below 25° scored weight 2.

The particle mean size and the size distribution are characteristics which can influence powder behavior. When the size distribution is wide, the *span* value is high. This characteristic helps to obtain satisfactory packing values, especially for tapped and bulk densities [35]. However, homogenization of the powder is affected when there is large particle size distribution [127, 128]. Thus, the minimum particle mean size chosen was 200 μm and the maximum value for the *span* was 2. Both values above the particle mean size of 200 μm and *span* below 2 received weight 1.

Chemical marker degradation was considered an important feature and scored weight 2 when it presented a value lower than 10%.

In order to select the excipient which provided good general characteristics for the *C. langsdorffii* dried extracts, a decision-making technique by criteria and weight was performed [147]. At the end, the rates for each dried extract were scored and summed as shown in Table 5. The dried extract with the best features was mannitol which scored the highest number (13) among other dried extracts.

In general, mannitol presented good powder packing and flowability and the degradation of the evaluated chemical constituents was less than 10%. It also presented good results of moisture content and moisture sorption as it is a nonhygroscopic excipient [145].

Bruschi (2003) studied spray dried propolis extract using gelatin with and without mannitol as an excipient. The gelatin microparticles containing mannitol presented a higher process yield and moisture content in the same conditions as the non-containing mannitol. Bruschi (2003) remarks that mannitol is used in spray dried formulations to improve its physical features and to avoid having a sticky powder [149].

Gonnissen (2007) used mannitol to co-spray dry acetaminophen formulations which provided free-flowing, high densities and low moisture sorption powders. In addition, mannitol increased the direct compressed tablet strength [150].

Table 5. Score for the decision-making of the product quality of the dried extracts

Samples	*Ms*	*Py*	ρ_t	*Ic*	θ	d_{50}	*S*	*Degradation*			*Score*
								δFT	δQ	δA	
Maltodextrin	*0*	*1*	*0*	*0*	*0*	*1*	*1*	2	2	2	*9*
Colloidal silicone dioxide	*1*	*1*	*1*	*0*	*2*	*1*	*1*	2	*0*	2	*11*
Corn strach	*1*	*1*	*0*	*0*	*0*	*1*	*1*	2	2	2	*10*
D-mannitol	*1*	*0*	*1*	*2*	*2*	*1*	*0*	2	2	2	*13*
Lactose monohydrated	*1*	*1*	*0*	*0*	*0*	*1*	*1*	2	2	2	*10*
Sorbitol	*0*	*0*	*0*	*0*	*0*	*1*	*0*	*0*	2	2	*5*
Microcrystalline cellulose	*0*	*1*	*0*	*0*	*0*	*1*	*0*	*0*	*0*	*0*	*2*
Modified corn starch	*0*	*0*	*0*	*0*	*0*	*1*	*1*	2	2	2	*8*
----	*0*	*0*	*0*	*0*	*0*	*1*	*1*	2	*0*	*0*	*4*

Py: process yield; Ms: moisture sorption; ρt: tapped density; Ic: Carr index; θ: angle of repose; d_{50}: particle mean size; δFT: total flavonoids degradation; δQ: quercitrin degradation; δA: afzelin degradation.

In another study, the formulation containing 50% (w/w) of mannitol and ciprofloxacin seemed to have the best aerosol performance, good stability and the lowest particle cohesion. Furthermore, mannitol did not seem to modify the effectiveness of the ciprofloxacin antimicrobial activity [151].

Mizoe (2007) obtained nanoparticles-containing microparticles of pranlukast hemihydrate (PLH) in a 4-fluid nozzle spray drying using mannitol (MAN) as a carrier. The absorption of PLH was enhanced by pulmonary delivery of PLH-MAN [152].

Thus, mannitol is a well-studied excipient for drug delivery systems especially for pulmonary ones, because it seems to be the ideal replacement for lactose because it does not have the risk of transmitting the transmissible spongiform encephalopathy. When mannitol is co-spray dried with drugs, it can obtain fine particles with enough flowability to ensure reproducible dosing as the powder flows from a reservoir into well defined orifices. Additionally, mannitol does not carry reducing groups, which may cause chemical interactions with drugs, such as proteins, and can be found crystalline when spray-dried, which is important for drug bioavailability [144, 153, 156].

In fact, mannitol has been used in food and pharmaceutical industries for a long time. It is considered safe for oral intake in the United States and Europe and a 20-g limit daily ingestion is suggested in the literature, an amount that is not reached in solid dosage forms [122].

REFERENCES

[1] Calixto, João Batista.2000. Efficacy, safety, quality control, marketing and regulatory guidelines for herbal medicines (phytotherapeutic agents). *Braz. J. Med. Biol. Res.,* Ribeirão Preto, v.33, p.179-189.

[2] Niazi, Sarfaraz K. 2007.Chapter 10: Characterization of Phytomedicines. *Handbook of preformulation: chemical, biological, and botanical drugs*. New York: Informa healthcare. Availablehttps: //muhammadcank.files.wordpress.com/2010/02/handbook-of-preformulation-chemical-biological-and-botanical-drugs.pdf.

[3] Barnes, Joanne.2003. "Quality, efficacy and safety of complementary medicines: fashions, facts and the future. Part I. Regulation and quality." *British Journal of Clinical Pharmacology* 55, no. 3 .226-33. doi:10.1046/j.1365-2125.2003.01810.x.

[4] *General Guidelines for Methodologies on Research and Evaluation of Traditional Medicine*. 2000. Pdf. World Health Organization.

[5] Bulletin of the World Health Organization. 1993. Research guidelines for evaluating the safety and efficacy of herbal medicine. Geneva, p.1-86.

[6] Bulletin of the World Health Organization.1998. Regulatory situation of herbal medicines. *A worldwide review*. Geneva, p.1-43.

[7] Runha, F. P., D. S. Cordeiro, Cláudia. Cordeiro Pereira, José Vilegas, and Wanderley Pereira Oliveira.2001. “Production of Dry Extracts of Medicinal Brazilian Plants by Spouted Bed Process.” *Food and Bioproducts Processing* 79, no. 3.p.160-68. doi:10.1205/09603080175042525 3.

[8] Banker, G.S., Rhodes, C.T., 2002. *Modern Pharmaceutics*, fourth ed. Marcel Dekker, New York, NY.

[9] Cortés-Rojas, D.F., Wanderley, Oliveira, Pereira. 2012. Physicochemical properties of phytopharmaceutical preparations as affected by drying methods and carriers. *Dry. Technol*. 30, 921–934.

[10] Cechinel-Filho, Valdir.2012. *Plant bioactives and drug discovery principles, practice, and perspectives*. Hoboken, NJ: John Wiley & Sons.

[11] Weiguang Yi and Hazel Y. Wetzstein.2011. Effects of Drying and Extraction Conditions on the Biochemical Activity of Selected Herbs. *Hort Science*. 46(1).p.70–73.

[12] Augsburger, Larry L., and Stephen W.2007. Hoag. *Pharmaceutical dosage forms. tablets*. New York: Informa Healthcare.

[13] Pawar, Pallavi Dadasaheb, Pooja Manohar Arane, Harshata Bhaidas Saindane, Swati Gokul Talele, Ganesh Shinde, and Ghanashyam Chaudhari.2015. “Review on Pharmaceutical Excipients.” *American Journal of pharmacy and health research* 3, no. 2. http://www.ajphr.com/archive/volume-3/february-2015-issue-2/302003.html.

[14] S. Shalini. 2012.”Advantages and Applications Of Nature Excipients –A Review.” *Asian Journal of Pharmaceutical Research* 2, no. 1.p. 30-40. http://www.ajpr journal.com/zip.php?file=File_Folder/30-39.pdf &id=66&quat=2.

[15] Chaudhari, Shilpa P., and Pradeep S. Patil.2012.”Pharmaceutical Excipients: A review.” *International Journal of Advances In Pharmacy, Biology And Chemistry* 1, no. 1.p.21-34. http://www.ijapbc.com/files/4.pdf.

[16] Jozsef Tópar. “Spray Drying Investigations on Medicinal Plant Based Pharmaceutical Products.1994.” *Periodica Polytechnica*, p. 157-64. Available: <https://pp.bme.hu/me/article/download /5522/4627>.

[17] MacCabe, Warren L., Peter Harriot, and Julian C. Smith. 1994. Unit operations of chemical engineering. 5ª ed. New York: McGraw-Hill.

[18] Mujumdar, Arun S. 2005. Guide to industrial drying: principles, equipment and new developments. Mumbai, India: Colour Publications Pvt. Ltda.

[19] Mujumdar, Arun S. 2006. *Handbook of industrial drying*. 3ª ed.New York: Marcell Dekker.

[20] Oliveira, P. Wanderley, Luis A. P. Freitas, and José T. Freire. 2009. In: José T. Freire, Ana Maria da Silveira. (Org.). Fenômenos de Transporte em Sistemas Particulados: Fundamentos e Aplicações. 1 ed. São Carlos: Editora da UFSCAR, no.1. 131-164.

[21] Bansal, Arvind K.2002, "Product Development Issues of Powders for Injection." Pharmaceutical Technology p.122-132. Available: <March 2002. Accessed January 18, 2017. http://images.alfresco.advanstar.com/alfresco_images/pharma/2014/08/22/ffc04161-23ba-4e79-b9cb-3631d92b4bcc/article-12518.pdf>.

[22] L. Zhu, L. Lu, S. Wang, J. Wu, J. Shi, T. Yan, C. Xie, Q. Li, M. Hu, and Z. Liu.2016. "Oral absorption basics: Pathways and Physicochemical and biologicl factors affecting absorption." In *Developing Solid Oral Dosage Forms: Pharmaceutical Theory and Practice*, 297-395. 2° ed.

[23] Gilhotra, Ritumehra, Kalpana Nagpal, and Dinanath Mishra. 2011."Azithromycin novel drug delivery system for ocular application." *International Journal of Pharmaceutical Investigation* 1, no. 1.doi:10.4103/2230-973x.76725.

[24] Masters, Keith. 1985. Spray Drying Handbook. 4ªEdition, Longman John Wiley, USA.

[25] *PEREIRA, J. A.M.*, Queiroz D.M., P*sicometria*. 1983. Vicosa, 27p.

[26] E Silva, Juarez De Souza, Roberto Precci Lopes, and Ricardo Caetano Resende. "Capítulo 3: Princípios básicos de psicrometria." In *Apostila do Professor Juarez de Souza e Silva*. Accessed December 12, 2016. ftp://ftp.ufv.br/dea/Disciplinas/Evandro/Eng671/Aulas/Aula03.Principios%20basicos%20de%20psicrometria.pdf.

[27] "Chapter 2: The measurement of temperature and humidity." Accessed November 23, 2016. Available:http://www.metoffice.gov.uk/media/pdf/4/k/Chapter2.pdf.

[28] Jangam, Sachin V, Chung Lim Law, and Arun S. Mujumdar. 2010."Chapter 1. Basic Concepts and Definitions." In *Drying of Foods, Vegetables and Fruits*. Vol. 1. Singapore. http://www.arunmujumdar.com/file/Publications/books/Drying%20of%20Foods%20Vegetables%20and%20Fruits%20Volume%201.pdf.

[29] Jones, E. B.1976. *Instrument technology*. London: Newnes-Butterworth.

[30] "Chapter 3: "Measurement of humidity." 1-20. Accessed October 12, 2016. Available:http://www.jma.go.jp/jma/jma-eng/jma-enter/ric/material/1_Lecture_Notes/CP3-Humidity.pdf.

[31] Rao, Dubasi Govardhana.2010. *Introduction to biochemical engineering*. New Delhi: Tata McGraw-Hill.

[32] "Physical Mechanism of Drying." NPTEL. Accessed December 02, 2016. Available:<http://nptel.ac.in/courses/103103027/module4/lec1/2.html>.

[33] Lachman, Leon. 1988. Theory and practice of industrial pharmacy. Philadelphia, Lea & Febiger.

[34] Mujundar, Arun S., Anllkumar S. Menon. 2014. "Drying of solids: principles, classification, and selection of dryers." In *Handbook of industrial drying,* 1-39. 4ª ed. New York.

[35] Walters, Robert H., Bakul Bhatnagar, Serguei Tchessalov, Ken-Ichi Izutsu, Kouhei Tsumoto, and Satoshi Ohtake. 2014. "Next Generation Drying Technologies for

Pharmaceutical Applications." *Journal of Pharmaceutical Sciences* 103, no. 9 2673-695. doi:10.1002/jps.23998.

[36] "Chapter 11: Drying." In *Bioseparations Science and Engineer*, 407-40. Accessed December 12, 2016. Available: <http://portal.unimap.edu.my/portal/page/portal30/Lecturer%20Notes/KEJURUTERAAN_BIOPROSES/Semester%202%20Sidang%20Akademik%20201520161/Bioprocess%20Engineering%20Program/Third%20Year/ERT%20320%20Bioseparation%20Engineering/Dr%20Mohd%20Irfan%20Hatim%20B%20Mohd%20Dzahir/Drying.pdf>.

[37] Dominguez, José Emanuel. 2011."Drying." Edited by Murray Moo Young. In Comprehensive *Biotechnology*, 727-35. Vol. 2. New York: Academic Press.

[38] "Solids Drying: Basics and Applications - Chemical Engineering." Chemical Engineering Solids Drying Basics and Applications Comments. Accessed november 24, 2016. http://www.chemengonline.com/solids-drying-basics-and-applications/?printmode=1.

[39] Cooper, Jack, Charles J. Swartz, and William Suydam.1961 "Drying of Tablet Granulations." *Journal of Pharmaceutical Sciences* 50, no. 1 67-75. doi:10.1002/jps.2600500116.

[40] Fontana, Antony. 2007. Measurement of Water Activity, Moisture Sorption Isotherms, and Moisture Content of Foods, in *Water Activity in Foods: Fundamentals and Applications* (eds G. V. Barbosa-Cánovas, A. J. Fontana, S. J. Schmidt and T. P. Labuza), Blackwell Publishing Ltd, Oxford, UK. doi: 10.1002/9780470376454.ch6.

[41] Labuza, Ted, Kaanane, and Jefferson Chen.1985. "Effect of Temperature on the Moisture Sorption Isotherms and Water Activity Shift of Two Dehydrated Foods." Journal of Food Science 50, no. 2, 385-92. doi:10.1111/j.1365-2621.1985.tb13409.x.

[42] Limousin, Guillaume.; J. P. Gaudet., L. Charlet., S. Szenknect., V. Barthes., M. Krimissa. 2007. Sorption isotherms: a review on physical bases, modeling and measurement. *Applied Geochemistry*. 22, no.2, 249-75. doi:101016/japgeochem 200609010.

[43] Blahovec, Jiří, and Stavros Yanniotis. 2009. "Modified classification of sorption isotherms"Journal of Food Engineering 91, no. 1, 72-77. doi:10.1016/j.jfoodeng.2008.08.007. [44] Chirife, Jorge, and Hector A. Iglesias. 2007. "Equations for fitting water sorption isotherms of foods: Part 1 - a review." *International Journal of Food Science & Technology* 13, no. 3, 159-74. doi:10.1111/j.1365-2621.1978.tb00792.x.

[44] Brunauer, Stephen, Lola Deming, Edwards Deming, and Edward Teller. 1940. "On a Theory of the van der Waals Adsorption of Gases." *Journal of the American Chemical Society* 62, no. 7, 1723-732. doi:10.1021/ja01864a025.

[45] Gerhardt, Armin H. "Moisture Effects on Solid Dosage Forms-Formulation, Processing, and Stability" *Journal of GXP Compliance*. Accessed December 2, 2016. Available:http://www.ivtnetwork.com/sites/default/files/MoistureEffects_01.pdf.

[46] Vippagunta, Sudha R., Harry G. Brittain, and David J.W. Grant. 2001. "Crystalline solids." *Advanced Drug Delivery Reviews* 48, no. 1 3-26. doi:10.1016/s0169-409x(01)00097-7.

[47] Yu, Lian. 2001 "Amorphous pharmaceutical solids: preparation, characterization and stabilization." *Advanced Drug Delivery Reviews* 48, no. 1 27-42. doi:10.1016/s0169-409x(01)00098-9.

[48] Padma, Ishwarya S., Chinnaswamy Anandharamakrishnan, and Andrew G.F. Stapley. 2015 "Spray-freeze-drying: A novel process for the drying of foods and bioproducts." *Trends in Food Science & Technology* 41, 2 161-81. doi:10.1016/j.tifs.2014.10.008.

[49] Barros de Araujo, Gabriel Lima, Altivo Pitaluga Junior, Selma Gutierrez Antônio Carlos O. P. Santos, and Jivaldo Do Rosário Matos. 2012 "Polimorfismo na produção de medicamentos." Revista de Ciências Farmacêuticas Básica e Aplicada, 27-36.

[50] Bronlund, John, and Tony Paterson. 2004 "Moisture sorption isotherms for crystalline, amorphous and predominantly crystalline lactose powders." *International Dairy Journal* 14, no. 3 247-54. doi:10.1016/s0958-6946(03)00176-6.

[51] De Haan, A. 2015. *Process Technology. An Introduction*. Berlin.: De Gruyter.

[52] "Classification of dryers." Classification of dryers. Accessed Oct. & nov., 2016.http://www.unido.org/fileadmin/import/32148_34ClassificationofDryers.17.pdf.

[53] Mujumdar, Arun S., and Chung Lim Law. 2010."Drying Technology: Trends and Applications in Postharvest Processing." *Food and Bioprocess Technology* 3, no. 6 843-52. doi:10.1007/s11947-010-0353-1.

[54] Vehring, Reinhard, Willard R. Foss and David Lechuga-Ballesteros. 2007 "Particle formation in spray drying." *Journal of Aerosol Science* 38, no. 7, 728-46. doi:10.1016/j.jaerosci.2007.04.005.

[55] "APV Dryer Handbook. 2006. University of Maryland, Baltimore." *APV Dryer handbook*. Accessed October 30, 2016. http://userpages.umbc.edu/~dfrey1/ench445/apv_dryer.pdf.

[56] Tadeusz Kudra, Arun S. Mujumdar Kudra, 2009. *Advanced drying technologies*. CRC press.

[57] Kunii, D.; Levenspiel, O. 1991. Fluidization Engineering, 2° ed, Butterworth-Heinemann: Newton, MA.

[58] Guerrero, Manuel Perez, Carlos Albet, Antonio Palomer, and Armando Guglietta. 2003. "Drying in Pharmaceutical and Biotechnological Industries." *Food Science and Technology International* 9, no. 3 237-43. doi:10.1177/1082013203035567.

[59] Freitas, A.P Luís; José Freire. 1997. Experimental Study on The Dynamics of a Spouted Bed with Particle Feed Through the Base. *Brazilian Journal of Chemical Engineering*, v. 14, p. 269-80.

[60] Gohel, Mukesh, Rajesh Parikh, Lalji Baldaniya, Bhavesh Subhashchandra Barot, Hardik Joshi, Punit Parejiya, Pritesh Mistry, Amirali Popat, Tushar Patel, Ramesh Parmar.2007. Fluidized Bed Systems: A Review. Pharmainfo. net, 1-41.

[61] Hovmand.199.S. Fluidized bed drying. In Handbook of Industrial Drying; Mujumdar, A. S., Ed.; Marcel Dekker: New York,p.195–248.

[62] Freire, José. 1992. Secagem de Pastas em Leito de Jorro; Grafica da UFSCar: São Carlos, Brazil.

[63] Marreto, N. Ricardo, Peixoto, M. P. G., Luciana Alves Tacon, Luis A. P. Freitas. 2007. Paste Residence Time in a Spouted Bed Dryer. I: The Stimulus Response Methodology. *Drying Technology*, 25, no 5. 821-30.

[64] Marreto, N. Ricardo, José T. Freire., Luis A. P. Freitas. 2006. Drying of pharmaceuticals: The applicability of spouted beds. *Drying Technology,* no.24 327–38.

[65] Mathur, Kishan B., and Norman Epstein.1974. "Developments in spouted bed technology." *The Canadian Journal of Chemical Engineering* 52, no. 2. 129-44. doi:10.1002/cjce.5450520201.

[66] John Barley. Basic Principles of Freeze Drying. 2016. Review of *SP SCIENTIFIC* Accessed December 1. Available:<Http://www.spscientific.com/freeze-drying-lyophilization-basics/>.

[67] R, Nireesha G., L. Dyvia, C. Sowmya, N. Venkateshan, N. Niranjan Babu, and V. Lavakumar. "Lyophilization/Freeze Drying - An Review.2013" *International Journal of Novel trends in Pharmaceutical Sciences*. Accessed December 2, 2016. Available: http://www.ijntps.org/File_Folder/0047.pdf.

[68] Liapis, Athanasios L., and Roberto Brutini. 1987 "Freeze Drying." In Handbook of Industrial Drying," Edited by Arun S. Mujundar. 309-42. Academic Press.

[69] Rankell S. Albert, Hebert A. Lieberman, Robert S. Schiffman. 1986. Drying. In: *The theory and practice of industrial pharmacy*, edited by Leon Lachman, H.A. Lieberman & J. Kanig, 3º edition, Lea & Fabiger, Philadelphia, PA, USA, chapter 3,47-65.

[70] Freitas, A. P. Luis., Cristiane C. Teixeira, Luciana A. Tacon, Tsukada, M. 2010. Innovative applications of spray drying. In: José, M. J. S. (Ed.). *Advances in Chemical Engineering*. Kerala, India, cap. 1, p.1-13.

[71] Filková, Iva, Xin Huang, 2006. Industrial spray drying systems." Edited by Arun S. Mujumdar, In *Handbook of industrial drying*, 155-254.CRC/Taylor & Francis, Boca Raton, FL, USA.

[72] Marquele, D. Franciane, KM Stracieri, Maria J. V. Fonseca, Luis A.P. Freitas. 2006. Spray-dried propolis extract. I: physicochemical and antioxidant properties. Die Pharmazie-An International Journal of Pharmaceutical Sciences.

[73] Araujo, Rafael Rodrigo, Cristiane C. Teixeira, Luís A.P. Freitas. 2010. The preparation of ternary solid dispersions of an herbal drug via spray drying of liquid feed. *Drying Technology* 28, no.3, p. 412-21.

[74] Khadka, Prakash, Jieun Ro, Hyeongmin Kim, Iksoo Kim, Jeong Tae Kim, Hyunil Kim, Jae Min Cho, Gyiae Yun, and Jaehwi Lee.2014. "Pharmaceutical particle technologies: An approach to improve drug solubility, dissolution and bioavailability." *Asian Journal of Pharmaceutical Sciences* 9, no. 6. p.304-16. doi:10.1016/
j.ajps.2014.05.005.

[75] Soares, Luiz Alberto Lira, George González Ortega, Pedro Ros Petrovick, and Peter Christian Schmidt. 2005."Optimization of tablets containing a high dose of spray-dried plant extract: A technical note." *AAPS PharmSciTech* 6, no. 3. doi:10.1208/pt060346.

[76] Neto, Youssef Ali Abou Hamin, Hamilton Cabral and Luís Alexandre P. Freitas "Fermentação, purificação, caracterização bioquímica e microencapsulação da protease produzida pelo fungo Eupenicillium javanicum." doi:10.11606 /d.60.2012.tde-01112012-151150.2014. Drying Technology, p.614–621.

[77] Oliveira, Olivia Werner, and Pedro Ros Petrovick. 2010."Secagem por aspersão (spray drying) de extratos vegetais: bases e aplicações." *Revista Brasileira de Farmacognosia* 20.(4): 641-50. Web.

[78] Jain Manu, Lohare Ganesh, Bari Manoj, Shah Chirag. 2012. Spray drying in pharmaceutical industry: *A review. Res. J. Pharm. Dos*. Forms Technol, 4, p.74-79.

[79] Patel, R. P., Patel, M. P., & Suthar, A. M. 2009. Spray drying technology: an overview. *Indian Journal of Science and Technology*, 2 no.10, p. 44-47.

[80] Gallo, Loreana, María Verónica Ramírez-Rigo, Juliana Piña, and Verónica Bucalá. 2015."A comparative study of spray-dried medicinal plant aqueous extracts. Drying performance and product quality." *Chemical Engineering Research and Design* 104.p.681-94. doi:10.1016/j.cherd.2015.10.009.

[81] Patil, Jagadevappa. 2016."Spray-Drying: An Emerging Technique for Pharmaceutical Product Development." *Journal of Pharmacovigilance* 04, no. 02.doi:10.4172/2329-6887.1000e150.

[82] Mehta, Piyush. 2016. "Dry Powder Inhalers: A Focus on Advancements in Novel Drug Delivery Systems." *Journal of Drug Delivery* 1-17. doi:10.1155 /2016/8290963.

[83] Teixeira, Cristiane Correa, L. M. Mendonça, M. M. Bergamaschi, R. H. C. Queiroz, G. E. P. Souza, L. M. G. Antunes, and Luis Alexandre Freitas. 2015. "Microparticles Containing Curcumin Solid Dispersion: Stability, Bioavailability and Anti-Inflammatory Activity." *AAPS PharmSciTech* 17, no. 2.p.252-61. doi:10.1208/s12249-015-0337-6.

[84] Nosari, Anna B.f.l., Juliana F. Lima, Osvaldo A. Serra, and Luis Alexandre P. Freitas.2015. "Improved green coffee oil antioxidant activity for cosmetical purpose by spray drying microencapsulation." *Revista Brasileira de Farmacognosia* 25, no. 3: 307-11. doi:10.1016/j.bjp.2015.04.006.

[85] Khadka, Prakash, Jieun Ro, Hyeongmin Kim, Iksoo Kim, Jeong Tae Kim, Hyunil Kim, Jae Min Cho, Gyiae Yun, and Jaehwi Lee.2014. "Pharmaceutical particle technologies: An approach to improve drug solubility, dissolution and bioavailability." *Asian Journal of Pharmaceutical Sciences* 9, no. 6 304-16. doi:10.1016/
j.ajps.2014.05.005.

[86] Martins, Rodrigo Molina, Marcela Olaia Machado, Simone Vieira Pereira, A. B. F. L. Nosari, Luciana Alves Tacon, and Luis Alexandre. Pedro Freitas. 2012."Engineering Active Pharmaceutical Ingredients by Spray Drying: Effects on Physical Properties and In Vitro Dissolution." *Drying Technology* 30, no. 9.p. 905-13. doi:10.1080/07373937.2012.679348.

[87] Mendonça, Leonardo Meneghin, Carla Da Silva Machado, Cristiane Cardoso Correia Teixeira, Luis Alexandre Pedro De Freitas, Maria Lourdes Pires Bianchi, and Lusânia Maria Greggi Antunes.2015 "Comparative study of curcumin and curcumin formulated in a solid dispersion: Evaluation of their antigenotoxic effects." *Genetics and Molecular Biology* 38, no. 4. 490-98. doi:10.1590/s1415-475738420150046.

[88] Chaves, Juliana Siqueira, Fernando Batista Da Costa, and Luís Alexandre Pedro De Freitas. 2009. "Development of enteric coated tablets from spray dried extract of feverfew (Tanacetum parthenium L)." *Brazilian Journal of Pharmaceutical Sciences* 45, no. 3.p.573-84. doi:10.1590/s1984-82502009000300024.

[89] Couto, Renê O., Frederico S. Martins, Luiza T. Chaul, Edemilson C. Conceição, Luis Alexandre P. Freitas, Maria Teresa F. Bara, and José R. Paula. 2013."Spray drying of Eugenia dysenterica extract: effects of in-process parameters on product quality." *Revista Brasileira de Farmacognosia* 23, no. 1.p115-23. doi:10.1590/s0102-695x2012005000109.

[90] Peixoto, Maria Paula G., and Luís Alexandre P. Freitas. 2013. "Spray-dried extracts from Syzygium cumini seeds: Physicochemical and biological evaluation." *Revista Brasileira de Farmacognosia* 23, no. 1. 145-52. doi:10.1590/s0102-695x 2012005000124.

[91] TEIXEIRA, Cristiane Cardoso Correia. Desenvolvimento tecnológico de fitoterápico a partir de rizomas de Curcuma longa L. e avaliação das atividades antioxidante, anti-inflamatória e antitumoral. 2009. Tese de Doutorado. Universidade de São Paulo.

[92] Paradkar, Anant, Anshuman A. Ambike, Bhimrao K. Jadhav, and K.r. Mahadik. 2004."Characterization of curcumin–PVP solid dispersion obtained by spray drying." *International Journal of Pharmaceutics* 271, no. 1-2.p.281-86. doi:10.1016/j.ijpharm.2003.11.014.

[93] Martins, Rodrigo Molina, Simone Vieira Pereira, Silvia Siqueira, Wellington Fioravante Salomão, and Luis Alexandre Pedro Freitas.2013. "Curcuminoid content and antioxidant activity in spray dried microparticles containing turmeric extract." *Food Research International* 50, no. 2.p. 657-63. doi:10.1016/ j.foodres.2011.06.030.

[94] Nosari, Anna B.f.l., Juliana F. Lima, Osvaldo A. Serra, and Luis Alexandre P. Freitas.2015. "Improved green coffee oil antioxidant activity for cosmetical purpose by spray drying microencapsulation." *Revista Brasileira de Farmacognosia* 25, no. 3:p.307-11. doi:10.1016/j.bjp.2015.04.006.

[95] S, Jain Manu, Lohare Ganesh B, Bari Manoj, Chavan Randhir, Barhate Shashikant D, and Shah Chirag. "Spray Drying in Pharmaceutical Industry: A Review." *Journal Pharma. Dosage Forms and Tech* 4, no. 2,p. 74-79.

[96] Vehring, Reinhard, Willard R. Foss, and David Lechuga-Ballesteros.2007 "Particle formation in spray drying." *Journal of Aerosol Science* 38.7.p. 728-746.

[97] Vehring, Reinhard. 2008. "Pharmaceutical particle engineering via spray drying." *Pharmaceutical research* 25.5.p 999-1022.

[98] Guimarães, Thiago Frances, Aurea D. Lanchote, Jéssica Silva Da Costa, Alessandra Lifsitch Viçosa, and Luís Alexandre Pedro De Freitas. 2015 "A multivariate approach applied to quality on particle engineering of spray-dried mannitol." *Advanced Powder Technology* 26, no. 4: 1094-101. doi:10.1016/j.apt.2015.05.004.

[99] Narang, A. S., R. V. Mantri, and K. S. Raghavan. 2016. "Excipient compability and functionality." In *Developing Solid Oral Dosage Forms: Pharmaceutical Theory and Practice*,p. 151-79. 2º ed. Elsevier.

[100] Yoshii, Hirokazu, Hidefumi Hioshi, Hisashi Ohe, Masahumi Yasuda,Takeshi Furuta,Hiroshige Kuwahara,Masaaki Ohkawara, and Pekka Linko.2004. Encapsulation of shiitake (Lenthinus edodes) flavors by spray drying. Bioscience, biotechnology, and biochemistry, 68 no.1, p. 66-71.

[101] Couto Renê, Rafael R. Araújo, Luciana A. Tacon, Maria T. F. Bara, Edemilson C Conceição, José R. de Paula, Luis A. P. Freitas. 2011. Development of a Phytopharmaceutical Intermediate Product via Spray Drying. *Drying Technology*, v. 29, p 709-18.

[102] Souza, João Paulo, Luciana Alves Tacon, Cristiane C. Correia, Jairo. K. Bastos, Luis A. P. Freitas. 2007. Spray dried propolis extract II: Prenylated components of green propolis. *Die Pharmazie* 62, p.488-92.

[103] Tacon, Luciana Alves. 2012 "Estudo da extração e secagem por spray dryer das cascas de Endopleura uchi (Huber) Cuatrec. Humiriaceae." Ribeirão Preto, 106p. Dissertação de Mestrado, Programa de Pós-graduação em Ciências Farmacêuticas, Universidade de São Paulo.

[104] Killeen, M. J. 1993.The process of spray drying and spray congealing, *Pharm. Eng.*1993, p.56–64.

[105] Martins, Rodrigo Molina; Simone Siqueira.; Marcela Olaia Machado; Luis Alexandre Pedro de Freitas. The effect of homogenization method on the properties of carbamazepine microparticles prepared by spray congealing. *Journal of Microencapsulation* 2013, v. 30, n. 7, p. 692-700.

[106] Martins, R. M; Siqueira, S.; Vieira Fonseca; Luis Alexandre Pedro de Freitas.2014 Skin penetration and photoprotection of topical formulations containing benzophenone-3 solid lipid microparticles prepared by the solvent-free spray-congealing technique. *Journal of Microencapsulation*, v. 31, n. 7, p. 644-653.

[107] Okuro, P. K.; Matos Junior, F. E.; Favaro-Trindade, C. S. 2003.Technological Challenges for Spray Chilling Encapsulation of Functional Food Ingredients. *Food Technol. Biotechnol.* 51 (2) p.171–182.

[108] Pereira, Simone Vieira; Fábio Colombo; Rodrigo Molina Martins.; Luis Alexandre Pedro de Freitas Spray Cooling Process Factors and Quality Interactions During the Preparation of Microparticles Containing an Active Pharmaceutical Ingredient. *Drying Technology* 2014, v. 32, n. 10, p. 1188-1199.

[109] Wong, P. C.; Heng, P. W.; Chan, L. W. 2015.Spray congealing as a microencapsulation technique to develop modified-release ibuprofen solid lipid microparticles: the effect of matrix type, polymeric additives and drug-matrix miscibility. *Journal Microencapsule* 32(8):p.725-36.

[110] Martins, Rodrigo Molina, Silvia Siqueira, and Luis Alexandre Pedro Freitas. 2012."Spray Congealing of Pharmaceuticals: Study on Production of Solid Dispersions Using Box-Behnken Design." *Drying Technology* 30, no. 9 p. 935-45. doi:10.1080/07373937.2011.633251.

[111] Ali, M. E.; Lamprecht, A. 2014. Spray freeze drying for dry powder inhalation of nanoparticles. *European Journal of Pharmaceutics and Biopharmaceutics* 87.p. 510–517.

[112] Ishwarya, S. P.; Anandharamakrishnan, C.; Stapley, A.G.F. 2015.Spray-freeze-drying: A novel process for the drying of foods and bioproducts. *Trends in Food Science & Technology*. Volume 41, Issue 2, p. 161–181.

[113] Wanning, S.; Süverkrüp, R.; lamprecht, A.2015. Pharmaceutical spray freeze drying. *International Journal of Pharmaceutics*, Volume 488, Issues 1–2, 5, p. 136–153.

[114] Wang, Z. L.; Finlay, W. H.; Peppler, M. S.; Sweeney, L.G.2006. Powder formation by atmospheric spray-freeze-drying. *Powder Technology.* Volume 170, Issue 1, 30 November p.45–52.

[115] Bansal, Arvind K.2002, "Product Development Issues of Powders for Injection." Pharmaceutical Technology p.122-132. Available: <March 2002. Accessed January 18, 2017. http://images.alfresco.advanstar.com/alfresco_images/pharma/2014/08/22 /ffc04161-23ba-4e79-b9cb-3631d92b4bcc/article-12518.pdf>.

[116] Passerini, N., B. Perissutti, B. Albertini, E. Franceschinis, D. Lenaz, D. Hasa, I. Locatelli, and D. Voinovich. 2012."A new approach to enhance oral bioavailability of Silybum Marianum dry extract: Association of mechanochemical activation and spray congealing." *Phytomedicine* 19.2.p 160-68.

[117] Khwanpruk, K., Anandharamakrishnan, C., Rielly, C. D., & Stapley, A. G. F. (2008). Volatiles retention during the sub-atmospheric spray freeze drying of coffee and maltodextrin. 16th International Drying Symposium IDS 2008, 9-12th November 2008, Hyderabad, India. Vol b p.1066-1072.

[118] Janyawat Vuthijumnok, Abdul-Lateef Molan, Julian A. Heyes. 2013. Effect of freeze-drying and extraction solvents on the total phenolic contents, total flavonoids and antioxidant activity of different Rabbiteye blueberry genotypes grown in New Zealand. *Journal of Pharmacy and Biological Sciences.* Volume 8, Issue 1,p.42-48.

[119] Mahanom, H. Azizah, AH and Dzulkifly, M. H. 1999. Effect of different drying methods on concentrations of several phytochemicals in herbal preparation of 8 medicinal plants leaves. *Journal of Nutrition* Vol 5:p. 47-54.

[120] Al-Qarawi AA, Al-Damegh MA, ElMougy SA. 2002. Effect of freeze dried extract of Olea europaea on the pituitary-thyroid axis in rats. *Phytother Res.* Vol 16(3):p. 286-7.

[121] Brunauer, Stephen, Lola Deming, Edwards Deming, and Edward Teller. 1940. "On a Theory of the van der Waals Adsorption of Gases." *Journal of the American Chemical Society* 62, no. 7, p.1723-732. doi:10.1021/ja01864a025.

[122] Couto, Rodigo O., R. R. Araújo, Luciana A. Tacon, Edemilson C. Conceição, M. T. F. Bara, J. R. Paula, and Luis A. P. Freitas. "Development of a Phytopharmaceutical Intermediate Product via Spray Drying." *Drying Technology* 29, no. 6 p.709-18. doi:10.1080/07373937.2010.524062.

[123] F. Sansone, T. Mencherini, P. Picerno, M. d'Amore, R.P. Aquino, M.R. Lauro, 2011.Maltodextrin/ pectin microparticles by spray drying as carrier for nutraceutical extracts, *J Food Eng,* 105.p. 468-476.

[124] Nayak, Chetan A., and Navin K. Rastogi. 2010."Effect of Selected Additives on Microencapsulation of Anthocyanin by Spray Drying." *Drying Technology* 28, no. 12.p.1396-404. doi:10.1080/07373937.2010.482705.

[125] Wang, Wei, and Weibiao Zhou. 2012"Characterization of spray-dried soy sauce powders using maltodextrins as carrier." *Journal of Food Engineering* 109, no. 3.p.399-405. doi:10.1016/j.jfoodeng.2011.11.012.

[126] Xu, Jianchen, Li Li Bovet, and Kang Zhao. 2008"Taste masking microspheres for orally disintegrating tablets." *International Journal of Pharmaceutics* 359, no. 1-2.p63-69. doi:10.1016/j.ijpharm.2008.03.019.

[127] Villanova, J.c.o., E. Ayres, and R.l. Oréfice. 2011."Design of prolonged release tablets using new solid acrylic excipients for direct compression." *European Journal of Pharmaceutics and Biopharmaceutics* 79, no. 3.p. 664-73. doi:10.1016/j.ejpb.2011.07.011.

[128] Gallo, Loreana, Juan M. Llabot, Daniel Allemandi, Verónica Bucalá, and Juliana Piña.2011. "Influence of spray-drying operating conditions on Rhamnus purshiana (Cáscara sagrada) extract powder physical properties." *Powder Technology* 208, no. 1.p. 205-14. doi:10.1016/j.powtec.2010.12.021.

[129] Donsì, F., M. Sessa, and G. Ferrari.2010. "Nanoencapsulation of essential oils to enhance their antimicrobial activity in foods." *Journal of Biotechnology* 150.p.67. doi:10.1016/j.jbiotec.2010.08.175.

[130] Soottitantawat, Apinan, Kohei Takayama, Kenji Okamura, Daisuke Muranaka, Hidefumi Yoshii, Takeshi Furuta, Masaaki Ohkawara, and Pekka Linko. 2005. "Microencapsulation of l-menthol by spray drying and its release characteristics." *Innovative Food Science & Emerging Technologies* 6, no. 2. 163-70. doi:10.1016/j.ifset.2004.11.007.

[131] Teixeira, Cristiane Correira, Guilherme A. Teixeira, and Luis Alexandre Pedro Freitas.2011."Spray Drying of Extracts from Red Yeast Fermentation Broth." *Drying Technology* 29, no. 3 p. 342-50. doi:10.1080/07373937.2010.497235.

[132] Yusof, Y.a., F.s. Mohd Salleh, N.l. Chin, and R.a. Talib. 2011. "The Drying and Tabletting Of Pitaya Powder." *Journal of Food Process Engineering* 35, no. 5.p. 763-71. doi:10.1111/j.1745-4530.2010.00625.x.

[133] Zareifard, Mohammad Reza, Mehrdad Niakousari, Zohre Shokrollahi, and Shahram Javadian.2011. "A Feasibility Study on the Drying of Lime Juice: The Relationship between the Key Operating Parameters of a Small Laboratory Spray Dryer and Product Quality." *Food and Bioprocess Technology* 5, no. 5 .p1896-906. doi:10.1007/s11947-011-0689-1.

[134] G.S. Schwartz SS, 1982. *Plastics Materials and Processes*, in, Van Nostrand Reinhold Company Inc., New York, EUA, p. 547.

[135] V. Ganesan, K.A. Rosentrater, K. Muthukurnarappan, 2008.Flowability and handling characteristics of bulk solids and powders: a review with implications for DDGS, *Biosyst Eng*, 101.p.425-435.

[136] D. Geldart, E.C. Abdullah, A. Hassanpour, L.C. Nwoke, I. Wouters.2006. Characterization of powder flowability using measurement of angle of repose, *China Particuology*, 4, p. 104-107.

[137] American Pharmacopeia. *USP XXX: United States Pharmacopeial Convention*, in: United States Pharmacopeial Convention, USP: Rockville, MD, 2008.

[138] Abdullah, E.c., and D. Geldart. 1999. "The use of bulk density measurements as flowability indicators." *Powder Technology* 102, no. 2.p.151-65. doi:10.1016/s0032-5910(98)00208-3.

[139] M.E. Aulton, *Pharmaceutics: the science of dosage form design*, Churchill Livingstone, Edinburgh, 2002.

[140] Liu, L.x., I. Marziano, A.c. Bentham, J.d. Litster, E.t.white, and T. Howes. 2008. "Effect of particle properties on the flowability of ibuprofen powders." *International Journal of Pharmaceutics* 362, no. 1-2 p. 109-17. doi:10.1016/j.ijpharm.2008.06.023.

[141] J. Broadhead, S.K.E. Rouan, C.T. Rhodes, 1992. The spray drying of pharmaceuticals, *Drug Development and Industrial Pharmacy*, 18.p.1169-1206.

[142] D.E. Walton, 2000.The morphology of spray-dried particles a qualitative view, *Dry Technol,* 18.p. 1943-1986.

[143] D.E. Walton, C.J. Mumford.1999.The morphology of spray-dried particles: the effect of process variables upon the morphology of spray-dried particles, Trans IChemE, 77 p. 442-460.

[144] Lee, Yan-Ying, Jian X. Wu, Mingshi Yang, Paul M. Young, Frans Van Den Berg, and Jukka Rantanen. 2011."Particle size dependence of polymorphism in spray-dried mannitol." *European Journal of Pharmaceutical Sciences* 44, no. 1-2.p.41-48. doi:10.1016/j.ejps.2011.06.002.

[145] Rowe, Raymond C. *Handbook of pharmaceutical excipients*. London: Pharmaceutical Press, 2012.

[146] J. Hauke, T. Kossowski, 2011.Comparison of values of pearson's and spearman's correlation coefficients on the same sets of data, *Quaestiones Geographicae*, 30.p 87-93.

[147] J.J. Wang, Y.Y. Jing, C.F. Zhang, J.H. Zhao.2009.Review on multi-criteria decision analysis aid in sustainable energy decision-making, *Renew Sust Energ Rev*, 13.p. 2263-2278.

[148] Simões.Cláudia Maria, E.P. Schenkel, G. Gosmann, J.C.P. Mello, L.A. Mentz, P.R. Petrovick, 2001.Farmacognosia: da planta ao medicamento, 1 ed., Editora da Universidade UFRGS/ Editora da UFSC, Porto Alegre/ Florianópolis.

[149] Bruschi, M.l, M.l.c Cardoso, M.b Lucchesi, and M.p.d Gremião.2003. "Gelatin microparticles containing propolis obtained by spray-drying technique: preparation and characterization." *International Journal of Pharmaceutics* 264, no. 1-2.p.45-55. doi:10.1016/s0378-5173(03)00386-7.

[150] Gonnissen, Y., J. p. Remon, and C. Vervaet. 2007."Development of directly compressible powders via co-spray drying." *European Journal of Pharmaceutics and Biopharmaceutics* 67, no. 1.p. 220-26. doi:10.1016/j.ejpb.2006.12.021.

[151] Adi, Handoko, Paul M. Young, Hak-Kim Chan, Helen Agus, and Daniela Traini.2010. "Co-spray-dried mannitol–ciprofloxacin dry powder inhaler formulation for cystic fibrosis and chronic obstructive pulmonary disease." *European Journal of Pharmaceutical Sciences* 40, no. 3.p. 239-47. doi:10.1016/j.ejps.2010.03.020.

[152] T. Mizoe, T. Ozeki, H. Okada.2007. Preparation of drug nanoparticle-containing microparticles using a 4-fluid nozzle spray drier for oral, pulmonary, and injection dosage forms, *Journal of Control Release,* 122.p. 10-15

[153] Littringer, E.m., A. Mescher, H. Schroettner, L. Achelis, P. Walzel, and N.a. Urbanetz.2012. "Spray dried mannitol carrier particles with tailored surface properties – The influence of carrier surface roughness and shape." *European Journal of Pharmaceutics and Biopharmaceutics* 82, no. 1.p. 194-204. doi:10.1016/j.ejpb.2012.05.001.

[154] Drop Trajectory predicitions and their inportance in the design of spray dryers.

[155] R. P. Patel, M. P. Patel, A. M. Suthar, 2009. Spray drying technology: an overview, *Indian Journal of Science and Technology*, 2. p. 44-47.

[156] Maas, Stephan G., Gerhard Schaldach, Eva M. Littringer, Axel Mescher, Ulrich J. Griesser, Doris E. Braun, Peter E. Walzel, and Nora A. Urbanetz. 2011. "The impact of spray drying outlet temperature on the particle morphology of mannitol." *Powder Technology* 213, no. 1-3,p. 27-35. doi:10.1016/j.powtec.2011.06.024.

[157] Costa, Ana Rita de Mello.2016.Lipossomas contendo ácido caurenoico ou extrato de Copaifera langsdorffii:desenvolvimento, caracterização e atividade antitumoral e tripanocida [thesis].Ribeirão preto:Faculdade de Ciências Farmacêuticas de Ribeirão Preto. Available from: http://www.teses.usp.br/teses/disponiveis/60/60137 /tde-17062016-151719/en.php.

In: Recent Developments in Phytomedicine Technology
Editors: L. A. Pedro de Freitas et al.
ISBN: 978-1-53611-977-0

Chapter 7

RECENT DEVELOPMENT IN PREPARATION METHODS OF POLYMERIC MICRO/NANOPARTICLE AND SOLID LIPID CARRIES TO PHYTOMEDICINE

Mariza A. Miranda, Margarete M. Araujo and Priscyla Daniely Marcato**

NanoBiolab, School of Pharmaceutical Science of Ribeirão Preto,
Universidade de São Paulo, Brazil

ABSTRACT

Phytomedicine has been used by human civilization for many years to treat different diseases showing to be a promising source of activity compounds. However, the phytomedicine shows some disadvantages as the reproducibility of biological activity of herbal extracts and isolated compounds, its toxicity and adverse effects, stability, low water solubility and bioavailability. The phytomedicine encapsulation in delivery systems can overcome these challenges. Different micro and nanoparticles can be used for phytomedicine encapsulation as polymeric and solid lipid nanoparticles. In this chapter, some methods of preparation to different kind of nanoparticles will be described. Examples of phytomedicine encapsulated and their main advantages are described. These nanostructures offer a feasible approach to modulating phytomedicine.

Keywords: phytomedicine, polymeric micro/nanoparticles, solid lipid nanoparticles

---

* Corresponding Author address. Email: pmarcato@fcfrp.usp.br.

INTRODUCTION

Delivery System of Phytomedicine

The plants have been extensively used for the treatment of several diseases. Nowadays, about 50% of the drugs used by the population are obtained from natural sources [1]. Advancements in phytochemistry made possible isolation of medicinally active plant constituents improving the phytomedicines. However, several challenges need to be overcome in the development of these medicines. In general, phytomedicines exhibit high *in vitro* activity but low *in vivo* efficacy due to their poor solubility, low bioavailability and instability in gastric environment. Furthermore, they show toxicity and adverse effects. These drawbacks can be overcome using nanotechnology. Nanophytomedicine is a new emerging area, which allows the development of innovative herbal drugs through the encapsulation of active phytocompounds of medicinal plants in nanoparticles [1, 2]. The nanoparticles definition has been highly debated in the world. Nowadays, particles with a size below 1000 nm are considered nanoparticle if these particles exhibit properties or phenomena, including physical or chemical properties or biological effects, that are attributable to its dimension [3, 4].

The phytomedicines encapsulation can improve the solubility and bioavailability in active constituents of medicinal plants, decrease toxicity, enhance pharmacological activity, improve stability during storage and in gastric environment, sustain release of the active encapsulated, etc. Different nanoparticles have been used in phytomedicine encapsulation to highlight polymeric micro/nanoparticles and solid lipid nanoparticles nanoparticles because of the easy and low cost production methods of these particles and low costs. The phytomedicine encapsulation efficacy depends on the physic-chemical properties of the herbal extracts or isolated compounds, the particles type, the nanoparticles composition, and the method of particles preparation. Therefore, understanding the particle preparation method is critical for the development of nanophytomedicines [3, 4, 5]. Thus, this chapter will describe the main methods available to prepare polymeric micro/nanoparticles and solid lipid nanoparticles for phytomedicine encapsulation.

Polymeric Micro/Nanoparticles

The polymer-based drug delivery system has been extensively studied in nanophytomedicine. Biodegradable and biocompatible polymers are used to form polymeric particles. The most commonly polymers used to form polymeric nanoparticles are shown in Table 1. Depending on the method and particle composition, nanospheres or nanocapsules can be obtained. Nanocapsules are vesicular structures with a core, surrounded by a polymer membrane, which can composite by oil, while nanospheres are matrix systems (Figure 1). The herbal drug can be entrapped, dispersed, dissolved within or adsorbed on nanoparticle surface [6, 7, 8].

Different methods are described in the literature to obtain polymeric nanoparticles. The most used methods are based on precipitation of pre-formed polymers, which include nanoprecipitation, emulsion evaporation method, ionic gelation and spray-drying method. These methods are described below.

Table 1. Synthetic and natural polymers used in the polymeric nanoparticles preparation

Polymers	Structure
Natural polymers	
Chitosan	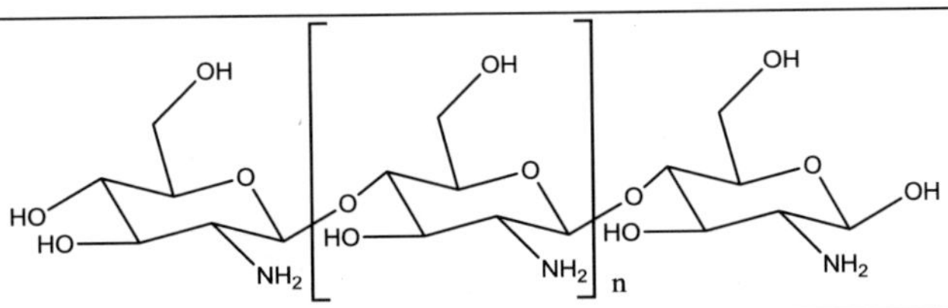
Alginate	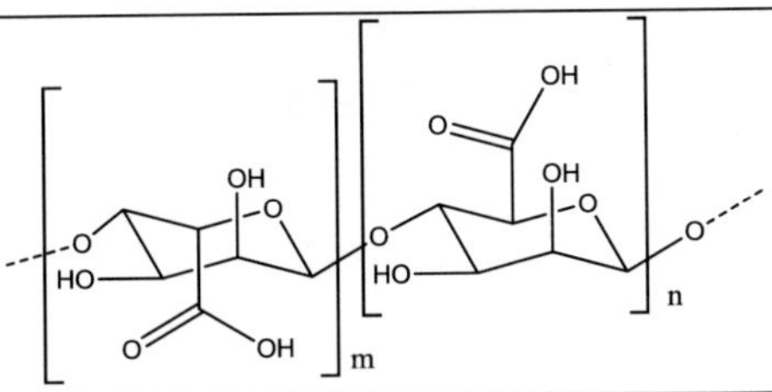
Hyaluronic acid	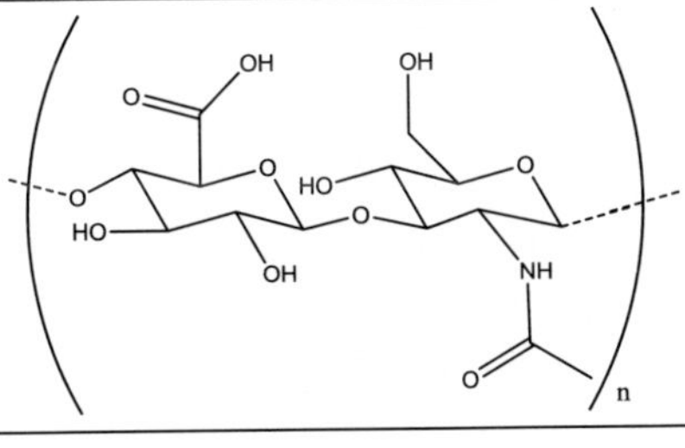
Carrageenan	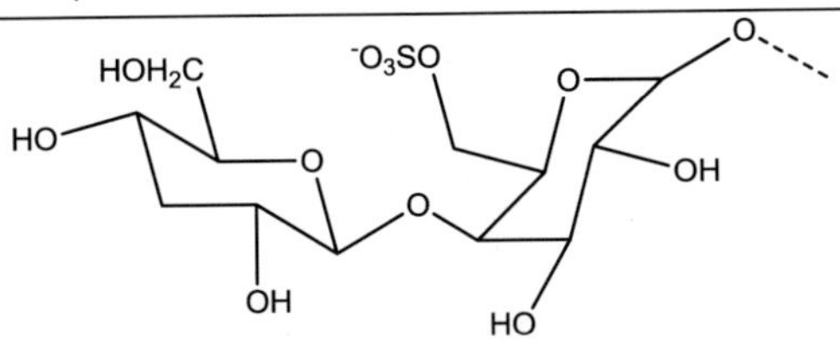 gamma- carrageenan

Table 1. (Continued)

Polymers	Structure
Synthetic polymers	
Poly(lactic acid) (PLA)	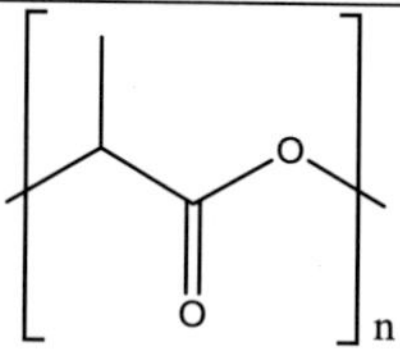
Poly(caprolactone) (PCL)	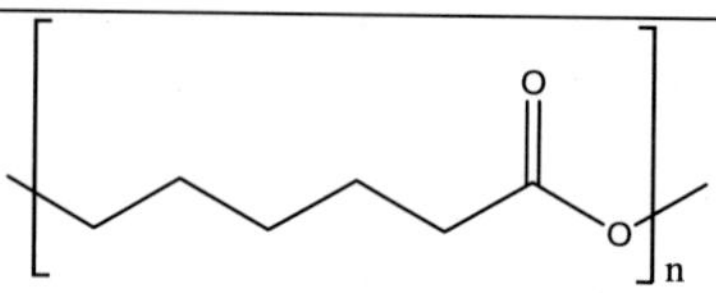
Poly Lactic-co-Glycolic Acid (PLGA)	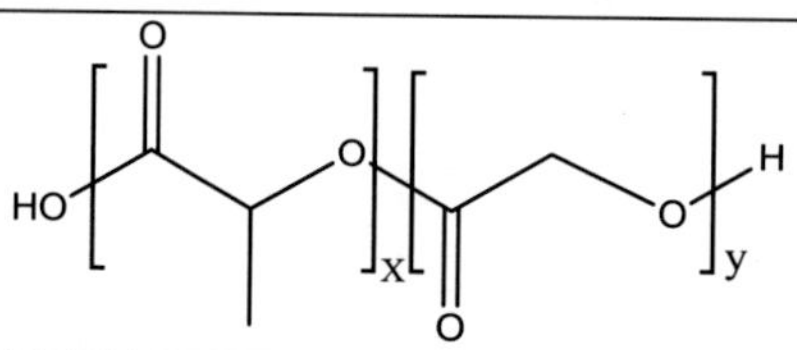
Poly(glycolic acid) (PGA)	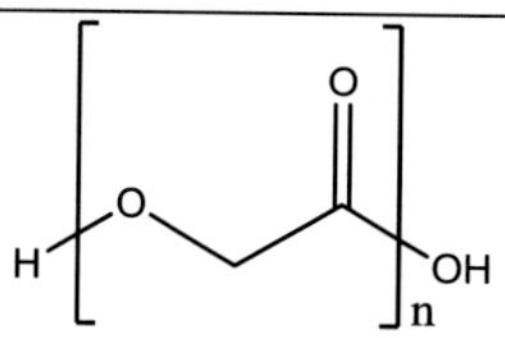
Poly (vinyl alcohol) (PVA)	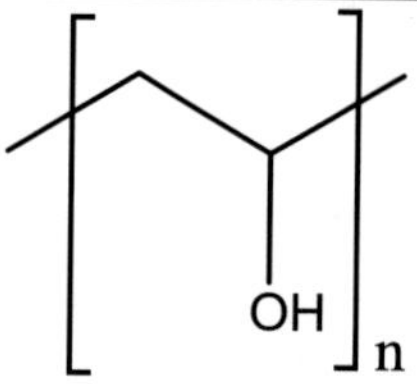
Ethyl cellulose	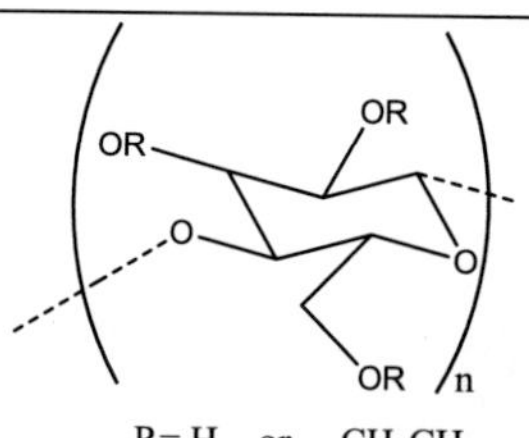 R= H or CH_2CH_3
polyhydroxybutyrate (PHB)	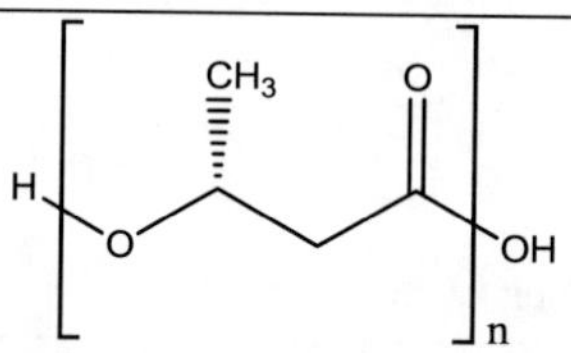

Nanoprecipitation

Nanoprecipitation was developed by Fessi's group [9] and is also called solvent displacement or interfacial deposition method. Nanoprecipitation is a reproducible, easy, fast, and economic method for the preparation of monodisperse polymeric nanoparticles or with low polydispersity index (very narrow particle size distribution). In this method, particles in a size range of 20–300 nm can be obtained [7, 9, 10].

Water miscible organic solvents (e.g., acetone, ethanol) are required for this method. First, organic and aqueous phases are prepared. The organic phase is composite by the organic solvent; polymer and herbal drug while aqueous phase is composite by water and surfactant. Different surfactants can be used, but in general Polysorbates and Poloxamer are employed. The organic phase is added to an aqueous phase under moderate stirring (e.g., magnetic) leading to the immediate formation of colloidal particles. Afterward, the organic solvent is removed under reduced pressure (Figure 2). If an oil is added in the organic phase, nanocapsule will be obtained. The key process variables are polymer concentration, type of organic solvent, type and concentration of surfactant. In general, a high polymer concentration can increases particle size because it increases the viscosity of the organic phase. On the other hand, the increased surfactant concentration can decrease the particles size due to interfacial tension reduction. However, high surfactant concentration may favor the particles aggregation. Usually, a surfactant concentration in the range of 0.5-1.5% is used in the nanoprecipitation method. Another important parameter in this method is velocity of diffusion of the organic solvent. The use of organic solvent with high diffusion coefficients (e.g., acetone) tends to form small nanoparticles due to faster solvent diffusion. Furthermore, conditions of adding the organic phase to the aqueous phase and aqueous phase agitation rate can influence the particles size and the polydispersity index, mainly when the organic phase is highly viscous [8, 10, 11].

This method is used mostly for encapsulation of hydrophobic drugs, but can also be employed to incorporate hydrophilic drugs with low encapsulation efficiency.

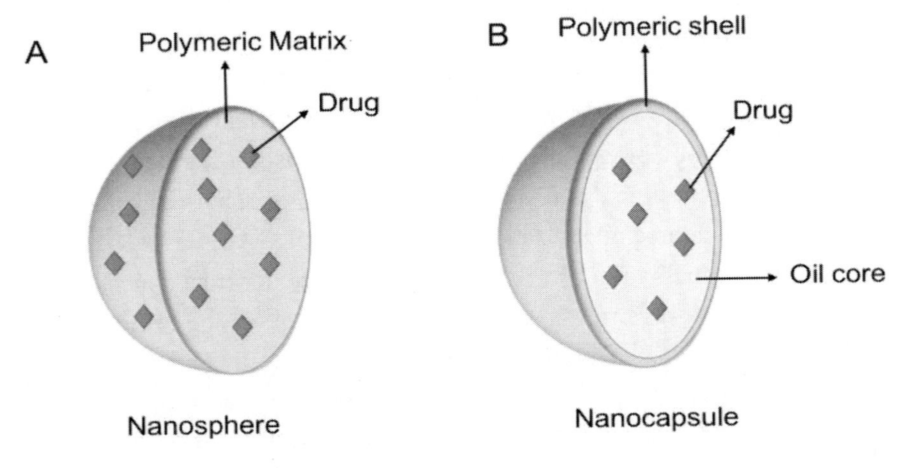

Figure 1. Polymeric particle structure: A) nanocapsule, B)nanospheres.

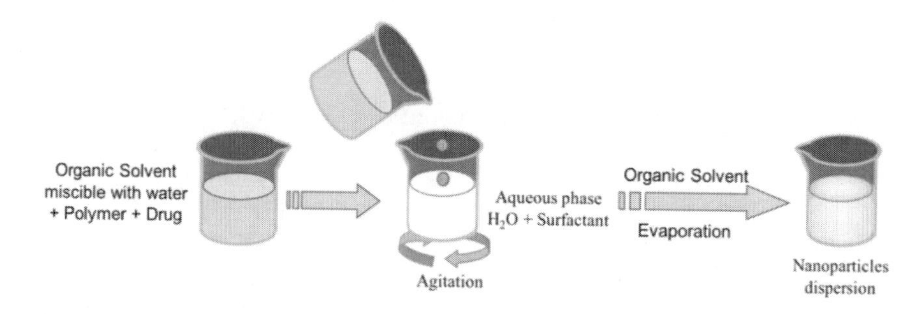

Figure 2. Scheme of polymeric nanoparticle preparation by nanoprecipitation method.

Nanoprecipitation method has been used by many authors to prepare nanophytodrug. To obtain controlled release and to preserve the antioxidant activity of the polyphenols, Sanna et al. [12] prepared polymeric nanoparticles with white tea (Pai Mu Tan) leaves extract using poly(ε-caprolactone) (PCL) and alginate. The nanoparticles were prepared using the nanoprecipitation method. The polymer PCL was dissolved in 3 mL of acetonitrile and added dropwise, under magnetic stirring (700 rpm), into a solution containing pluronic F-127 (0.5% w/v), alginate (0.1%, 0.5%, and 1.0% w/v), white tea extract, and water, to give a final polymer concentration of 6.0 mg/mL. The resulting colloidal suspension was evaporated under stirring (500 rpm) at room temperature for 1 h to remove the organic solvent. The optimal alginate concentration was found to be 0.5% w/v that produced nanoparticles spherical, a mean diameter of 380.80 ± 37.97 nm with unimodal distribution (PDI 0.15 ± 0.06). The nanoparticles selected demonstrated the effectiveness of the nanoencapsulation to control the white tea extract release in gastrointestinal fluids and to preserve the antioxidant activity of the polyphenols. Also, the encapsulation increased stability preventing the loss of total polyphenol content and catechins. This work showed that the use of the nanotechnology could offer interesting perspectives for the potential use of white tea extract-loaded nanoparticles for nutraceutical applications.

Polymeric nanoparticles encapsulating the polyphenol trans-resveratrol (RSV) was proposed by Sanna et al. [13] as novel prototypes for prostate cancer treatment. The nanosystem composed of a biocompatible blend of poly(epsilon-caprolactone) (PCL) and poly(D,L-lactic-co-glycolic acid)-poly(ethylene glycol) conjugate (PLGA-PEG-COOH) were prepared by a nanoprecipitation method. The PCL:PLGA-PEG-COOH blend based nanoparticules, with a mass ratio of 1.5:1 and RSV at three different concentrations (2, 3, and 4%, w/w), were dissolved in acetonitrile and added into water, under soft stirring, giving a final polymer concentration of about 7.0 mg/mL. The resulting colloidal suspension was stirred at room temperature to remove the organic solvent. The formulation loaded with 4% w/w of RSV was chosen based on encapsulation efficiency results (98%), average diameter (150 nm), and its abitiy to control the RSV release, supporting its potential use as chemoprevention/ chemotherapy for prostate cancer.

Teixeira et al. [14] developed PLGA nanospheres and nanocapsules containing the natural products xanthone (XAN) and 3-methoxyxanthone (3-MeOXAN). These two different nanosystems had the goal of improving the delivery of these poorly water-soluble compounds. Nanospheres were prepared using solvent displacement technique. An organic solution of PLGA (63 mg) and different amounts of XAN or 3-MeOXAN in acetone (10 mL) were poured, under magnetic stirring, into 10 mL of an aqueous solution of Pluronic F-68 0.25% (w/v). Following 5 minutes of stirring, the volume of nanosphere dispersion was concentrated under reduced pressure. The nanocapsules were prepared by the interfacial polymer deposition technique. 50 mg of polymer and 100 mg of soybean lecithin were dissolved in 10 mL of acetone. Different amounts of XAN or 3-MeOXAN were dissolved in 0.5–0.6 mL of Myritol 318 and then added to the previously prepared acetone solution. This mixture was poured into 20 mL of an aqueous solution of Pluronic F-68 0.5% (w/v) under stirring, leading to the formation of the nanocapsules. Then, acetone was removed under vacuum. This process allowed nanospheres of a mean diameter < 170 nm and nanocapsules of a mean diameter < 300 nm to be obtained. Nanocapsules appear to be more appropriate carriers for both xanthones, as once encapsulated compounds concentrations in the final dispersions were higher than nanospheres. This difference can be related to the xanthones solubility in the oil. 3-MeOXAN release from nanocapsules was governed mainly by its partition between the oil core and the external aqueous medium. The release profile of XAN from nanocapsules suggests an interaction of the drug with the polymer.

Nanoprecipitation was the technique adopted to prepare poly (lactide-co-glycolide) (PLGA) nanoparticles encapsulating the phytodrug called grape seed extract (GSE)-'NanoGSE'. NanoGSE was prepared by selecting various ratios of PLGA:GSE ranging from 5:2 to 5:5. Summarizing, 50 mg PLGA and 20 mg of GSE were dissolved in acetone. The resulting blend was added using a syringe directly dipped into MilliQ water (1:4v/v) under sonication. An additional volume of water was added to this mixture under stirring to enable the formation of a homogeneous nanocolloid. The organic phase was then evaporated under reduced pressure at 37°C. The nanosystem was conjugated with folic acid (FA) to increase the potential cancer targeting ligand, once the folate receptor is over-expressing in cancer cell membranes. The drug-loaded nanoparticles approximately 100nm in size exhibited high colloidal stability at physiological pH. The FA-NanoGSE showed substantially enhanced bioavailability to the tumor cells, sparing the normal ones [15].

Emulsion Evaporation Method

The emulsion evaporation method can be used to encapsulate hydrophobic and hydrophilic drugs. Furthermore, micro or nanoparticles can be obtained depending on the method conditions. In this method, water-immiscible organic solvents are used (e.g., chloroform, ethyl acetate). For hydrophobic herbal drug encapsulation, an oil/water emulsion is formed first. For this, the organic phase (organic solvent + polymer + herbal drug) is dropped into aqueous phase (water + surfactant) under high-shear forming an oil/water emulsion. Afterwards, the organic solvent is removed by reduceding pressure, leading to polymer precipitation and nanoparticle formation (Figure 3). For hydrophilic herbal drug encapsulation, a double emulsion of water/oil/water is used. The double emulsions are usually prepared using two-step process: 1) an aqueous phase with herbal drug is dripped into an organic phase composed of organic solvent, polymer and surfactant under high-shear, forming a W/O emulsion; 2) The W/O emulsion is quickly added in the second aqueous phase, comprised of water and surfactant, under high homogenization, thereby obtaining a W/O/W emulsion. Afterward, the organic solvent is removed using reduced pressure (Figure 4). Two different surfactants can be used: a hydrophobic one to stabilize the W/O internal emulsion interface and a hydrophilic one to stabilize the external interface of the oil globules [7, 8, 16].

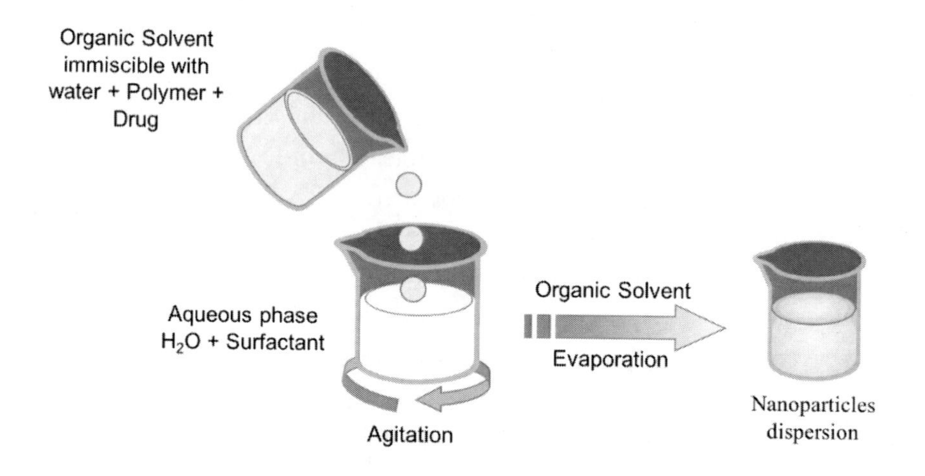

Figure 3. Scheme of polymeric nanoparticle preparation by emulsion (O/W) evaporation method for hydrophobic herbal drug encapsulation.

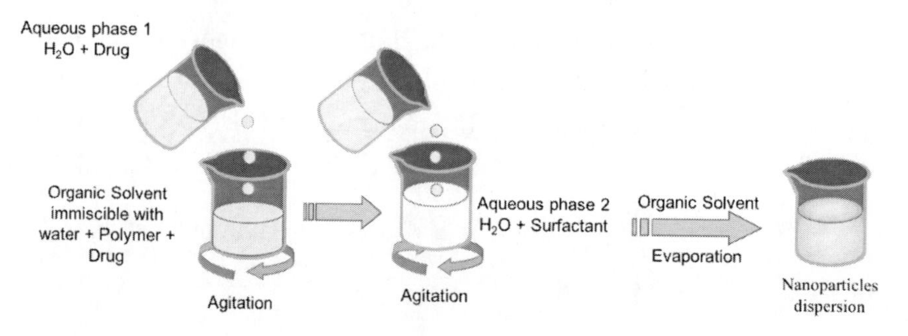

Figure 4. Scheme of polymeric nanoparticle preparation by emulsion (W/O/W) evaporation method for hydrophilic herbal drug encapsulation.

The most common surfactants used in emulsion evaporation method are poly(vinyl alcohol) (PVA), Polysorbate and Sorbitan. The critical parameters in this method are the polymer concentration, and the type and concentration of surfactant, as described in the nanoprecipitation method. However, the most important process variables for affecting the size and the polydispersity index are adding the organic phase to the aqueous phase, and aqueous phase stirring. The slow dripping of the organic phase into the aqueous phase with high-shear tends to reduce the size of the emulsion droplet and consequently, also reduce the particle size. Thus, these parameters will largely determine the final particle size. Homogenization using Turrax or Tip sonication is usually employed in this method [7, 8, 11, 16, 17].

Dubey et al. [18] encapsulated the pentacyclic triterpenediol (TPD) isolated from Boswellia serrata in a biocompatible and biodegradable PLGA polymer using emulsion–diffusion–evaporation technique. 50 mg of PLGA and 5 mg of TPD was dissolved in 2.5 mL of dichloromethane (DCM) at room temperature. The organic phase was added drop-wise in 5 mL of an aqueous phase containing varying concentration of PVA as a stabilizer under different homogenization speed. The resulting o/w emulsion was sonicated at 60% amplitude through ultrasonicator and then poured into 5 mL of water under stirring for 3 h in order to evaporate the organic phase and form of nanoparticles. The TPD-loaded nanosystem exhibited an average particle size of about 161 nm demonstrate enhanced *in vitro* cytotoxicity and, apoptosis, and generated higher reactive oxygen species (ROS) as compared with free TPD. In addition, the nanoparticles with TPD showed superior *in vivo* anticancer activity in Ehrlich solid tumor model. Further, no hematological or biochemical toxicity was observed after the treatment, thereby improving its anticancer potential.

Proanthocyanidins (PAs) extracted from grapes have several bioactive properties, including protection from cancer, cardiovascular disorders, obesity, diabetes, and neurodegenerative disorders. However, PAs are unstable in the digestive tract and must be stabilized to allow oral administration. Fernández et al. [19] proposed stabilizing grape seed and skin extracts with high content in PAs using poly-D,L-lactide (PLA) and the emulsion-evaporation method. 50 mg of PLA and dried PAs extract (5 mg) in 2 mL dichloromethane (DCM) were sonicated at 40% amplitude for 30 s at room temperature. PVA (4 mL of 3%, w/v) was added and sonicated similarly to form an emulsion. The emulsion was diluted by 0.1% (w/v) PVA solution to a final 80 mL solution. The organic solvent was evaporated under vacuum. The process was optimized to achieve higher encapsulation efficiency (EE = 82.7%) and a smaller size (256 nm). The *in vitro* release studies using stomach and intestine simulation showed sustained release of PAs from PLA nanoparticles.

Curcumin (CUR) is a natural polyphenolic antioxidant and is typically obtained from the rhizome of Curcuma longa Linn. Many biological activities are described to CUR. However, its biopharmaceutical properties limit its feasibility as a therapeutic agent. It is poorly absorbed due its low aqueous solubility and its degradability in alkaline conditions. Also, the possibility of photo-degradation should be considered when designing and optimizing CUR delivery systems. Yoon et al. [20] produced poly(D,L-lactic acid)-glycerol (PDLLA-G)-based nanoparticles (NPs) for the intravenous delivery of curcumin (CUR). CUR-loaded PDLLA-G nanoparticles were prepared using the emulsification-solvent evaporation technique. Briefly, PDLLA-G (30 mg) and CUR (2 mg) were dissolved in dichloromethane (1 mL), and the solution was transferred to a PVA solution (5 mL; 2%, weight per volume (w/v)). The resulting emulsion was sonicated for 20 min using a probe sonicator. The organic solvent was then evaporated under stirring for 30 min. The nanoparticles showed a mean diameter of approximately 200 nm, a narrow size distribution, and high efficiency drug encapsulation (95.82%). The encapsulation of CUR was shown to enable prolonged circulation of the drug in the blood stream and improved anticancer activity after intravenous injection.

Costunolide is a sesquiterpene lactone extracted from *Saussurea lappa* Clarke (Compositae) that has shown cytotoxicity on different cancer cell lines. Eight nanoparticles of poly (D,L-lactic-co-glycolic acid) (PLGA) containing costunolide were prepared with the goal of analyzing the release behavior *in vitro* in model anticancer. The costunolide loaded nanoparticles were prepared by a modified oil in water single emulsion solvent evaporation technique. A solution of PLGA (21 mg) in 3.5 mL of ethyl acetate containing costunolide (16.6% w/w of polymer) was prepared first. An aqueous phase containing Tween 80 (0.86% w/v) that was homogenized for 1 min by vortex was also prepared. Afterwards, 2 mL of organic phase was added to 10 mL of the aqueous phase. Then, the solution was sonicated using a microtip probe sonicator set at 50W of energy output during 4 min to produce the oil-in-water emulsion. The formed O/W emulsion was stirred at room temperature (22°C) by a magnetic stirrer at 800 rpm for 2 h to remove the organic solvent. Nanoparticles showed mean diameter of 112.1 ± 6.4 nm with low polydispersity index. The formulation containing surfactant Tween 80 showed maximum *in vitro* costunolide release compared to the formulation produced with surfactant PVA [21].

Ionic Gelation

Ionic gelation is based on the cross-link between polyelectrolytes and counter ions, leading to a hydrogel particles formation. This method is mostly used to prepare particles with biopolymers, especially charged polysaccharides, such as alginate, and, chitosan. The use of biopolymer has been highlighted in the nanophytomedicine due to its interesting properties, such as pH sensitive (e.g., alginate) or mucoadhesive (e.g., chitosan). For example, alginate particles can protect acid-sensitive herbal drugs from the gastric juice, and chitosan nanoparticle can enhance the drug absorption due to adhesion of the particles in the intestinal mucous. This method is preferably used for encapsulation of hydrophilic drugs [22].

The ionic gelation is a simple and mild method that can only be conducted in aqueous phase without the use of any organic solvent and preferably used to encapsulation of hydrophilic drugs. The disadvantage of this method is high diluted conditions, which limit the yield of production of particles. For the particles preparation, the biopolymer is dissolved in water with a concentration below the gel point with herbal drug. Then, this polymer solution is dropped into the polyvalent ions aqueous solution, forming a three-dimensional lattice ionically cross-linked. Micro or nanoparticles are obtained; depending on the process conditions. These particles can be subsequently stabilized with oppositely charged polyelectrolytes. For example, alginate nanoparticles can be obtained by adding alginate solution into a calcium ions solution, leading to a pre-gel phase which is then stabilized by chitosan (Figure 5). The key process variables are biopolymer concentration, type and concentration of polyvalent ions, aqueous phase stirring, conditions of adding the polymer phase to the polyvalent ions phase, and the molecular weight of the opposite charged macromolecule [7, 23].

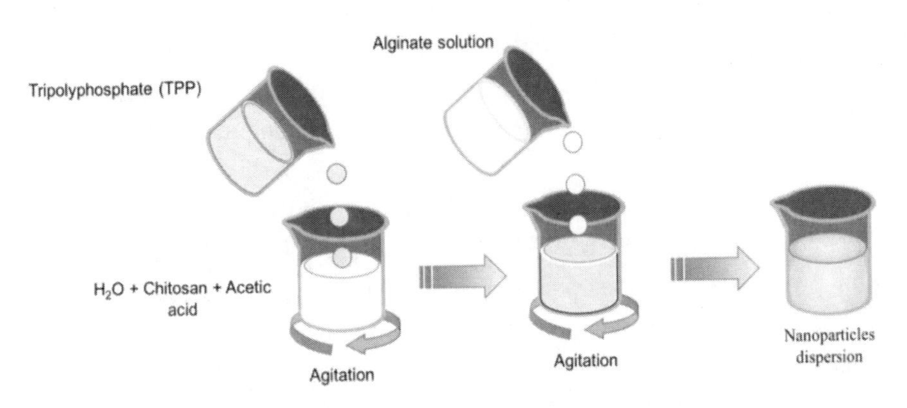

Figure 5. Scheme of chitosan nanoparticle preparation by ionic gelation.

Harangozo et al. [24] used 4-sulfonatocalixarenes (SCX8) that induce supramolecular crosslinking of protonated chitosan to produce nanoparticles capable of carrying important pharmaceutical alkaloids with anticancer properties such as beberine and coralyne. Chitosan and SCXn were separately dissolved in 0.01 M HCl solution. After the adjustment of the pH by NaOH solution to the desired value, the necessary amounts of the two stock solutions (Chitosan and SCXn) were mixed under magnetic stirring at 200 rpm. The counterions of SCXn were H3O+ and/or Na+ depending on pH. For alkaloid encapsulation, the alkaloid was added in the SCX8 solution. The most stable nanoparticles with 160 nm diameter and narrow size distribution were obtained at pH 4 using low molecular weight chitosan. The larger aggregates were produced when chitosan concentration was increased. The most stable nanoparticles with 160 nm diameter and narrow size distribution were obtained at pH 4 using low molecular weight chitosan. These nanoparticles encapsulated coralyne with more than 90% entrapment efficiency and loading capacity of 15%.

Polycationic chitosan and polyanionic gum katira were used to prepare nanoparticles aiming enhancement the anti-inflammatory activity of glycyrrhizic acid, a triterpene saponin obtained from *Glycyrrhiza glabra*. Glycyrrhizic acid loaded chitosan-katira gum nanoparticles were prepared by ionic complexation method using Pluronic-F68 as a stabilizer. Briefly, an aqueous solution of katira gum (0.005–0.01%, w/v) containing Pluronic F-68 (1%, w/v) and glycyrrhizic acid (25–50%, w/w of polymer) was prepared. To this, chitosan solution (0.005–0.03%, w/v) was added under sonication for 15 min to prepare ionically crosslinked nanoparticles. Particle size and encapsulation efficiency of optimized formulation were 175.8 nm and 84.77%, respectively. *In vivo* anti-inflammatory efficacy of the triterpene was improved upon by encapsulation in nanoparticles, by overcoming the limited bioavailability of its other forms [25].

Zhang et al. [26] prepared chitosan nanoparticles with broadleaf holly leaf (Chinese herbal) with high concentration of flavoinoids. Chitosan nanoparticles with broadleaf holly leaf were prepared using the ionic gelation method. Chitosan was dissolved in 1% acetic acid to acquire chitosan solutions at different concentrations. In the following step, tripolyphosphate (TPP) was dissolved in distilled water at different concentrations. A specific volume of chitosan solution was slowly added into the total flavonoids of the broadleaf holly leaf solution at room temperature with magnetic stirring (600 rpm). This solution was slowly placed into the TPP solution using a syringe needle for 45 min until an blue opalescence appeared. The nanoparticles showed spherical shape, and the size ranged between 100 and 600 nm. The polydispersity index was 0.137. The optimal preparation process of the nanoparticles was: chitosan concentration 1 mg/mL, TPP concentration 1 mg/mL, and concentration of broadleaf holly leaf total flavonoids 1 mg/mL. In the *in vitro* assay, the total flavonoids release from the nanoparticles exhibited sustained release, showing that the chitosan nanoparticles are a potential broadleaf holly leaf delivery system.

Spray-Drying Method

Spray drying technique is a low-cost commercial process in a single-stage that can be conducted continuously to prepare microparticles in powder form. In this technique, a mixture solution of drug and excipient is atomized into fine droplets into a chamber with a stream of hot air. The particle is formed by solvent evaporation with the contact of the droplets with the hot drying gas. The particle size prepared by spray drying is <10 µm, with a large size distribution due to the variety of droplet sizes formed in the spray. However, nowadays, the Buchi® developed a Nano Spray Dryer that allowed production of nanoparticles by spray drying technique due to piezoelectric driven vibrating mesh atomizer and a high-efficiency electrostatic dry powder collector that allow collection of the submicron particles [27]. Hydrophilic and hydrophobic heat-resistant herbal drug can be encapsulated by this method. Heat-sensitive drugs can also be encapsulated by cooling spray drying. In this case a cool air stream is used into a chamber to dry the atomized droplets [28, 29].

The critical parameters that affect the size and the polydispersity index of the particles are atomization pressure, spray flow rate, the nozzle size, inlet air temperature, and polymer concentration (solution viscosity).

Sun-Waterhouse, Wadhwa, Waterhouse [30] proposed to encapsulate polyphenol bioactives, such as quercetin and vanillin, by spray-drying using natural fibre polymers such as sodium alginate and methyl β-cyclodextrin, hydroxypropylmethyl cellulose (HPMC) or inulin, as encapsulants agents. The type of encapsulant agent has an important impact on the encapsulation efficiency of the polyphenols. In the technique, the encapsulant agent solutions containing sodium alginate (0.2% w/w), methyl β-cyclodextrin (0.2% w/w), HPMC (0.2% w/w), or inulin (2% w/w) were prepared by dissolving the required amount of each encapsulant in Milli-Q water at 60°C. The obtained solutions were cooled and kept overnight at 4 ± 2°C. Quercetin or vanillin (30 mg) was first mixed with PEG (0.73 g) and then added into the encapsulant agent solutions and pre-homogenized in a shear homogenizer (3,000 rpm × 5 min). Soy lecithin was added as an additional emulsifier to improve the homogenization process at a ratio of 0.1g/1g encapsulant agent. A spray dryer (Büchi mini B-290, Büchi Labortechnik AG, Switzerland) equipped with a 0.7-mm standard diameter nozzle was used to prepare the spray-dried powders. The inlet and outlet temperature were 165 ± 2°C and 89 ± 2°C, respectively. The air flow rate, rate of liquid feed, atomization pressure, and pump speed were 600 L/h, 10 mL/min, 20 psi, and 30% respectively. The mean size of the formed particles, measured by scanning electron microscopy (SEM), was in the range of 0.5–15 micron. The encapsulation efficiency of vanillin was higher (36-53%) than for quercetin (9-19%), independent on encapsulant agent. This difference can be attributed to the low thermal stability of this polyphenol. Microparticles containing quercetin or vanillin produced in this study exhibited acceptable water activity and excellent dissolution properties in water. The results showed that spray-drying microencapsulation using natural fiber polymer encapsulants is a possible approach to deliver the dual health benefits of polyphenols microencapsulated and dietary fibre to consumers.

Laurel (Litsea glauscescens) is a tree or shrub belonging to the Lauraceae family. It is one of the most used spices in the world for, food additive, providing flavor, scents, colors and even help in food preservation. The species has been reported to give antimicrobial and antioxidant properties to food. Also, it has been used as an aid in gastrointestinal disorders, inflammation problems and atherosclerosis. All these benefits are related to phenolic compounds (polyphenols) such as phenolic acids and flavonoids. However, these compounds are extremely labile at ambient conditions (ultraviolet, radiation, temperature, oxygen, stomach digestion, etc.); affecting their stability and consequently, reducing the antioxidant benefits. Thus, to overcome these problems, Medina-Torres et al. [31] proposed the use of maltodextrin as a wall material in the spray dried encapsulation of laurel infusions, searching for the best drying conditions in relation to the preservation of the phenolic content and antioxidant capacity. Dispersions were prepared using the laurel infusion with 10% (w/v) of maltodextrin. The mixture was homogenized under magnetic stirrer at 300 rpm for 1 h at 25°C. Dispersions were than spray dried using a mini Spray Dryer B-290 Buchi (Flawil, Switzerland). The results evidenced that the best conditions for laurel encapsulation by spray dried were 160°C inlet temperature and 8 mL/min feed rate. The efficiency of encapsulation of laurel infusion was achieved with ~70%. The samples dried at 160°C have smaller particle size around 6 μm (D50 6.32 μm), quasimodal particle size distribution, and semi-spherical morphology. In the antioxidant activity evaluation by DPPH method, the microparticles with laurel infusions powder showed higher antioxidant activity (EC50 =1.3-3.1 mg/mL) than the laurel infusions free (EC50 = 0.45 mg/mL). The best antioxidant property was obtained using the powder with high phenolic and flavonoid content. Furthermore, prolonged release of laurel infusion was observed when exposed under conditions similar to that of the digestive tract.

Soy isoflavones, especially daidzein and genistein, showed different pharmacological activities and have been correlated with the decrease of osteoporosis, breast cancer, cardiovascular disease, and colon cancer in people who consume soya. However, despite the high biological activity, their poor water solubility has a negative effect on bioavailability. Trying to improve the solubility, Gaudio et al. [32] used nano spray drying to obtain nanoparticles loading soybean dry extract using carboxymethyl cellulose as excipient. The formulations were spray-dried with the Nano Spray Dryer B- 90 (Büchi Laboratoriums-Technik). The process parameters and conditions were as follows: inlet temperature 60°C, feed rate 9.5 mL/min; nozzle diameter 5.5 μm, air flow 100 L/min, relative spray rate 100%. The optimization of the process conditions allowed for the production of stable nanoparticles with a mean size of around 650 nm, a narrow size distribution and a high encapsulation efficiency (78% - 89%). The carboxymethyl cellulose was able to stabilize the isoflavone extract and enhance its affinity with water increasing its permeation through biological membranes up to 4.5 fold higher than pure soy isoflavone extract. These results can help the administration of the isoflavones extract, either topically or orally, once that the nanoparticulate powder obtained has great potential to enhance extract bioavailability.

Solid Lipid Carriers

Solid lipid nanoparticles (SLN) are composite by solid lipid at room and corporeal temperature. This particle was developed by Müller group's in 1996 and is an innovative carrier system that combine the advantages and avoids the drawbacks of several colloidal carriers such as high biocompatibility and bioavailability, drug controlled release, high physical stability, protection of incorporated labile drugs from degradation, and its production process is easily scalable. Hydrophobic drug are mostly encapsulated in SLN, but hydrophilic drugs have also been encapsulated in SLN in specific conditions [33, 34].

The first SLN structure developed showed some problems due to its high crystallinity or its crystallinity change during the storage. This problem is associated with the composition of the particles. SLN is composite only by solid lipid, forming particles with high crystallinity and consequently, low space for drug encapsulation (Figure 6A). Furthermore, the encapsulated drug can be expelled from the particles if there is a change in the polymorphic forms. Lipids show three different polymorphic forms: α form, β' form, and β form. The crystallinity degree of these forms is α form < β' form < β form. Thus, SLN in α form show lower crystallinity than the other polymorphic forms and, consequently, more drug is encapsulated. However, the α form can be changed to β form, causing the drug expulsion from the SLN (Figure 6B) [35, 36].

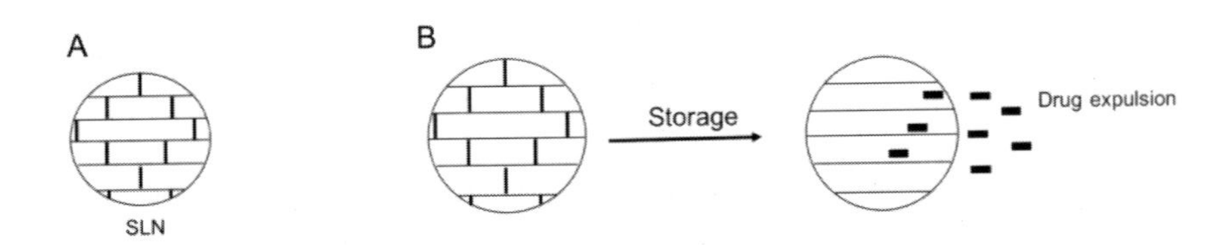

Figure 6. A) Solid lipid nanoparticles (SLN); B) Crystallization process during storage and drug expulsion from SLN.

Due to these limitations, nanostructured lipid carrier (CLN) was developed and is known as second solid lipid nanoparticle generation. There are three different CLNs: CLN imperfect that is composite by lipid blends using lipids with different fatty chain (e.g., mixture of different lipid with length of carbon chain or/and mixture of saturated and unsaturated fatty chain); CLN amorphous and CLN multiple, which are composite by the mixture of solid lipid and liquid lipid (oils). In the CLN multiple preparation, a higher oil amount is used than the CLN amorphous, causing the formation of oil nanocompartments (Figure 7). All CLN types are solid but exhibit lower crystallinity than the SLN, leading to a higher drug encapsulation and avoiding the drug expulsion during the storage.

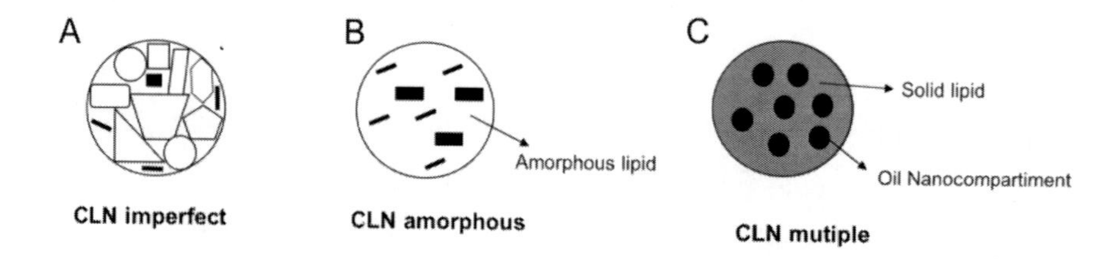

Figure 7. CLN structures: A) CLN imperfect, B) CLN amorphous and C) CLN multiple.

Several synthetic and naturals lipid can be used to prepare SLN and CLN. Some examples are showed in Table 2.

Table 2. Solid and liquid lipid used in the SLN and CLN preparation

Lipids	Structure
Solid lipids	
Precirol® ATO-5(Glyceryl distearate/ Glyceryl palmitostearate)	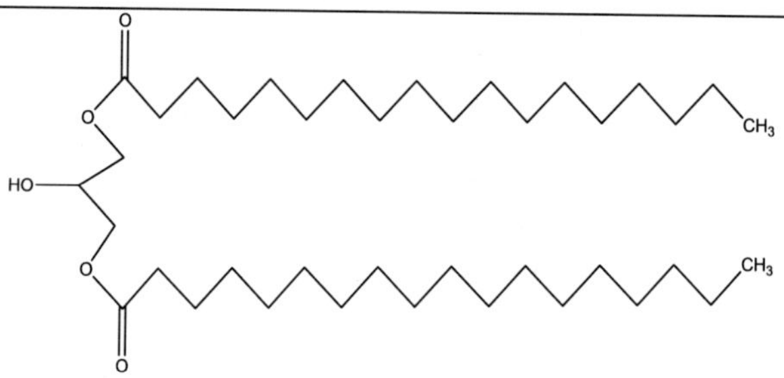
Glyceryl monostearate (monostearin)	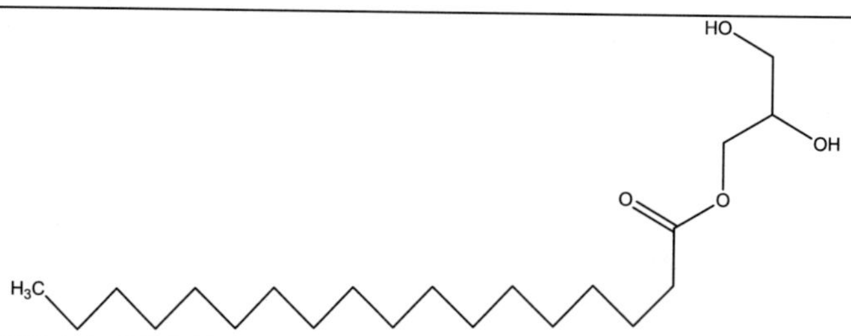
Glyceryl monooleate	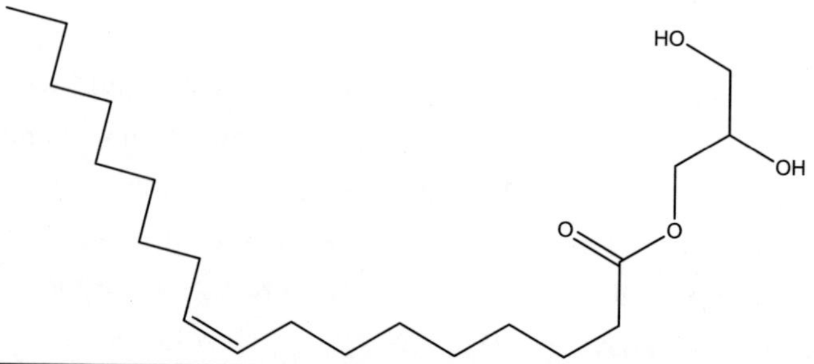
Stearic acid	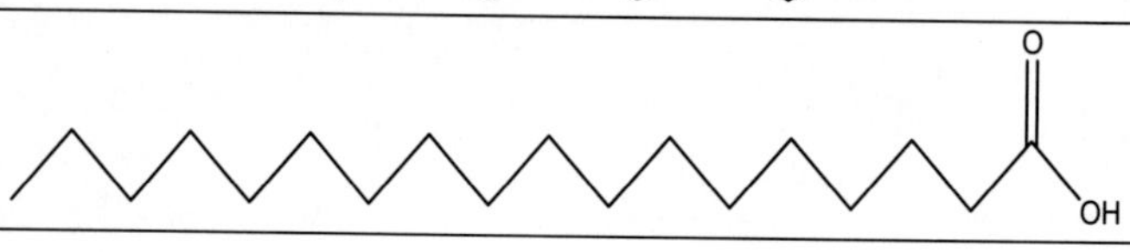

Table 2. (Continued)

Lipids	Structure
Cetylpalmitate	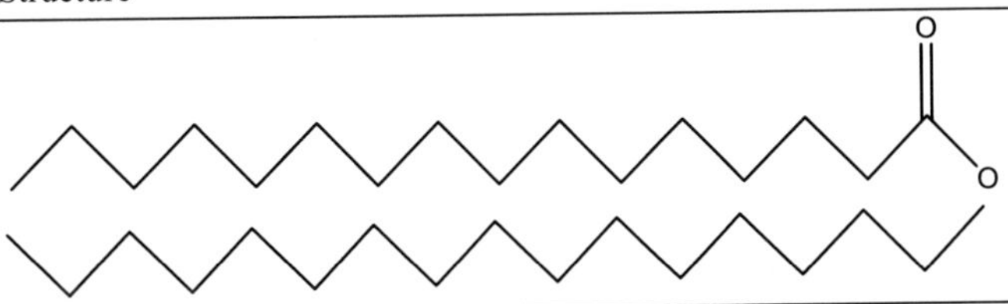 O, O
Trimyristin	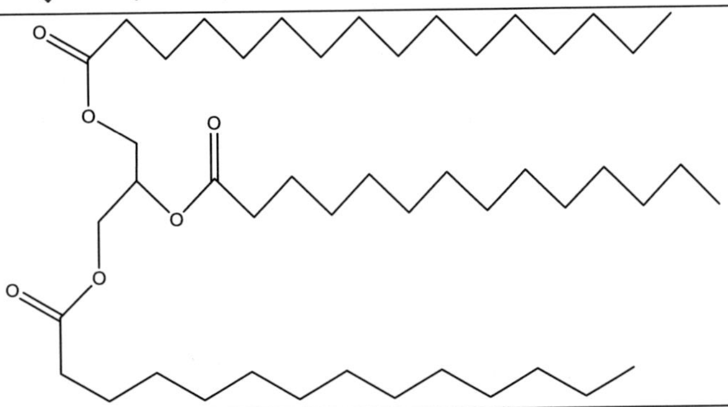 O, O, O, O, O, O
Compritol® 888 ATO (Glyceryldibehenate)	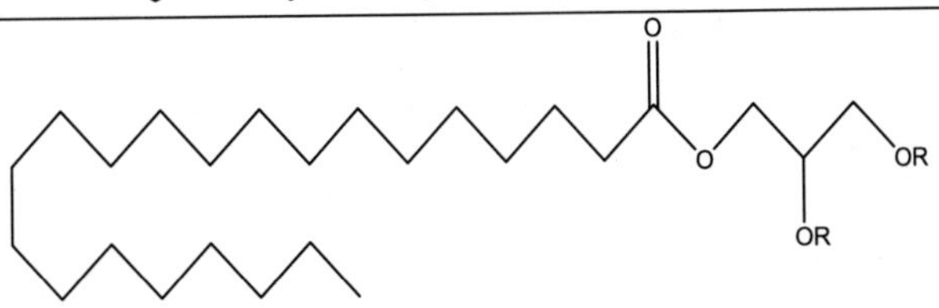 O, O, OR, OR R = H or 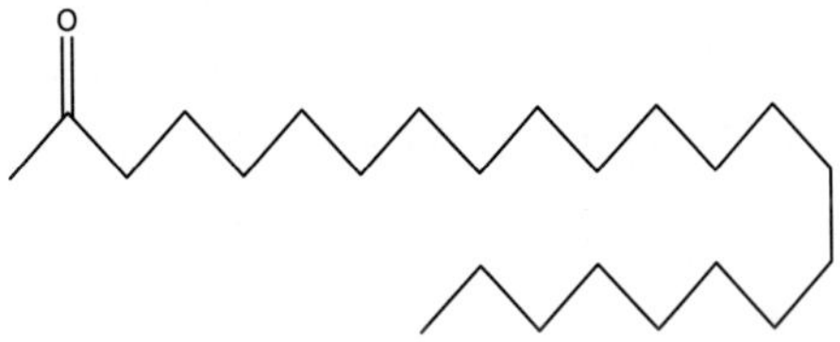 O
Liquid lipids	
Oleic acid	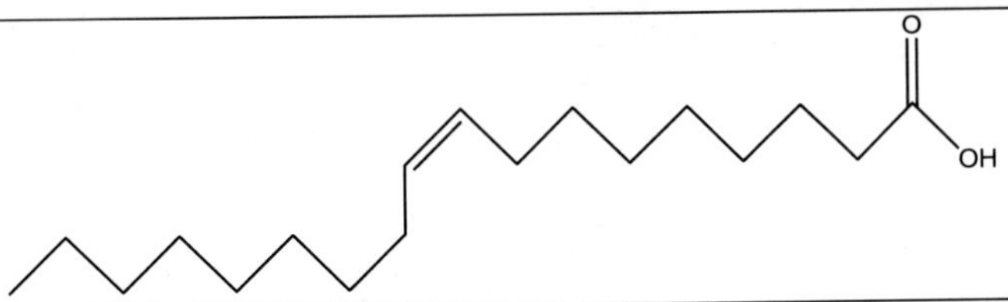 O, OH
Medium chain triglyceride	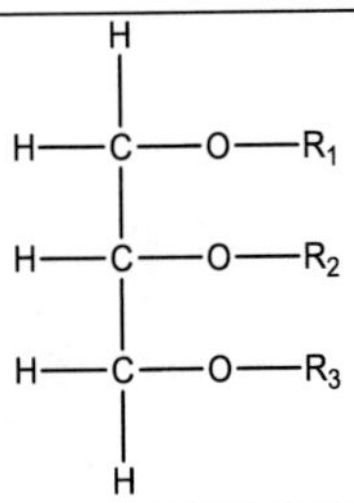 H, H—C—O—R_1, H—C—O—R_2, H—C—O—R_3, H where R1, R2 and R3 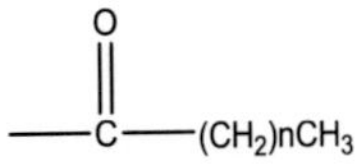 = —C(=O)—$(CH_2)nCH_3$ n= 6-8

Different methods are described in the literature to obtain solid lipid carriers. Some are described below:

High-Pressure Homogenization

High-pressure homogenization (HPH) is a technique used in the industry for the production of nanoemulsions for parenteral foods, homogenization of milk, ice cream and others. This method is interesting to SLN production because it is easily scalable and done without organic solvent. In this technique, the dispersion is pushed under high pressure (in the range of 100-2000 bar) through a narrow gap, causing a high shear stress and cavitation forces, which disrupt particles/drops. Particles in the nanometer range are obtained using this method. As the process occurs, there is an increase in the temperature (10°C for every 500 bar) due to the high acceleration (~1000 km/h) and friction inside the equipment. But it is possible to use a refrigeration accessory at the end of the equipment when labile molecules are used. For SLN and CLN production by HPH method usually 2-30% of lipid and between 0.5-2% of surfactant are used. However, the amount and type of lipid influence the particle size. The surfactant concentration also influences the particle size and stability. High surfactant concentrations reduce the surface tension, thereby decreasing the particle size. Furthermore, the surfactant increases the particles stability because it covers the particle surfaces and avoid its agglomeration. The most common surfactant used are phospholipids (e.g., soybean lecithin, egg lecithin, etc), bile salts (sodium cholate, sodium taurocholate, etc) and poloxamers [33, 34]. There are two approaches of HPH: hot homogenization and cold homogenization.

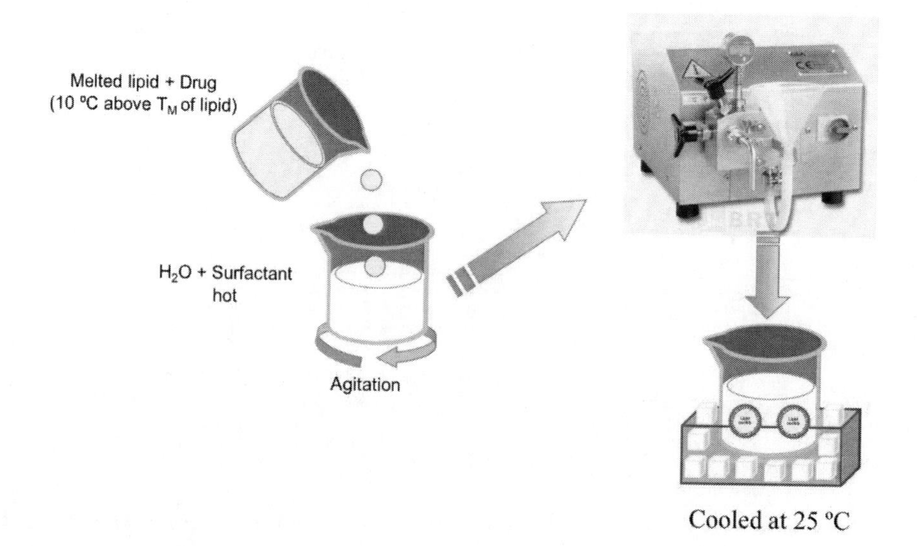

Figure 8. Scheme of SLN preparation by hot high-pressure homogenization.

Hot Homogenization

Hot homogenization method is used for encapsulation of lipophilic drugs. In this method, all phases are maintained at temperatures above the melting point of the lipid. The lipid or mixture of solid lipids or solid and liquid lipid is heating until 10°C above solid lipid melting temperature. Then, the drug is adding in the lipid molten. Afterwards, hot aqueous phase composited by water and surfactant is added in the lipid phase under high shear (e.g., using ultraturrax), forming a pre-emulsion. The pre-emulsion is transferred to homogenization equipment and homogenized under pressure by 1 or more cycles (Figure 8). Pressure and number of cycle will influence the size and polydispersity index of the nanoparticles. The increase of pressure or number of cycles tends to decrease the particle size up to a certain limit. High pressure or several cycles leads to particle coalescence due to increase in kinetics energy. In general, two or three homogenization cycles at 500-1000 bar are applied. Furthermore, high temperature tends to decrease viscosity of the lipid phase, and consequently decrease particle size [33, 34, 37].

Cold Homogenization

Cold homogenization overcome some problems of hot homogenization, such as drug degradation due to high temperature, loss of drug into the aqueous phase, and crystallization step of the nanoemulsion leading to supercooled melts. Thus, this method is adequate for encapsulation of temperature-sensitive drug and/or hydrophilic drugs. Firstly, the drug is dispersed in the lipid(s) molten and immediately cooled using liquid nitrogen or dry ice forming drug-loaded lipid. This solid lipid is ground until lipid microparticles (50–100 microns) by means of ball or mortar milling. Then, these microparticles are dispersed in a cold aqueous surfactant solution. This dispersion is homogenized under pressure by 1 or more cycles (Figure 9). Larger particle sizes with broader size distribution are typically obtained in cold homogenization in comparison with the hot homogenization. In order to reduce the particle size and the polydispersity index, high pressure and/or several cycles are used in homogenization process [34, 37].

Phytomedicine has been encapsulated in SLN and CLN using high-pressure homogenization method. Silymarin has been used clinically to treat several hepatic disorders. However, because of poor water solubility and low permeability, and consequently low and variable bioavailability, its clinical application is limited. To improve oral absorption of silymarin, Shangguan et al. [38] encapsulate silymarin in CLNs. CLNs were prepared by hot high-pressure homogenization method with minor modifications. Precirol ATO-5 (2.0 g, solid lipid), oleic acid (0.9 g, liquid lipid), sylamarin (400 mg) and lecithin (1.0 g, surfactant) were the oil phase that was heated at 80 °C. The melted mixture was dispersed into water phase (30 mL) containing Tween 80

(1.0 g) and ultrapure water at 80ºC under high shear at 8000 rpm/min for 1 min. The obtained pre-emulsion was homogenized using homogenizer under 20,000 lbf/in2 for five cycles. The resulting hot O/W nanoemulsions were cooled down to room temperature to form CLNs. The silymarin nanostructured lipid carrier prepared under optimum conditions was spherical in shape with mean particle size of about 78.87 nm, zeta potential of - 65.3 mV, loading capacity of 8.32% and entrapment efficiency of 87.55%. The bioavailability of silymarin encapsulated in CLNs was, respectively, 2.54 and 3.10 fold greater than that commercial silymarin (LEGALON®) and than that solid dispersion pellets with silymarin.

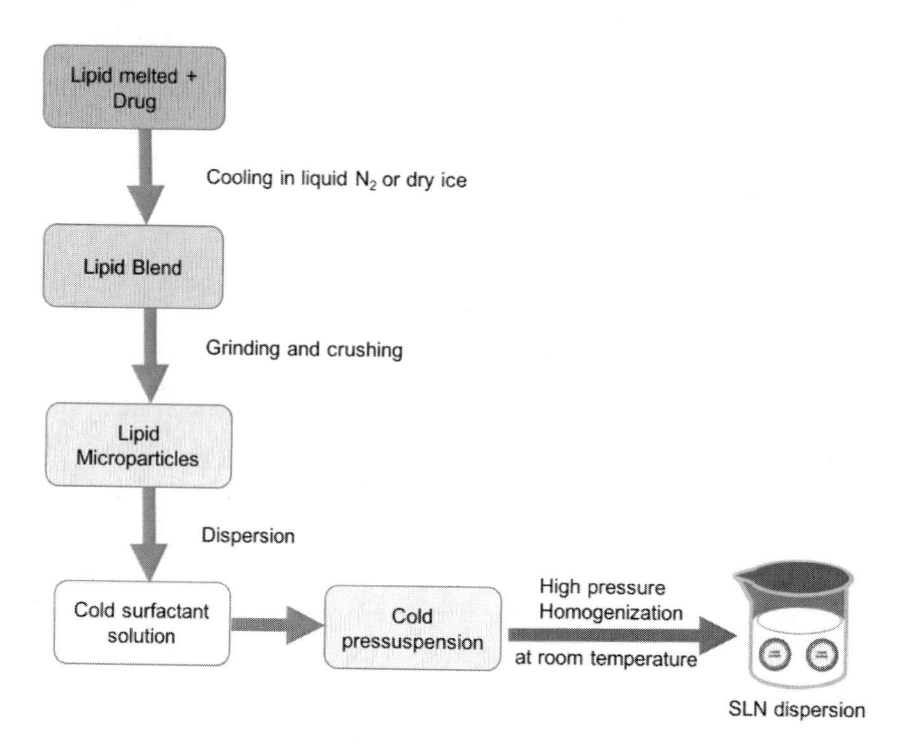

Figure 9. Scheme of SLN preparation by cold high-pressure homogenization.

Aqueous extract of *Spirogyra* spp., freshwater macro-algae in the north and northeast of Thailand, has been widely described as an antioxidant agent. Hydrophilic drugs have not been completely investigated about incorporated into CLN. In this way, Chimsook [39] investigated the potential of CLNs as carriers for aqueous extract of *Spirogyra spp.* The oil phase, melted at 70 ºC, consisted of glyceryl monostearate (2.0% W/V, GMS) as solid lipid, medium chain triglyceride (1.5% W/V, MCT) as liquid lipid and soy lecithin (1.5% W/V, SL) as surfactant. The water phase was composite by Cremophor® ELP (3.0% W/V), Spirogyra spp. extract and deionized water, which was heated at the same temperature of oil phase. The water phase was dispersed in the oil phase using a mechanical agitate at 2000 rpm for 5 min. Afterwards, the hot pre-emulsion was further processed by high-pressure homogenization applying five homogenization cycles at 800 bar and 60 °C. The nanodispersion were freeze-dried to obtain dried product used for further analysis. The CLNs showed spherical morphology with smooth surface under transmission electron microscope (TEM), with mean particle size of about 120 nm. The encapsulation efficiency was 61.23 ± 6.25%. The aqueous extract of Spirogyra spp. released from the CLN exhibited a biphasic pattern with burst release at the initial stage, and sustained release subsequently over 24 h. The results indicated that the CLN obtained in this study was a potential carrier for the delivery of aqueous extract of *Spirogyra* spp.

High Shear Homogenization or Ultrasonication

High shear homogenization method is widespread and easy to handle and applied to prepare SLN and CLN in laboratory scale. However, metal contamination from the turrax or ultrasound tip is commonly observed in the final formulation. Furthermore, broader particle size distribution in micrometer range is usually obtained that can lead physical instabilities by particle growth upon storage [34].

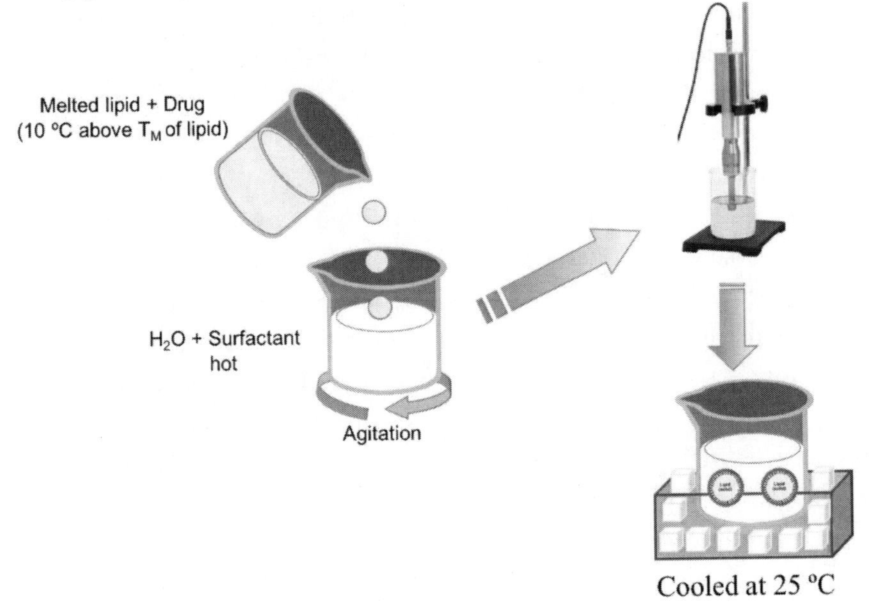

Figure 10. Scheme of SLN preparation by ultrasonication method.

All phases are maintained at temperature above the melting point of the lipid. The lipid or mixture of solid lipids or solid and liquid lipid is heating until 10°C above solid lipid melting temperature. Then, the drug is adding in the lipid molten followed by the addition of hot aqueous surfactant solution under high shear using ultra-turrax or probe sonication (ultrasonication) forming a pre-emulsion. The pre-emulsion is cooled at room temperature (25°C) obtaining a SLN or CLN [33] (Figure 10). To reduce particle size and mainly produce particles with narrow distribution (low polydispersity index) more sonication time or high homogenization speed is necessary. However, this strategy can increase metal contamination [33, 40].

Kundu et al. [41] studied the antiglioma activity of curcumin loaded in solid lipid nanoparticles, in order to overcome the low bioavailability of curcumin (CUR). The SLN was prepared with glyceryl monooleate (GMO) (solid lipid) and as stabilizers were used Pluronic F-68 and vitamin E D-α-tocopherol polyethylene glycol 1000 succinate (TPGS). The lipid nanoparticles were produced by sonication using a microtip probe sonicator. Curcumin (300 mg) was added to melt GMO (1.75 mL about 40 °C) and was emulsified with water phase (10 mL) containing Pluronic F-68 (10% w/v) by sonication for 2 min at an amplitude of 30% over an ice bath. Further, TPGS (5% w/v) was added in the dispersion and the nanodispersion was again sonicated by 2 min. The nanoemulsion obtained was frozen and lyophilized. The size of SLN-CUR was in the range of 90 nm with a negative zeta potential -19,7 mV and entrapment efficiency about 90%. *In vivo* assay in rats, the CUR-loaded in SLN showed higher bioavailability in the serum (about 20 fold) and in the brain tissue (about 10 fold) than the CUR free. This result indicates that SLN is a potent vehicle to transport drug across the BBB and it is interesting to treatment of glioma. Further studies are underway to enhance the *in vivo* performance of curcumin after systemic delivery in an animal model with glioblastoma.

Tiyaboonchai et al. [42] produced curcuminoids loaded in amorphous CLNs using a microemulsion and high shear homogenization method. The water phase consisted of curcuminoids extract (0.1% w/w), Poloxamer F-68 (5-15%, w/w), dioctyl sodium sulfosuccinate (5-20%, w/w AOT), ethanol and deionized water. The oil phase consisted by the mixture of solid lipid stearic acid (5-12.5% w/w) and glyceril monoestearate (4% w/w). Both (water and oil phase) were heated about 75 °C, then water phase was added to the oil phase under high-speed homogenization at 8000 rpm for 15 min. Afterwards, the warm emulsion was dispersed in cold water (1:20) under agitation. The process parameters, such as the amount of lipid and emulsifier, were crucial factors that affected the mean particles size and the efficacy of drug incorporation. At optimal conditions; stearic acid (5%, w/w); poloxamer 188 (5%, w/w); AOT (5%, w/w); ethanol (15%, w/w), the mean particle size of SLN with curcuminoids was 447 nm and the incorporation efficacy of curcuminoids was 70% (w/w). The light and oxygen sensitivity of curcuminoids was strongly reduced by incorporating curcuminoids into CLNs. In an *in vivo* study with healthy volunteers, a significant reduction of skin wrinkles was observed when creams with SLN-curcuminoids was used. Besides that, the cream with CLN-curcuminoids improved skin moisture and the firmness, elasticity, and viscoelasticity of the skin of the volunteers after 3 weeks of application; with a 95% confidence level.

Bufadienolides are the principal biologically active components of toad venom. These compounds exhibit different biological activities, as antineoplastic effects, stimulation of myocardial contraction and blood pressure, anti-inflammatory effects.

However, they are highly lipophilic. To overcome this issue, Li et al. [43, 44] developed bufadienolide-loaded CLNs by a modified melt-emulsification and ultrasonic method. Lipoid E-80® (1.5g), Pluronic F68 (1.0 g), sodium deoxycholate (0.25 g) and Tween 80 were dissolved in distilled water at 75°C and were further dispersed in the melted lipid phase, containing glyceryl monostearate (1.8 g), medium-chain triglyceride (0.75 g), oleic acid (0.45 g) and bufadienolides, under magnetic stirring. The resultant pre-emulsion was ultrasonicated using probe sonication at 30% amplification for 10 min. The nanoemulsion obtained was cooled in an ice bath. The particle size was 104.1 ± 51.2 nm and the zeta potential of CLNs was between −15 to −20 mV. The entrapment efficiency of the bufadienolides was all above 85%. The pharmacokinetic profile of bufadienolides was improved when bufadienolides was encapsulated in CLN resulting in a higher plasma concentration and lower clearance after its intravenous administration compared with bufadienolides solution. Moreover, bufadienolide-loaded CLNs showed enhanced antitumor efficacy, good hemocompatibility and reduced the adverse effects compared with that of bufadienolides suspensions. Therefore, the CLN system is a promising approach for the intravenous delivery of bufadienolides.

Emulsification-Solvent Evaporation

Water-immiscible organic solvent is used in this method to solubilize the lipid and drug. This organic solution is added in an aqueous surfactant phase under high agitation. Thereafter, the organic solvent is evaporated under reduced pressure leaving lipid precipitates of SLN or CLN (Figure 11). The concentration of lipid in organic phase, conditions of adding the organic phase to the aqueous phase and aqueous phase stirring are the most important process parameters that influence the size and the polydispersity index of the SLN or CLN. The slow dripping of organic phase into aqueous phase with high-shear tends to reduce the size of the emulsion droplet and consequently the SLN or CLN size. Further, high lipid concentration increase the viscosity of organic phase, increasing the particles size [33, 34, 37].

Puerarin is prescribed for patients with cardiocerebrovascular diseases in China. However, it is hardly water-soluble and shows a very poor oral absorption. Luo et al. [45] and Luo et al. [46] investigated puerarin-loaded SLNs following oral administration, including pharmacokinetics, tissue distribution, and bioavailability in rats. Puearin (20 mg), monostearin (150 mg) and soya lecithin (150 mg) were mixed in methanol and ethanol (1:9), forming the organic phase. The water phase consisted of Poloxamer F-68 (0.5% w/v) in ultrapure water, heated at 75 ± 2°C. The organic phase was injected into the water phase under mechanical agitation. The pre-emulsion, further, was injected into Poloxamer F-68 at 0-2°C to form SLN. The mean particle size of Puearin loaded-SLNs was 160 nm with a zeta potential of −35.43 ± 5.19 mV. When incorporated into the

SLNs, puerarin was rapidly and well absorbed, and its bioavailability improved more than 3-fold compared with the puerarin suspensions. In addition, SLNs produced increased the puerarin tissue concentrations in target organs, particularly in the heart and brain.

Yuan and co-workers [47] studied the antitumor effect of tripterine encapsulated in CLN functionalized with cell-penetrating peptide on prostate tumor cells in *in vitro* and *in vivo* models. Precirol ATO-5 and Labrafil M 1944CS (3:1, w/w) were chosen as solid and liquid lipid, respectively. Soybean lecithin and D-α-tocopherol polyethylene glycol succinate 1000 were used as surfactants. The organic phase consisted of tripterine, surfactants and lipids dissolved in acetone and ethanol (3:1). The water phase consisted of Poloxamer F-68 (0,5% w/v), Ste-R6-L2 (30 mg) (cell-penetrating peptide) and ultrapure water. The organic phase was injected into the stirred water phase at 60ºC and 400 rpm for 4 hours. The resulting nanoemulsion was stirred in an ice bath for 2 hours to stabilize the CLNs. Tripterine loaded CLNs was spherical in shape with mean particle size of about 126.7 nm, zeta potential of 28.7 mV and entrapment efficiency of 72.40%. Tripterine encapsulated in CLN functionalized with cell-penetrating peptide effectively suppressed proliferation in prostate carcinoma cells (PC-3 and RM-1) *in vitro*. Tripterine encapsulated in CLN functionalized with cell-penetrating peptide effectively suppressed the proliferation of PC-3 and RM-1 cells *in vitro*. Besides, this formulation showed higher antitumor activity and fewer side effects in a mouse model of prostate cancer than tripterine free.

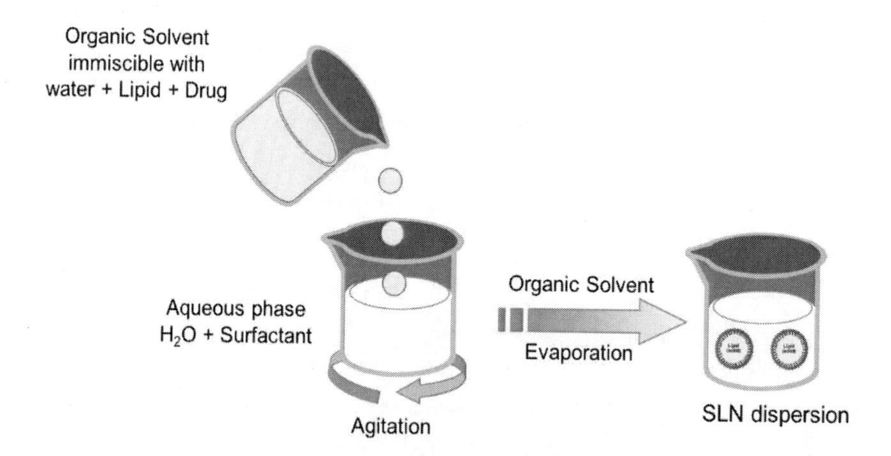

Figure 11. Scheme of SLN preparation by emulsification-solvent evaporation method.

Phase Inversion Temperature (PIT) Method

PIT method is commonly used for the preparation of nanoemulsions and was recently adapted for the SLN preparation. The PIT method is based on changes in the properties of non-ionic surfactants (e.g., molecular geometry, packing, and oil-water partitioning) when temperature is changed. Thus, in this method, surfactants that can leads to an emulsion inversion from O/W macroemulsion to a W/O emulsion when temperature is increased above the PIT. O/W nanoemulsion is formed when the temperature is next lowered below the PIT [48]. This is an easy and scalable method interesting to produce SLN.

An oil phase, constituted by solid lipids and non-ionic surfactants and a surfactant aqueous phase are separately heated above the PIT. Then, the aqueous phase is added dropwise to the oil phase, at constant temperature and under agitation, forming an opaque W/O emulsion. The opaque appearance of the W/O emulsion can be attributed to strong light scattering due to large droplets of the emulsion. Thereafter, this emulsion is cooled to room temperature under stirring. At the PIT, the turbid mixture becomes translucent, which is indicative of the bicontinuous microemulsion formation. Then, below the PIT, an O/W nanoemulsion is formed, which turns in SLN when cooled below the lipid melting point [48, 49].

Gomes and co-workers [50] encapsulates beta-carotene in CLN composed by *Theobroma grandiflorum* butter via PIT method. Cremophor RH 40 (12 g) and Span 80 (40.8 g) were used as surfactants. A hot surfactant solution was dispersed in melted *Theobroma grandiflorum* (10 g) butter through mechanical stirring at 500 rpm. The pre-emulsion was then submitted to two heating and cooling cycles. Beta-carotene and alpha-tocopherol (essential for carotenoid preservation) were added to the mixture in the second heating cycle. The inversion temperature of the nanoparticles was 74ºC and their average diameter was 35 nm. Beta-carotene loaded CLN had physicochemical stability regarding of size and polydispersity index over a storage period of 100 days and 85% of the initial amount of beta-carotene remained in the nanoparticles after this period. In conclusion, the results showed that the lipid nanoparticles produced can potentially be used in the controlled release of bioactives.

Beta-carotene was also used as a model lipophilic bioactive compound by Zhang et al. [51]. They produced CLNs as vehicles to incorporate bioactive compounds in transparent functional beverages by PIT method. Anhydrous milk fat (1-15% w/w) and beta-carotene (6.25 mM) was melted and then mixed with warm water phase (composed of NaCl (0 – 1.0 M) and Tween 80 (5-40% w/w) dissolved in deionized water at 60 ºC) under agitation at 1000 rpm. The pre-emulsion was transferred to glass vials that were heated for 30 min in a water bath maintained at a constant temperature (75, 80, 85, 90 and 95 ºC) without stirring. After thermal treatment, these samples were first cooled at ambient conditions with had shaking until a homogeneous appearance, followed by quenching in an ice bath under static conditions. At 0.8 M NaCl and phase inversion by heating at 90°C for 30 min, transparent CLN dispersions were observed at lipid levels higher than 10% (w/w), with particle size about 25 nm. They observed that β-Carotene was successfully encapsulated in CLNs using the PIT method and had much better stability in CLNs than in soybean-oil-based nanoemulsions.

REFERENCES

[1] Gunasekaran, Thirumurugan, Tedesse Haile, Tedele Nigusse, Magharla Dasaratha Dhanaraju. 2014. "Nanotechnology: An Effective Tool for Enhancing Bioavailability and Bioactivity of Phytomedicine." *Asian Pacific Journal of Tropical Biomedicine* 4:S1-S7. Accessed December 5, 2016. doi:10.12980/APJTB.4.2014C980.

[2] Gopi, Sreeraj, Augustine Amalraj, Józef T. Haponiuk, Sabu Thomas. 2016. "Introduction of Nanotechnology in Herbal Drugs and Nutraceutical: A Review." *Journal of Nanomedicine & Biothera-peutic Discovery* 6:1–8. Accessed December 5, 2016. doi:10.4172/ 2155-983X.1000143.

[3] Watkins, Rebekah, Ling Wu, Chenming Zhang, Richey M Davis, Bin Xu. 2015. "Natural Product-Based Nanomedicine: Recent Advances and Issues." *International Journal of Nanomedicine* 10:6055–74. Accessed December 5, 2016. doi:10.2147/IJN.S92162.

[4] ManishaYadav, Vidhi. J. Bhatia, Gaurav Doshi, Keyur Shastri. 2014. "Novel Techniques in Herbal Drug Delivery Systems." *International Journal of Pharmaceutical Sciences Review and Research* 28:83–89.

[5] Saraf, Swarnlata, Anshita Gupta, Amit Alexander, Junaid Khan, Manmohan Jangde, Shailendra Saraf. 2015. "Advancements and Avenues in Nanophytomedicines for Better Pharmacological Responses." *Journal of Nanoscience and Nanotechnology* 15:4070–79. Accessed December 5, 2016. doi:10.1166/jnn.2015.10333.

[6] Guterres, Sílvia S, Marta P Alves, Adriana R Pohlmann. 2007. "Polymeric Nanoparticles, Nanospheres and Nanocapsules, for Cutaneous Applications." *Drug Target Insights* 2:147–57.

[7] Wang, Yichao, Puwang Li, Thao Truong-dinh Tran, Juan Zhang, Lingxue Kong. 2016. "Manufacturing Techniques and Surface Engineering of Polymer Based Nanoparticles for Targeted Drug Delivery to Cancer." *Nanomaterials* 6:1–18. Accessed December 5, 2016. doi:10.3390/nano6020026.

[8] Mora-Huertas, C E, H Fessi, A Elaissari. 2010. "Polymer-Based Nanocapsules for Drug Delivery." *International Journal of Pharmaceutics* 385:113–42. Accessed December 5, 2016. doi:10.1016/j.ijpharm.2009.10.018.

[9] Fessi, H., F. Puisieux, J.Ph. Devissaguet, N. Ammoury, Simon Benita. 1989. "Nanocapsule formation by interfacial polymer deposition following solvent displacement." *International Journal of Pharmaceutics* 55:R1-R4. Accessed December 5, 2016. doi:10.1016/ 0378-5173(89)90281-0.

[10] Beck-Broichsitter, Moritz, Erik Rytting, Tobias Lebhardt, Xiaoying Wang, Thomas Kissel. 2010. "Preparation of Nanoparticles by Solvent Displacement for Drug Delivery: A Shift in the 'Ouzo Region' upon Drug Loading." *European Journal of Pharmaceutical Sciences* 41:244–53. Accessed December 5, 2016. doi:10.1016/ j.ejps.2010.06.007.

[11] Bohrey, Sarvesh, Vibha Chourasiya, Archna Pandey. 2016. "Polymeric Nanoparticles Containing Diazepam : Preparation, Optimization, Characterization, *in vitro* Drug Release and Release Kinetic Study." *Nano Convergence* 3:1–7. Accessed December 5, 2016. doi:10.1186/s40580-016-0061-2.

[12] Sanna, Vanna, Giuseppe Lubinu, Pierluigi Madau, Nicolino Pala, Salvatore Nurra, Alberto Mariani, Mario Sechi. 2015. "Polymeric Nanoparticles Encapsulating White Tea Extract for Nutraceutical Application." *Journal of Agricultural and Food Chemistry* 63:2026-32. Accessed December 5, 2016. doi:10.1021/jf505850q.

[13] Sanna, Vanna, Imtiaz A Siddiqui, Mario Sechi, Hasan Mukhtar. 2013. "Nanoformulation of Natural Products for Prevention and Therapy of Prostate Cancer." *Cancer Letters* 334:142–51. Accessed December 5, 2016. doi:10.1016/j.canlet.2012.11.037.

[14] Teixeira, Maribel, Maria J. Alonso, Madalena M. M. Pinto, Carlos M. Barbosa. 2005. "Development and Characterization of PLGA Nanospheres and Nanocapsules Containing Xanthone and 3-Methoxyxanthone." *European Journal of Pharmaceutics and Biopharmaceutics* 59:491–500. Accessed December 5, 2016. doi:10.1016/j.ejpb.2004.09.002.

[15] Narayanan, Sreeja, N S Binulal, Ullas Mony, Koyakutty Manzoor. 2010. "Folate Targeted Polymeric 'Green' Nanotherapy for Cancer." *Nanotechnology* 21:1-13. Accessed December 5, 2016. doi:10.1088/0957-4484/21/28/285107.

[16] Mccall, Rebecca L, Rachael W Sirianni. 2013. "PLGA Nanoparticles Formed by Single- or Double-Emulsion with Vitamin E- TPGS." *Journal of Visualized Experiments* 27:1–8. Accessed December 5, 2016. doi:10.3791/51015.

[17] Iqbal, Muhammad, Jean-pierre Valour, Hatem Fessi, Abdelhamid Elaissari Abdelhamid Elaissari. 2015. "Preparation of Biodegradable PCL Particles via Double Emulsion Evaporation Method Using Ultrasound Technique." *Colloid and Polymer Science* 293:861–87. Accessed December 5, 2016. doi:10.1007/s00396-014-3464-9.

[18] Dubey, Ravindra Dhar, Ankit Saneja, Arem Qayum, and Amarinder Singh, Girish Mahajan, Gousia Chashoo, Amit Kumar, Samar S. Andotra, Shashank K. Singh, Gurdarshan Singh, Surinder Koul, Dilip M. Mondhe, Prem N. Gupta. 2016. "PLGA Nanoparticles Augmented the Anticancer Potential of Pentacyclic Triterpenediol *in vivo*." *RSC Advances* 6:74586–97. Accessed December 5, 2016. doi:10.1039/C6RA14929D.

[19] Fernández, Katherina, Javiera Aburto, Carlos Von Plessing, Marlene Rockel, Estrella Aspé. 2016. "Factorial Design Optimization and Characterization of Poly-Lactic Acid (PLA) Nanoparticle Formation for the Delivery of Grape Extracts." *Food Chemistry* 207:75–85. Accessed December 5, 2016. doi:10.1016/j.foodchem.2016.03.083.

[20] Yoon, In-soo, Ju-hwan Park, Hyo Jin, Ji Hyeong, Min Su, Dae-duk Kim, Hyun-jong Cho. 2015. "Poly (D,L -lactic acid)-Glycerol-Based Nanoparticles for Curcumin Delivery." *International Journal of Pharmaceutics* 488:70-7. Accessed December 5, 2016. doi:10.1016/j.ijpharm.2015.04.046.

[21] Vineeth, P, P R Rao Vadaparthi, K Kumar, B Dileep J Babu, A Veerabhadra Rao, K Suresh Babu. 2014. "Influence of Organic Solvents on Nanoparticle Formation and Surfactants on Release Behaviour *in vitro* Using Costunolide as Model Anticancer Agent." *International Journal of Pharmacy and Pharmaceutical Science* 6:638-45.

[22] Patil, J S, M V Kamalapur, S C Marapur, and D V Kadam. 2010. "Ionotropic Gelation and Polyelectrolyte Complexation: The Novel Techniques to Design Hydrogel Particulate Sustained, Modulated Drug Delivery System: A Review." *Digest Journal of Nanomaterials and Biostructure* 5:241–48.

[23] Patil, Poonam, Daksha Chavanke, Milind Wagh. 2012. "A Review on Ionotropic Gelation Method: Novel Approach for Controlled Gastroretentive Gelispheres." *International Journal of Pharmacy and Pharmaceutical Sciences* 4:27-32.

[24] Harangozó, József G, Véronique Wintgens, Zsombor Miskolczy, Catherine Amiel, László Biczók. 2016. "Nanoparticle Formation of Chitosan Induced by 4-Sulfonatocalixarenes: Utilization for Alkaloid Encapsulation." *Colloid and Polymer Science* 294:1807–14. Accessed December 5, 2016. doi:10.1007/s00396-016-3947-y.

[25] Bernela, Manju, Munish Ahuja, Rajesh Thakur. 2016. "Enhancement of Anti-Inflammatory Activity of Glycyrrhizic Acid by Encapsulation in Chitosan-Katira Gum Nanoparticles." *European Journal of Pharmaceutics and Biopharmaceutics* 105:141–47. Accessed December 5, 2016. doi:10.1016/j.ejpb.2016.06.003.

[26] Zhang, Hongliang, Qiuyan Huang, Zhenguang Huang, Taotao Liu, Yuanhong Li. 2015. "Preparation and Physicochemical Properties of Chitosan Broadleaf Holly Leaf Nanoparticles." *International Journal of Pharmaceutics* 479:212–18. Accessed December 5, 2016. doi:10.1016/j.ijpharm.2014.12.010.

[27] Oliveira, Adriano M, Kleber L Guimarães, Natália N P Cerize, Ariane S Tunussi, João G R Poço. 2013. "Nano Spray Drying as an Innovative Technology for Encapsulating Hydrophilic Active Pharmaceutical Ingredients (API)." *Journal of Nanomedicine & Nanotechnology* 4:1-6. Accessed December 5, 2016. doi:10.4172/2157-7439.1000186.

[28] Jyothi Sri. S, A. Seethadevi, K. Suria Prabha, P. Muthuprasanna, P. Pavitra. 2012. "Microencapsulation: A Review." *International Journal of Pharma and Bio Sciences* 3:509-31.

[29] Munin, Aude, Florence Edwards-Lévy 2011. "Encapsulation of Natural Polyphenolic Compounds; a Review." *Pharmaceutics* 3:793-829. Accessed December 5, 2016. doi:10.3390/pharmaceutics 3040793.

[30] Sun-waterhouse, Dongxiao, Sandhya S Wadhwa, Geoffrey I N Waterhouse. 2013. "Spray-Drying Microencapsulation of Polyphenol Bioactives: A Comparative Study Using Different Natural Fibre Polymers as Encapsulants." *Food Bioprocess Technology* 6:2376-88. Accessed December 5, 2016. doi:10.1007/s11947-012-0946-y.

[31] Medina-Torres, L., R. Santiago-Adame, F. Calderas, J.A. Gallegos-Infante, R.F. González-Laredo, N.E. Rocha-Guzmán, D.M. Núñez-Ramírez, M.J. Bernad-Bernad, O. Manero. 2016. "Microencapsulation by Spray Drying of Laurel Infusions (Litsea glauscescens) with Maltodextrin." *Industrial Crops & Products* 90:1-8. Accessed December 5, 2016. doi:10.1016/j.indcrop.2016.06.009.

[32] Gaudio, Pasquale Del, Francesca Sansone, Teresa Mencherini, Felicetta De Cicco, Paola Russo, Rita Patrizia Aquino. 2016. "Nanospray Drying as a Novel Tool to Improve Technological Properties of Soy Isoflavone Extracts." *Planta Medica.* Accessed December 15, 2016. Accessed December 5, 2016. doi: 10.1055/s-0042-110179.

[33] Parhi, Rabinarayan, Padilama Suresh. 2012. "Preparation and Characterization of Solid Lipid Nanoparticles-A Review." *Current Drug Discovery Technologies* 9:2–16. Accessed December 5, 2016. doi:10.2174/157016312799304552.

[34] Garud, Akanksha, Deepti Singh, Navneet Garud. 2012. "Solid Lipid Nanoparticles (SLN): Method, Characterization and Applications." *International Current Pharmaceutical Journal* 11:384–93. Accessed December 5, 2016. doi: 10.3329/icpj.v1i11.12065.

[35] Marcato, Priscyla D. 2009 "Preparation, Characterization and Application in Drugs and Cosmetics of Solid Lipid Nanoparticles." *Revista Eletrônica de Farmácia* 2: 1–37.

[36] Müller R. H., M. Radtke, S.A. Wissing. 2002. "Nanostructured Lipid Matrices for Improved Microencapsulation of Drugs." *International Journal of Pharmaceutics* 242:121–28. Accessed December 5, 2016. doi:10.1016/S0378-5173(02)00180-1.

[37] Mukherjee, S, S Ray, R S Thakur. 2009. "Solid Lipid Nanoparticles: A Modern Formulation Approach in Drug Delivery System." 71 :349-358. *Indian Journal of Pharmaceutical Sciences* 71:349–58. Accessed December 5, 2016. doi:10.4103/0250-474X.57282.

[38] Shangguan, Mingzhu, Yi Lu, Jianping Qi, Jin Han, Zhiqiang Tian, Yunchang Xie, Fuqiang Hu, Hailong Yuan, Wei Wu. 2014. "Binary Lipids-Based Nanostructured

Lipid Carriers for Improved Oral Bioavailability of Silymarin." *Journal of Biomaterials Applications* 28:887–96. Accessed December 5, 2016. doi:10.1177/0885328213485141.

[39] Chimsook, Thitiphan. 2014. "Preparation and Characterization of Nanostructured Lipid Carriers Loaded Spirogyra Spp. Extract." *Advanced Materials Research* 894:323–27. Accessed December 5, 2016. doi:10.4028/www.scientific.net/AMR.894.323.

[40] Wolfgang Mehnert, Karsten Mader. 2001. "Solid lipid nanoparticles: Production, characterization and applications." *Advanced Drug Delivery Reviews* 47: 165–196. Accessed December 5, 2016. doi: 10.1016/s0169-409x(01)00105-3.

[41] Kundu, Paromita, Chandana Mohanty, Sanjeeb K. Sahoo. 2012 "Antiglioma activity of curcumin-loaded lipid nanoparticles ant its enhanced bioavability in brain tissue for effective glioblastoma therapy." *Acta Biomaterialia* 8:2670-78. Accessed December 5, 2016. doi:10.1016/j.actbio.2012.03.048.

[42] Tiyaboonchai, Waree, Watcharaphorn Tungpradit, Pinyupa Plianbangchang. 2007. "Formulation and Characterization of Curcuminoids Loaded Solid Lipid Nanoparticles." *International Journal of Pharmaceutics* 337:299–306. Accessed December 5, 2016. doi:10.1016/j.ijpharm.2006.12.043.

[43] Li, Fang, Yanjiao Wang, Zitong Liu, Xia Lin, Haibing He, Xing Tang. 2010. "Formulation and Characterization of Bufadienolides-Loaded Nanostructured Lipid Carriers." *Drug Development and Industrial Pharmacy* 36:508–17. Accessed December 5, 2016. doi:10.3109/03639040903264397.(a)

[44] Li, Fang, Yan Weng, Lihui Wang, Haibing He, Jingyu Yang, Xing Tang. 2010. "The Efficacy and Safety of Bufadienolides-Loaded Nanostructured Lipid Carriers." *International Journal of Pharmaceutics* 393:204–12. Accessed December 5, 2016. doi:10.1016/j.ijpharm.2010.04.005.

[45] Luo, Cheng-Feng, Mu Yuan, Min-Sheng Chen, Shi-Ming Liu, Liu Zhu, Bi-Yun Huang, Xia-Wen Liu, Wen Xiong. 2011. "Pharmacokinetics, Tissue Distribution and Relative Bioavailability of Puerarin Solid Lipid Nanoparticles Following Oral Administration." *International Journal of Pharmaceutics* 410:138–44. Accessed December 5, 2016. doi:10.1016/j.ijpharm.2011.02.064.

[46] Luo, Cheng Feng, Ning Hou, Juan Tian, Mu Yuan, Shi Ming Liu, Long Gen Xiong, Jian Dong Luo, Min Sheng Chen. 2013. "Metabolic Profile of Puerarin in Rats after Intragastric Administration of Puerarin Solid Lipid Nanoparticles." *International Journal of Nanomedicine* 8:933–40. Accessed December 5, 2016. doi:10.2147/IJN.S39349.

[47] Yuan, Ling, Congyan Liu, Yan Chen, Zhenhai Zhang, Lei Zhou, Ding Qu. 2013. "Antitumor Activity of Tripterine via Lipid Carriers in a Prostate Cancer Model." *International Journal of Nanomedicine* 4339–50. Accessed December 5, 2016. doi:10.2147/IJN.S51621.

[48] Gao, Songran, David Julian McClements. 2016. "Formation and Stability of Solid Lipid Nanoparticles Fabricated Using Phase Inversion Temperature Method." *Colloids and Surfaces A: Physicochemical and Engineering Aspects* 499:79-87.

[49] Sarpietro, Maria Grazia, Maria Lorena Accolla, Giovanni Puglisi, Francesco Castelli, Lucia Montenegro. 2014. "Idebenone Loaded Solid Lipid Nanoparticles: Calorimetric Studies on Surfactant and Drug Loading Effects." *International Journal of Pharmaceutics* 471:69–74. Accessed December 5, 2016. doi:10.1016/j.ijpharm. 2014.05.019.

[50] Gomes, Graziela V L, Mirella R Sola, Luís F P Marostegan, Camila G Jange, A Vicente, Samantha C Pinho, Camila P S Cazado, Ana C Pinheiro. 2017. "Physico-Chemical Stability and *in vitro* Digestibility of Beta-Carotene-Loaded Lipid Nanoparticles of Cupuacu Butter (*Theobroma grandiflorum*) Produced by the Phase Inversion Temperature (PIT) Method." *Journal of Food Engineering* 192:93–102. Accessed December 5, 2016. doi:10.1016/j.jfoodeng. 2016.08.001.

[51] Zhang, Linhan, Douglas G. Hayes, Guoxun Chen, Qixin Zhong. 2013. "Transparent Dispersions of Milk-Fat-Based Nanostructured Lipid Carriers for Delivery of ß-Carotene." *Journal of Agricultural and Food Chemistry* 61: 9435–43. Accessed December 5, 2016. doi:10.1021/jf403512c.

In: Recent Developments in Phytomedicine Technology ISBN: 978-1-53611-977-0
Editors: L. A. Pedro de Freitas et al.

Chapter 8

RECENT DEVELOPMENTS IN EXPERIMENTAL METHODS OF LIPOSOMAL PRODUCTION

Stephânia F. Taveira, Ellen C. P. Alonso, Priscila B. R. da Rocha and Ricardo N. Marreto [*]
Laboratory of Nanosystems and Drug Delivery Devices (NanoSYS), School of Pharmacy, Federal University of Goiás, Goiânia, GO, Brazil

ABSTRACT

Liposomes are self-assembled vesicles consisting of one or more phospholipid bilayers, which have been widely used as safe and effective carriers for drugs. Encapsulation in liposomes can improve drug stability, enhance its bioavailability, promote controlled drug release, and change the in vivo distribution of the loaded drug. There is a great variety of liposome's preparation methods. However, the implementation of these techniques for large-scale production still needs improvements, as it requires, for instance, process optimization and scale-up, in order to develop products with high quality. Process development has been attempted through trial and error, which involves changing one variable at a time, which is uneconomical, time-consuming and, occasionally, unsuccessful. On the contrary, the use of experimental design requires fewer experiments to achieve an optimum formulation and process, representing a cost-effective tool to develop liposomes and other drug delivery systems. This chapter attempts to provide information about these experimental tools, covering the conventional and the novel methods of liposome preparation.

Keywords: phytosomes, stimuli-responsive liposomes, factorial design, plant extracts, novel methods

---

[*] Corresponding Author address. Email: ricardomarreto@ufg.br.

I. General Considerations and Concepts

1. Introduction

Liposomes (Figure 1A) are self-assembled spherical vesicles with particles ranging in size from 20 nm to several micrometers that have been widely used as safe, effective carriers for drug delivery. Liposomal systems were first described in the 1960s by Bangham, Standish [1]. Although the first formulations were composed of natural lipids only, currently they can include lipids and surfactants that are natural or synthetic. Their internal aqueous compartments are involved by one or more concentric lipid bilayers, which allows hydrophilic or lipophilic drug encapsulation [2], as shown in Figure 1B. The liposomal structure can improve drug stability, enhance its bioavailability, promote controlled release, and change its *in vivo* distribution.

Despite various methods by which to prepare liposomes, their implementation for large-scale production requires process optimization and scaling up in order to develop high-quality products. To date, however, the development of the process has been achieved by trial and error, which has involved the uneconomical, time-consuming, and sometimes ineffective changing of one variable at a time. By contrast, experimental designs require fewer trials in order to optimize the formulation and process and thereby represent cost-effective tools for developing liposomes and other drug delivery systems. In this chapter, we provide information about those tools while elucidating both conventional and novel methods of liposome preparation.

2. Liposome Structure and Composition

Liposomes form spontaneously when phospholipids are exposed to excess water [3, 4], given the amphiphilic property of the substances. Phospholipids are biocompatible molecules with a hydrophilic head and two apolar hydrophobic chains [3, 5]. Once dispersed in aqueous media, phospholipids give rise to lamellar layers, with the polar head group facing outward to the aqueous region and the long apolar chains interacting with each other, in a process that forms spherical vesicles [6, 7].

The unique structure of liposomes depends on the occurrence of hydrophobic interactions and van der Waals forces between two adjacent hydrocarbon chains. Hydrogen bonds and polar interactions are also responsible for connecting the polar heads of the phospholipids with the surrounding water [6, 8]. The formation of two layers is necessary to reduce the high free-energy differences between the hydrophobic and hydrophilic environments, thereby ensuring the structure's stability due to its supramolecular self-assembled structure [9].

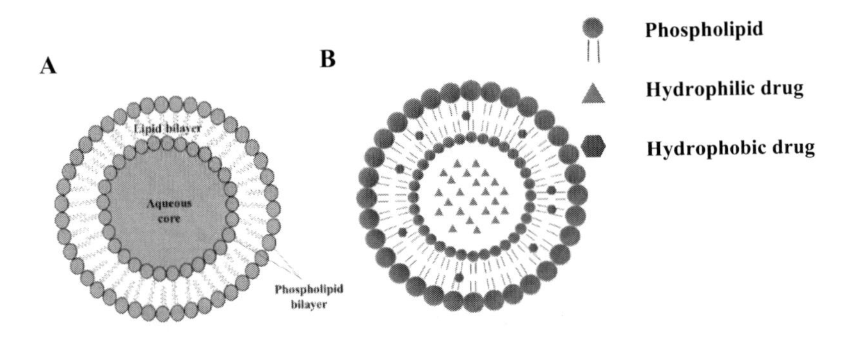

Figure 1. Liposome structure (A) and possible drug location in liposomal drug delivery systems (B).

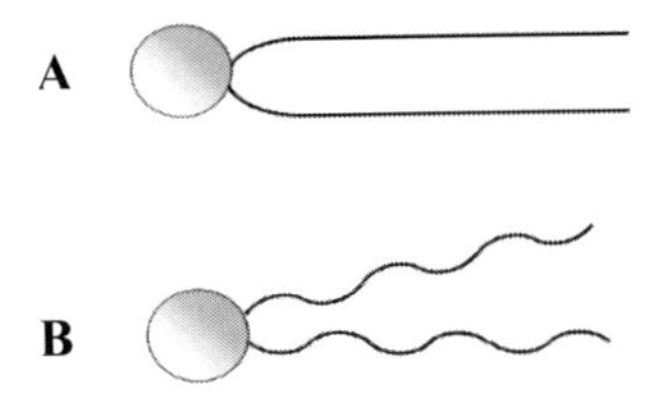

Figure 2. Representation of a phospholipid (A) in the gel state (i.e., at a temperature below the transition temperature) and (B) in the liquid crystalline state (i.e., at a temperature above the transition temperature).

Though the chemical compositions of vesicles can vary, they generally include natural or synthetic phospholipids (uncharged or charged), if not both, such as phosphatidylcholine, phosphatidylethanolamine, phosphatidylserine, and phosphatidylglycerol, as well as cholesterol and water [10, 11]. These components have low toxicity and are biocompatible and weakly immunogenic [12].

The phase transition temperature [13] of phospholipids can provide information about the gel or fluid phase of the system (Figure 2). Below Tc phospholipids are more rigid and ordered, whereas they are more fluid and disorganized above Tc [9, 14].

Temperature and other physical and chemical factors can influence phase transition. Shifting from the gel to fluid phase induces drug leakage, which could be problematic depending on the route of administration. For intravenous administration, drug leakage means that the system will lose its controlled release and targeting properties. Although the uptake by the reticuloendothelial system is greater when liposomes are in the fluid state [15], for topical drug delivery, more fluid bilayers can increase the drug's permeation to deeper skin layers, and in some cases, those liposomes can be deemed absorption enhancers. Although the gel state at physiological conditions can be required to stabilize liposomes, the fluid state can be exploited in order to encapsulate drugs more efficiently during liposome production [9, 10].

Cholesterol is one of the most widely used ingredients to produce liposomes. In concentrations in the formulation up to 50% (w/w), cholesterol can decrease membrane fluidity and improve bilayer stability in the presence of biological fluids [14, 16, 17]. Cholesterol can also be used to anchor other molecules such as polyethylene glycol

(PEG) or DNA [6] and thereby plays an important role in liposome composition [10, 11, 18].

The presence of charged components is important to improve the physical stability of the systems [19]. Negatively charged lipids such as phosphatidylserine and cholesterylsulfate and positively charged detergents such as stearylamine can prevent rapid aggregation in storage due to electrostatic repulsion between vesicles. At the same time, cationic liposomes are usually more convenient for loading nucleic acids given their negative charge, which allows them to be loaded electrostatically [10].

3. Classification and Types of Liposomes

Among the several classification systems available to categorize liposomes, most are based on liposome size or number of bilayers, if not both (Figure 3). Liposomes can also be classified in terms of their preparation method (see Section II) and applicability (Figure 4).

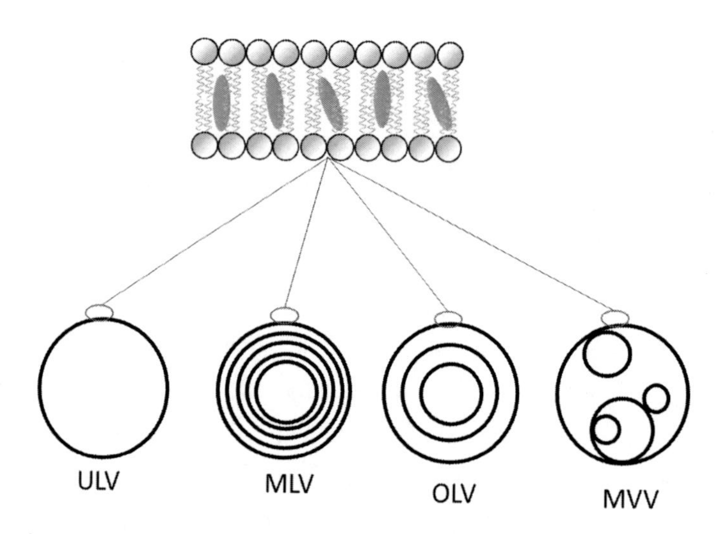

Figure 3. Classification of liposomes based on their structure. ULV: Unilamellar vesicles; MLV: Multilamellar vesicles; OLV: Oligolamellar vesicles; MVV: Multivesicular vesicles.

By size, unilamellar liposomes are classified as giant unilamellar vesicles (GUVs, >1 μm), large unilamellar vesicles (LUVs, 500–1000nm), medium unilamellar (MUVs, 100–500 nm), and small unilamellar vesicles (SUVs, 20–100 nm) [20].

The number of bilayers influences drug loading and release, stability during storage, interaction with cells, internalization, and the addition of surface-bound molecules [18, 21, 22]. Although these classifications are quite didactic, liposomes are currently classified according to their applicability, primarily because most systems for drug delivery are SUVs.

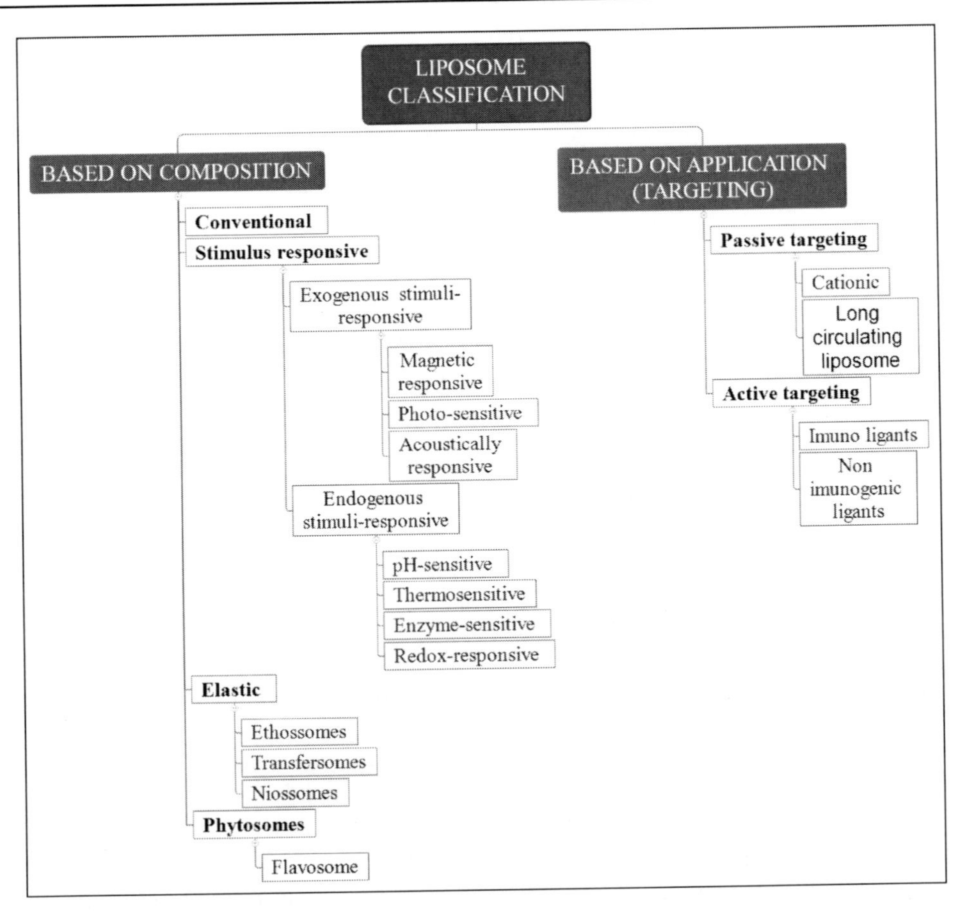

Figure 4. Classification of liposomes based on composition and application [6, 19, 23-25].

Over the years, conventional liposomes have demonstrated their ability to enhance therapeutic effects and reduce toxicity, yet have also been less efficient in controlling drug delivery. To circumvent that problem, trigger-responsive (i.e., stimulus-responsive) liposomes have been reported in the literature; these liposomes change their structure or conformation when subjected to endogenous (e.g., pH, enzyme, and temperature) or exogenous (e.g., magnetic field, light, and ultrasound) stimuli, thereby releasing the drug in a controlled manner and at the target site [25].

Developed to release drugs specifically at tumor sites using local hyperthermia, thermosensitive liposomes are a highly promising strategy for cancer treatment [24]. To do so, a liposomal system is produced with lipids exhibiting a phase transition just above physiological temperature [26].

pH-sensitive liposomes are prepared in order to allow drugs to avoid degradation into inactive compounds by enzymes following endocytosis [24]. A pH-sensitive liposome is commonly stable at physiological pH, but can be destabilized and acquire fusogenic properties under acidic conditions, in which it releases its aqueous content [27]. To achieve the pH-sensitive release of liposome content, vesicles are formulated with pH-sensitive components, typically by using dioleoyl phosphatidyle-thanolamine [28].

Redox-responsive liposomes take advantage of the major difference of redox potential that can exist, for instance, between normal and tumor tissues. These liposomes can be prepared by linking a small portion of bilayer lipids with disulfide bonds. Accordingly, with a drastic difference in potential, the disulfide bond is destabilized and releases the entrapped drug [25]. Enzyme-sensitive liposomes can be triggered by an enzyme that can cleave liposomes composed of the enzyme substrate mixed in lipid bilayers [25].

Exogenous stimuli have been used to trigger drug release by using light, the magnetic field, and ultrasound. The most common are magnetic liposomes, which are a combination of liposomes and magnetic elements (i.e., Fe_3O_4 or Fe_2O_3) that can be employed for diagnostic purposes and to treat cancer [29] The presence of magnetic nanoparticles allows liposomes to be driven to a specific site when an external magnetic field is applied at a specific area to release, for example, an antineoplastic drug. Magnetic liposomes can also act as contrast agents in magnetic resonance imaging [25].

Elastic liposomes have been proposed with an aim to prepare flexible structures for topical and transdermal application. There are three basic types of elastic liposomes: niosomes, transfersomes, and ethosomes. First, niosomes are highly stable vesicles produced with a single-chain surfactant molecule in combination with cholesterol that can modify the structure of the stratum corneum due to their surfactant properties [30-33]. Second transfersomes are ultraflexible lipid vesicles that, still intact, penetrate the stratum corneum [34, 35]; they consist of phospholipids, 10–25% of the surfactant and 3–10% ethanol [36]. Third, ethosomes represent the third generation of elastic lipid carriers; they are comprised mainly of phospholipids, ethanol in relatively high concentrations (20–50%), and water [37]. The high concentration of ethanol disturbs the skin lipid bilayer, as well as provide a more flexible liposome structure [38, 39].

Also attracting the attention of researchers are phytosomes, which are composed of plant extract associated with phospholipids, which often significantly enhance the bioavailability of plant constituents. A more detailed discussion of those systems appears in Section II.

Some modifications in conventional liposomes have been made to better target vesicles to specific organs, cells, or even organelles, especially in the treatment of solid tumors. The passive vectoring of nanosystems to solid tumors is based on the enhanced permeability and retention effect [40], which requires long-lasting circulating liposomes. To do so, conventional liposomes have been coated with PEG; PEGylated or stealth liposomes can reduce the adsorption of plasma proteins, which decreases the uptake of liposomes by the reticular endothelial system [41]. Passive targeting can also be achieved by cationic liposomes, since positively charged lipids can interact with the negative charges of tumor cells. They are also used for gene delivery [42].

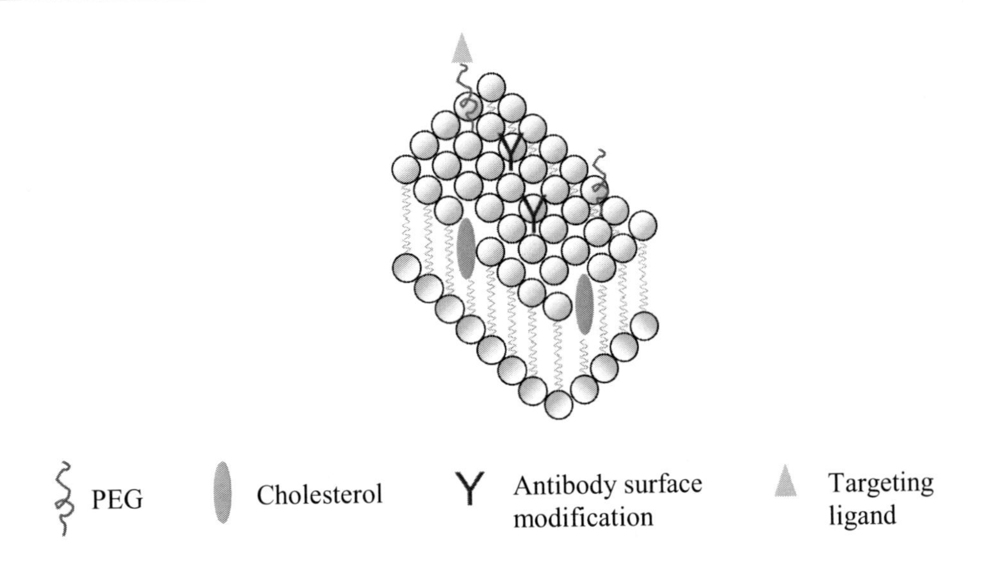

Figure 5. Portion of a typical lipid bilayer with multifunctional surface modifications.

By contrast, active targeting is characterized by the use of linkers at the liposome's surface to specifically interact with some cells (e.g., tumor cells). Monoclonal antibodies or fragments and other nonimmunogenic ligands can be attached to the liposome surface. Figure 5 demonstrates multifunctional surface modifications that a conventional liposome may have.

All of those surface modifications have been used to better enable liposomes to mediate the intracellular delivery of biologically active molecules. Therefore, several other lipid carrier-mediated vesicular systems, including cochleates, cryptosomes, archaeosomes, virosomes, sphingosomes, and ufasomes have emerged [43].

In sum, diverse new liposomes have emerged in order to improve the drug delivery performance of systems. Recently, the production of liposomes with plant extracts has gained in popularity, due to the great efficacy of those active materials, even compared to the neatness of synthetic drugs [44].

II. Liposomes as Phytomedicines: Liposomes versus Phytosomes

Despite the many nanostructures proposed for loading plant extracts, liposomes remain among the most studied, chiefly because plant extracts show different physical–chemical characteristics depending on the extraction and purification methods used [45]. As such, liposomes are quite interesting, for they can encapsulate both hydrophilic and lipophilic molecules.

Regarding the encapsulation of different extracts, some extracts are encapsulated more efficiently than others. For instance, more lipophilic substances such as essential oils could be dispersed in lipid bilayers, thereby resulting in greater entrapment efficiency [45]. Phytoconstituents, including some flavonoids, exhibit good water solubility and low bioavailability due to their great size and poor passive diffusion through lipid membranes [46, 47]. Recently, it has been widely proposed that the complexation of herbal extract constituents with phospholipids, or phytosomes, can significantly enhance the bioavailability of plant constituents and extracts such as silymarin [48], curcumin [49], *Ginkgo biloba* [50], ginseng, grape seed, green tea, and olive oil [51]. Phytosomes that encapsulate flavonoids are also called flavosomes or flavanosomes.

Although liposomes and phytosomes have some similarities, in liposomes phospholipid molecules surround the plant extract or active ingredient. Meanwhile, in phytosomes, the phospholipid makes H-bonds with active compounds at the polar region. To do so, different molar ratios can be used, usually about 1:1 or 2:1 phospholipid to active ingredient [52].

Phytosome represent a technology patented by Indena SPA (Milan, Italy). There are also patents for phytosomes with curcumin (i.e., Mariva®) and with olive pulp extract (i.e., Oleaselect®), as Shakeri and Sahebkar [53] report. On their heels, many other patents have emerged for different plant extracts.

Given the variety of plants the citation of all published literature on plant extract-loaded liposomes is quite difficult. Thus, the most studied and popular standardized herbal extracts in the last 15 years have been chosen for discussion in this section. For a better understanding, Table 1 describes some important liposome formulations divided according to plant extract encapsulated.

Ginkgo biloba is a plant that has existed on Earth for more than 200 million years. It is reported to have several properties beneficial to health, including scavenging radical (i.e., antioxidant properties), antitumor, and protective effects in the central nervous system [50]. One of the first studies to report the plant appeared in 2000, with the production of hybrid liposomes (i.e., micellar systems with liposomes).

Silybum marianum is a plant extract widely used in the treatment of liver and gallbladder diseases [54]. Due to its low solubility and bioavailability, some strategies have been applied to overcome these drawbacks, such as the preparation of liposomal formulations [55]. Table 1 presents some reports on liposome and phytosome preparations aimed at improving the oral bioavailability of *Silybum marianum* constituents [56-58]. Phytosomes for parenteral administration [59] and liposomes targeted to the liver [60] have also been developed.

Centella asiatica (L.) Urban, also known as gotu kola and Indian pennywort, is an herbaceous plant characterized as a creeper plant with rooted nodes [61] used for centuries in traditional Asia medicine to treat wounds [62], burns, leprosy, and lupus [63, 64]. Its major components are triterpenic saponins and the corresponding aglycones, such as madecassoside, madecassic acid, asiatic acid, and asiaticoside (AS), the latter being the most active constituent in the plant [65].

Due to its high molecular weight (959.12 Da) and low bioavailability, AS encapsulated in liposomes can improve therapeutic value. Wang, Ma [66] used the ethanol injection method to produce *Centella* total glucosides (CTG)-loaded liposomes and observed a higher cumulative absorption in the ileum of rats than of non-encapsulated CTG. Using flexible nanoliposomes, Ren, He [67] encapsulated AS and improved its transdermal absorption.

Panax ginseng exhibits antioxidant properties, activities in modulating vascular tone and ability to increase energy and vitality [68, 69]. However, as most plant extracts, it has low bioavailability and low permeability through skin and the use of nanosystems has shown to be promising for the encapsulation of this extract; besides the possibility of improving its antioxidant activity. Choi, Cho [70] developed ginsenoside transfersomes to improve the topical delivery of this extract. They obtained a significantly higher skin permeation profile when compared with conventional liposomes. Other studies also demonstrated the advantages of encapsulating *Panax ginseng* in vesicles [71, 72], improving its bioavailability or increasing its therapeutic properties.

Extensively studied due to its therapeutic efficacy in numerous chronic diseases and some types of cancer, curcumin exhibits several activities, including antioxidant, anti-inflammatory, antimicrobial, and antiviral ones. Despite those important characteristics, it has not been approved as a therapeutic agent due to its low bioavailability, instability at physiological pH, low water solubility and cellular uptake, and rapid metabolism inside cells [73]. To overcome some of those disadvantages, liposomal formulations have been studied with the aim to entrap curcumin [74]. Table 1 describes some interesting studies, including those about the production and evaluation of liposomal curcumin as antimalarial and antileishmanial preparations [75, 76]. For anticancer activity, different strategies have been studied with the aim to enhance curcumin bioavailability, including the development of liposomes for passive targeting via surface modification [77], as well as curcumin and doxorubicin coencapsulation [78]. To improve liposomal stability and curcumin's sustained release, Eudragit S100 was used to achieve intestinal curcumin delivery [79], and chitosan was used to coat liposomes in order to enhance lipid bilayer stability [80].

To better understand the process development of the different types of liposomes, and its scale-up, it is important to discuss the conventional and novel methods of liposomes preparation.

Table 1. Different types of liposomal formulations loaded plant extracts

	Liposome Type	Method	Diameter (nm)	Encapsulation efficiency (%)	Refe-rence
Ginkgo biloba	Proliposomes	SD	211	91	[81]
	Niosomes	FDH / SD / FD	141	FD 50; SD 77	[50]
Silybum marianum	Phytosomes	RPE	165	100	[59, 82]
	Liposome	EM	95.5	83	[83]
	Liposome	FHM	329	55	[58]
	Liposome and Ethosome	FHM	272 321	60 69	[57]
	Liposome	FHM	155	70	[60]
	Proliposome	Film dispersion	7 – 50	81	[56]
	Hibrid liposome	RPE	660	69	[84]
	Proliposome	Film deposition	239	90	[85]
	Liposome	*	---	65 – 83	[48]
Panax ginseng	Prolipossome	EIM / SD	275	69 - 71	[86]
	Ethosomes and transfersomes	Microflui-dization	90 – 286	47 – 66	[87]
	Liposome	FHM / HPH	200 – 450	*	[88]
	Hybrid liposome	FHM / SON	147	27 – 67	[89]
	Hybrid liposome	FHM / SON	99 – 106	*	[90]
Centella asiatica	Liposome	EIM	137	12 – 47	[66]
	Liposome	FHM	293	41	[91]
	Elastic liposomes	RPExt / lyophilization	70	31	[57]
	Elastic liposomes	TLE	100	25-60	[92]
	Elastic liposomes	FHM /homogenization	150-495	25 – 35	[93]
Curcuma longa	Prolipossome	FHM	280	78 – 82	[79]
	Stimulus responsive liposome	EIM	93 - 333	41 – 53	[80]
	Liposome	FHM	110	70	[94]
	Liposome	FHM	*	45	[76]
	Liposome for passive targeting	FHM	161 - 252	35 – 70	[77]
	Liposome for passive targeting	FHM	190 – 230	74 – 86	[78]
	Liposome	SON	110 – 135	63 – 67	[95]
	Liposome	FHM	176	84 – 94	[75]
	Liposome, Transfersome Ethosome	FHM	212 – 262 175 – 199 167 – 195	43 – 47 80 – 84 68 - 72	[96]

FHM: film hydration method; RPE: reverse-phase evaporation; SD: spray drying; FD: freezing drying; EM: Extrusion method; EIM: Ethanol injection; HPH: high pressure homogenization; RPEx: reserve phase extrusion;TLE Thin layer evaporation; SON: sonication.

* Data not informed.

III. LIPOSOME PREPARATION METHODS

Each of the several methods to prepare liposomes (Figure 6) can influence liposome properties, including size, number of bilayers, drug loading, and entrapment efficiency. The choice of the appropriate method depends on many factors, including (1) physicochemical characteristics of both drug and liposome ingredients [97], toxicity and the concentration of the drug in the formulation, (3) type of medium in which the liposomes are intended to be disperse, (4) desired size and half-life, (5) administration route [97], type of liposome (e.g., elastic or phytosome), and (7) costs, reproducibility, and applicability [6].

Methods of liposome preparation can be categorized as conventional or novel. Although some techniques are simple, others are more complex and require special equipment to be useful for large-scale production [10]. Notably, many variations and adaptations of production methods are available. Moreover, many authors have combine methods in order to find suitable characteristics of a final formulation for a specific application.

1. Conventional Methods

As shown in Figure 7, conventional methods can be classified as three techniques: mechanical dispersion, solvent dispersion, and detergent removal [12]. Simple preparation methods such as the formation of MLVs by mechanical dispersion are often used due to their simplicity and potential to produce liposomes without sophisticated equipment [98]. However, such preparation requires a subsequent reduction in size, typically performed by sonication, extrusion through a polycarbonate membrane, homogenization (e.g., French pressure cell or high-pressure homogenization), or freeze–thaw cycles [98].

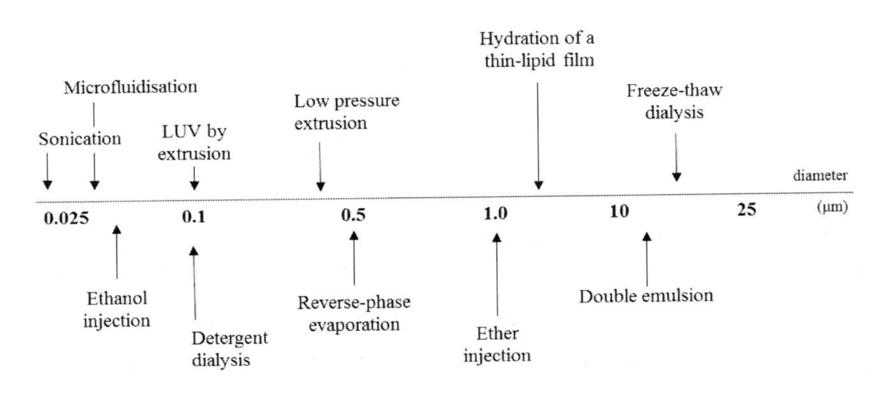

Figure 6. Methods of liposome preparation and size range of final liposomes [9, 11, 98].

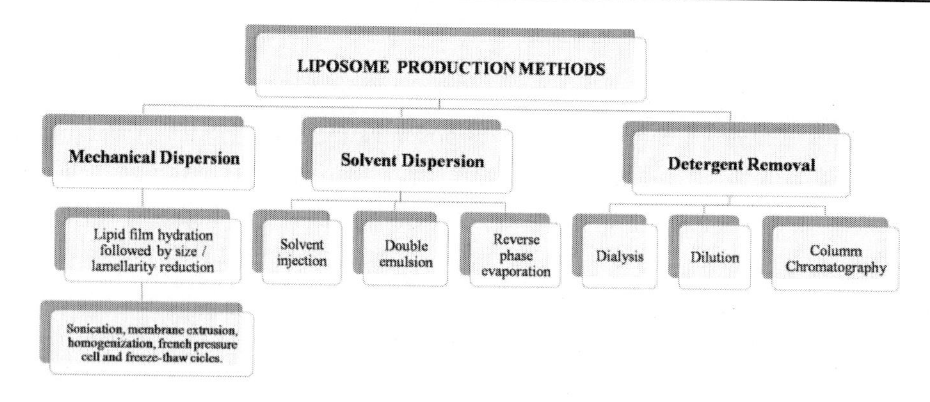

Figure 7. Classification of conventional methods of liposome preparation.

Other conventional methods such as solvent injection (i.e., ether or ethanol), reverse-phase evaporation, and detergent removal by dialysis are also widely used, as discussed below [10, 11, 99].

1.1. Mechanical Dispersion: Preparation and Hydration of a Thin Lipid Film Followed by Size and Lamellarity Reduction

Thin-film hydration, or the Bangham method, is one of the most widely used techniques for liposome preparation. It comprises the formation of a lipidic thin film in a round-bottomed flask by dissolving the lipid in an organic solvent, followed by solvent evaporation. Liposomes form after rehydration with aqueous solvents or buffers [1, 100]. Lipophilic drugs are included in the lipid film, whereas hydrophilic ones are dissolved in the aqueous media.

The hydration of the lipid film induces the swell and growth of the thin lipid layer, and mechanical stirring causes the formation of liposomes [101]. With vigorous shaking during hydration, MLVs with heterogeneous size distribution form, while gentle stirring gives rise to GUVs [20]. SUVs with a narrow size distribution (i.e., low PdI) can be achieved by sonication, extrusion through a polycarbonate membrane, or homogenization [20, 102, 103].

Sonication can reduce MLVs in size to 30–50nm; however the PdI can remain quite high. In addition, ultrasound energy can promote phospholipid and drug degradation [98]. The method of the French pressure cell allows the extrusion of the formulation through a small orifice [100], whereas high-pressure homogenization is more common in large-scale production, since they are commonly used for the large-scale production of parenteral emulsions. In this latter technique, the formulation is continuously pumped through an orifice or very thin channels at a very high pressure. The most used method is membrane extrusion, due to its simplicity at laboratory scale and initial development. Formulations are extruded several times through a membrane with a defined pore size. The average size of vesicles decreases with increased pressure and number of extrusion cycles or with smaller membrane pores [98].

Mechanical dispersion techniques have some disadvantages, however, such as low entrapment efficiency (5–15%) for hydrophilic drugs [6, 10, 11]. The multiple steps of these production methods can complicate the control of variables and upscaling. For example, how the solvent is evaporated and how quickly evaporation occurs significantly influences liposomal production [104]. However, when parameters are established well, the techniques can be useful, reproducible, and applicable [105].

1.2. Solvent Dispersion: Reverse-Phase Evaporation

An alternative to mechanical methods is reverse-phase evaporation, which was introduced by Szoka and Papahadjopoulos [106] and consists of forming a water-in-oil emulsion by sonication. One phase contains the drug in an aqueous buffer and another contains the phospholipids dispersed in an organic solvent. After emulsification, the slow removal of the organic solvent is performed under reduced pressure, which induces a viscous, gel-like state [106]. The gel state breakdown and some inverted droplets become disturbed, and the excess of phospholipids in the mixture forms a complete bilayer around the residual droplets, thereby forming liposomes [12].

The liposomes formed exhibit a large internal aqueous space and can entrap a great number of hydrophilic drugs, with an entrapment efficiency of up to 65% [100]. The major disadvantage of the technique is the interaction of the remaining solvent with the drug and lipids [10, 107]. By contrast, considerable improvement in the entrapment of the hydrophilic drugs occurs [108] with substantially increased drug bioavailability [84].

1.3. Solvent Dispersion: Solvent Injection

The dissolution of phospholipids into an organic phase (i.e., ethanol or ether) and their injection into aqueous media containing the drug prompts liposome formation [107]. When ethanol is injected, it generally forms unilamellar vesicles with a low polydispersity index and high entrapping volume, which results in the great efficiency of entrapment of hydrophilic drugs [109]. By contrast, when ether is injected, it generates a heterogeneous population of liposomes.

The size and homogeneity of the resulting vesicles can be controlled by including ethanol in the aqueous phase or by controlling the stirring level [110]. Stano, Bufali [111] used ethanol injection to obtain gimatecan-loaded (i.e., a novel camptothecin analogue) liposomes that varied in several parameters in order to obtain a final suitable formulation. They observed, for instance, that different liposome sizes were obtained when the aqueous solutions were pure water or saline solution (0.9% NaCl).

1.4. Detergent Removal via Dialysis

Detergents have been used to solubilize lipids at their critical micellar concentrations [112]. In that technique, phospholipids are solubilized by detergents at their micellar concentration in aqueous media, after which the removal of detergents, mostly by dialysis, results in the coalescence of the phospholipid and formation of LUVs [100]. Dialysis allows the production of homogenous populations in a reproducible manner [113, 114], although detergent traces are retained. Chromatographic techniques and extensive dilutions have also been used to remove detergents.

In general, some problems are associated with conventional methods, including (1) large mean diameter or broad distribution of liposomes [115, 116, 97] low entrapment efficiency [117, 118], (3) low reproducibility [119], and (4) presence of traces of solvents or detergents, which can influence the stability and toxicity, as well as complicate their use at industrial scales due to the great amount of residues [120, 121].

To solve those problems, novel methods have been used to efficiently prepare liposomes with easier upscaling that can be applied to an array of liposome constituents and drugs.

2. Novel Methods of Liposome Production

New techniques for liposome production have gained relevance given their ability to overcome drawbacks of conventional methods, including the necessary rational use of an organic solvent, high energy consumption, and difficulties in upscaling [99, 122, 123]. The supercritical fluid technique, freeze drying, dual asymmetric centrifugation, membrane contactor technology, and microfluidics are some of the new methods used to prepare liposomes, all of which are briefly discussed in what follows.

2.1. Dual Asymmetric Centrifugation Method

Dual asymmetric centrifugation was first used for liposome preparation by Massing, Cicko [124]. It differs from traditional centrifugation because the sample rotates on its own vertical axis, which prompts a counter-rotating movement resulting in more effective homogenization (Figure 8). In their pioneering study, the authors reported the preparation of liposomes with diameters 60 nm on average and an encapsulation efficiency of 56% for calcein [124]. Hirsch, Ziroli [125] used the technique to produce a sterile liposomal formulation containing siRNA, which resulted in small (70–120 nm), stable liposomes (at least 3 months), with a high entrapment efficiency of up to 71%.

The method allows the production of small batches in sterile conditions at low temperatures, which is especially important for some thermolabile drugs and biological compounds [124]. The technique also avoids the use of organic solvents for dispersing lipid, which results in small liposomes with a high encapsulation efficiency for water-soluble drugs [99].

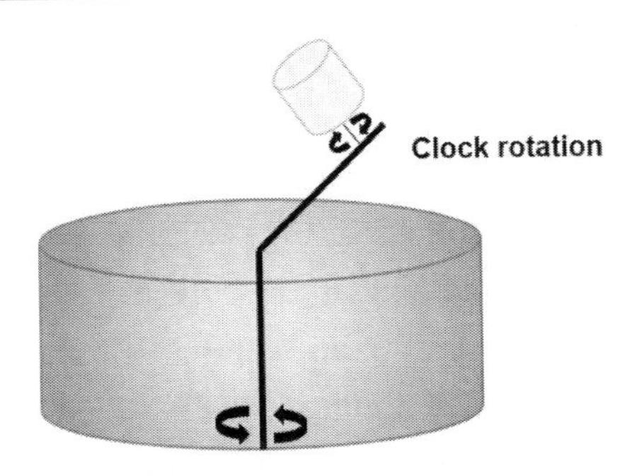

Figure 8. Dual asymmetric centrifuge operation.

Table 2. Liposome production by membrane contactor method

Drug	Diameter (nm)	Encapsulation efficiency (%)	Rerefences
Indomethacin	50 – 160	63	[127]
Beclomethasone dipropionate		98	
Spironolactone	120	93	[128]
Caffeine	82	10	[129]
Spironolactone	95	86	

2.2. Membrane Contactor Method

Charcosset [126] defined membrane contactor as the connection of two phases through membrane pores, in which an external phase is pressurized and forced to permeate through a membrane into a continuous internal phase, which flows tangentially to the membrane surface. In this process, some parameters are responsible for particle size and size distribution, including pore size, distribution of the membrane, and degree of coalescence, both at the membrane surface and in the bulk solution [126]. Jaafar-Maalej, Charcosset [127] used the technique to produce liposomes for the first time by forcing a pressurized phospholipid solution in ethanol through a membrane into an aqueous phase, after which the organic solvent was removed by rotary evaporation.

Other researchers have used the membrane contactor method to produce liposomes (Table 2) and generally highlighted the advantages of the continuous process, including control of the particle size, high encapsulation efficiency, and the potential for upscaling [98].

2.3. Freeze-Drying Double Emulsion

The drying process is an interesting alternative that can overcome a primary drawback of liposomal formulations namely, low physical stability. Freeze-drying, or lyophilization, ranks among the most commonly used drying methods [130, 131]. Freeze-drying double emulsion was proposed by Wang, Deng [132] with the objective to produce sterile submicron unilamellar liposomes. The method was based on the preparation of double emulsion with disaccharides as lyoprotectants in the inner and outer aqueous phases, after which double emulsion was sterilized by passing it through a 0.22-μm membrane pore filter and lyophilizing it for solvent removal. The final liposome produced in that work was small (<200 nm) and showed both a high entrapment efficiency and excellent stability for 12 months [132].

After optimization, the technique was successfully used to produce topotecan-loaded liposomes, which dried were stable for 6 months and after rehydration formed unilamellar liposomes with particles of about 200 nm and entrapment encapsulation greater than 80% [133]. Another interesting study reported the preparation of liposomes with flurbiprofen, ketoprofen, topotecan, ciprofloxacin, and 5-fluorouracil (i.e., amphiphilic, hydrophilic, and lipophilic drugs) by freeze-drying water-in-oil-in-water double emulsion using disaccharides as lyoprotectants. The authors reported the formation of unilamellar liposomes with 200 nm average diameter and high encapsulation efficiency for amphiphilic and lipophilic drugs (around 90%). The systems were stable for 10 months [134].

Other drying processes have been used for liposomal formulation with good results, including spray drying [135, 136], spray-freeze drying [137] and supercritical fluid technology [122].

2.4. Supercritical Fluid Technique

A supercritical fluid (SCF) is any substance at a temperature and pressure above its critical point. In such conditions, dense gas has properties between those of the liquid and gas phases, including high compressibility, diffusivity, and evaporation rate, thereby making it possible to modulate the solvent power, adapting pressure, and temperature rating [122, 138, 139]. The supercritical state is defined as a region in which the material exhibits properties of the liquid and gas state: like a gas shows low viscosity and high diffusivity; as a liquid exert solvation effect due to high density.

The most common substance used as SCF is carbon dioxide (CO_2) because it is available, inexpensive, and nontoxic and needs a low critical temperature and pressure (31°C and 74 bar). Supercritical CO_2 also has a solvation force similar to organic solvents and can thus replace them. After depressurization, all CO_2 is released, and no solvent remains in the final product [140]. Given those characteristics, CO_2 SCF has aroused interest for use in liposome production.

The use of SC technologies for liposome production was first published by Frederiksen, Anton [141] using an anti-solvent technique. Phospholipids and cholesterol were dissolved in CO_2 SCF using ethanol as a co-solvent and then rapidly expanded in the water phase that contained the substance to be entrapped. The chief limitation of that method was low encapsulation efficiency (15%), although that first attempt also used 15-fold less organic solvent, unlike conventional methods.

Recently, Campardelli, Baldino [142] reviewed the application of SCF in nanomedicine and compared two optimized techniques: the depressurization of an expanded solution into aqueous media (DESAM), developed by Meure, Foster [143], and supercritical assisted liposome formation (SuperLip), develop by Santo, Campardelli [144]. In DESAM, an ethanolic solution containing phospholipids is introduced into the chamber and expanded with CO_2 SC. The resulting solution is then injected in a water bath to form small unilamellar liposomes with a 200 nm diameter on average and an encapsulation efficiency of 29% [143]. With the SuperLip method, water droplets are produced by atomization directly inside a high-pressure vessel with expanded liquid containing phosphatidylcholine, ethanol as a cosolvent, and CO_2 SCF. Liposomes were formed because the lipids in the expanded liquid could spontaneously organize themselves in a layer around the water droplets [144]. That technique showed a high encapsulation efficiency for bovine serum albumin (85–90%) and a size distribution in the range of 130–290 nm.

SCF is a novel technology that can be broadly applied to achieve better results for liposome production. At once, it is a versatile process in which changes in the supercritical substance, process parameters, and design of the apparatus can generate new methods with better results. SCF techniques can also upscale more easily than conventional methods [98].

2.5. Microfluidics

Microfluidics is the manipulation of fluids in channels with micrometers in dimension and is an interesting emerging technology with several applications in chemical synthesis and biological analysis [145]. The method was proposed for the early stages of drug development, given the small-scale of devices used, the little material it needs, all of which prompt smaller residue formation and lower process costs [146]. Other benefits to producing liposomes by microfluidics systems include the reproducible control of particle size in a process operating in a continuous flow [98, 147]. van Swaay and deMello [148], described and compared different methods using microfluidics systems for forming liposomes (Figure 9).

Droplet emulsion transfer ranks among the most interesting microfluidic techniques developed initially for macroscale production [149]. Later, Matosevic and Paegel [150] developed a y-shaped microfluidic assembly line with two input channels and one output where liposomes were collected. For vesicle formation, uniform water-in-oil lipid-stabilized droplets are generated in the left channel, and the oil flow containing the droplets merges with the water flow from the right channel to form a continuous central flow. In the middle of the central channel is a triangular apparatus where the oil is skimmed and the lipid-stabilized droplets are displaced for the water flow; once the second lipid layer is completed, giant unilamellar liposomes are formed with a high encapsulation efficiency of 83% [150].

Numerous studies have used microfluidic devices for liposome production (Table 3). Microfluidic technology is a new, promising technology, and there are clearly many opportunities to improve the techniques for liposome production by focusing on their different drawbacks and applications. The most challenging issue for microfluidics is to develop a system on a chip that results in a process with high yield and encapsulation efficiency [151]. Furthermore, the upscaling of the microfluidic method needs to be achieved if large-scale production is the goal [147].

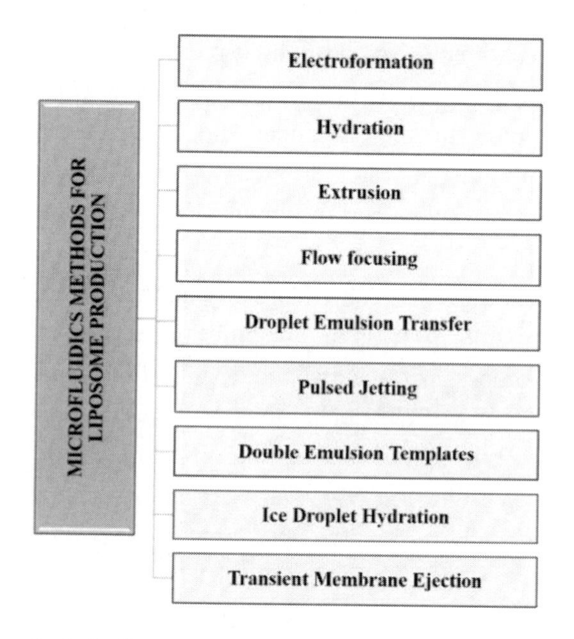

Figure 9. Microfluidic methods for liposome production.

Table 3. Liposome production by microfluidic techniques

Method	Diameter (nm)	Reference
Ultrasound-enhanced microfluidic method	66	[99]
Rapid Freezing Continuous-Flow	100 – 300	[152]
Hydrodynamic flow focusing method	100 – 130	[153]
	< 500	[154]

As shown, several methods are available for liposome production, upon which researchers have based new formulations by applying factorial designs.

IV. Factorial Design for Liposome Production

Drug development is an expensive, time-consuming process [155] that often involves the trial-and-error approach, which precludes the evaluation of interactions between factors [156]. Experimental designs are important tools used to overcome that drawback, since it allows the evaluation of different factors at the same time by using statistical models. Moreover, the methods can logically correlate lots of experiments, thereby resulting in more accurate data with fewer tests [157].

There are many advantages of using experimental designs for product development, including (1) the possibility of evaluating all important factors and their possible interactions [97], achieving ideal product performance with fewer tests, (3) predicting product and process behavior using mathematic models, (4) improving yield and robustness among studies, and (5) saving time, raw material, effort, and money [156]. Given those advantages, statistical tools have been more widely used, and in pharmaceutical research, experimental designs have been more frequently applied [156], as shown in Figure 10.

Thus, the choice of experimental design is an important consideration and depends on the nature of factors, models, and the strategy [156]. For liposome production, some researchers have applied different experimental designs (Table 4). Alund, Smistad [158] highlighted the importance of using experimental designs to systematically investigate multivariate factors by performing fewer experiments. Alund, Smistad [158] and Loukas [159] additionally showed that the tool offers useful conclusions regarding the primary effects and interactions of evaluated factors that clarify complex interactions otherwise indiscernible with factor-by-factor evaluation.

Lastly, the success of any designed experiment depends on the planning, appropriate choice of the design, statistical analysis of data and teamwork skills, initially defined in the project scope [165].

Conclusion

In this chapter, liposomes' preparation methods were evaluated. Comprehensively understanding the current progress of these methods will be helpful for developing new formulations and novel liposome applications.

Table 4. Experimental design applied for liposome production

Design	Drug	Factors	Rerefence
3^3	Cytarabine	Sodium deoxycholate concentration Cytarabine Concentration Sonication time	[160]
2^{4-1}	Coated liposomes with pectin	Pectin concentration Lipid concentration Lipid charge Speed of addition	[158]
3^2	Vitamin E	Cholesterol concentration Phospholipids concentration	[161]
2^3	Silymarin	Charge inducer Tween 20 Tween 80 (presence and absence)	[84]
3^3	Idoxuridine	Organic phase volume Aqueous phase volume Drug/ phosphatidylcoline/ cholesterol molar ratio	[162]
3^3	Acyclovir	Organic phase volume Aqueous phase volume Drug/ phosphatidylcoline/ cholesterol molar ratio	[162]
Box-BehnKen (2^{5-1})	Primaquine	Phospholipid type, Cholesterol concentration Charge concentration Citrate concentration Drug concentration	[163]
2^4	Vitamin C	α-cyclodextrin Oil red O Oxybenzone Sulisobenzone (presence and absence)	[159]
2^4	Thioguanine	pH Cholesterol concentration Lipid charge Sonication time	[164]

Experimental design	Factorial designs, fractional–factorial designs
	Plackett–Burman designs
	Star designs
	Central composite designs
	Box–Behnken designs
	Center-of-gravity designs
	Equiradial designs
	Mixture designs
	Taguchi designs
	Optimal designs
	Rechtschaffner designs
	Cotter designs

Figure 10. Types of experimental design used in pharmaceutical product design.

REFERENCES

[1] Bangham, A. D., M. M. Standish, and J. C. Watkins. 1965. "Diffusion of univalent ions across the lamellae of swollen phospholipids". *J Mol Biol* 13(1): 238-IN27.

[2] Gregoriadis, Gregory. 1976. "The Carrier Potential of Liposomes in Biology and Medicine". *New England Journal of Medicine* 295(14): 765-770.

[3] Tyrrell, D. A., T. D. Heath, C. M. Colley, and B. E. Ryman. 1976. "New aspects of liposomes". *Biochimica et Biophysica Acta* 457: 259-302.

[4] Gregoriadis, G. 2007. *Liposome Technology: Liposome preparation and related techniques*. 3th ed. Vol. I, New York: Informa Healthcare USA.

[5] El Maghraby, G. M., A. C. Williams, and B. W. Barry. 2006. "Can drug-bearing liposomes penetrate intact skin?". *J Pharm Pharmacol* 58(4): 415-29.

[6] Bozzuto, G. and A. Molinari. 2015. "Liposomes as nanomedical devices". *Int J Nanomedicine* 10: 975-99.

[7] Lasic, D. D. 1988. "The mechanism of vesicle formation". *Biochemistry Journal* 256: 1-11.

[8] Frolov, V. A., A. V. Shnyrova, and J. Zimmerberg. 2011. "Lipid polymorphisms and membrane shape". *Cold Spring Harb Perspect Biol* 3(11): a004747.

[9] Kalepu, S., K. T. Sunilkumar, B. Sudheer, and M. Mohanvarma. 2013. "Liposomal drug delivery system: A comprehensive review". *International Journal of Drug Development & Res.* 5(4): 62-75.

[10] Pattni, B. S., V. V. Chupin, and V. P. Torchilin. 2015. "New Developments in Liposomal Drug Delivery". *Chem Rev* 115(19): 10938-66.

[11] Laouini, A., C. Jaafar-Maalej, I. Limayem-Blouza, S. Sfar, C. Charcosset, and H. Fessi. 2012. "Preparation, Characterization and Applications of Liposomes: State of the Art". *Journal of Colloid Science and Biotechnology* 1(2): 147-168.

[12] Akbarzadeh, A., R. Rezaei-Sadabady, S. Davaran, S. W. Joo, N. Zarghami, Y. Hanifehpour, M. Samiei, M. Kouhi, and K. Nejati-Koshki. 2013. "Liposome-classification, preparation and applications". *Nanoscale Research Letters* 8(102).

[13] Thiago Frances Guimarães, Aurea D. Lanchotea, Jéssica Silva da Costab, Alessandra Lifsitch Viçosa, and Luís Alexandre Pedro de Freitas. 2015. "A multivariate approach applied to quality on particle engineering of spray-dried mannitol". *Advanced Powder Technology* 26(4): 1094-1101.

[14] Anderson, M. and A. Omri. 2004. "The effect of different lipid components on the in vitro stability and release kinetics of liposome formulations". *Drug Deliv* 11(1): 33-9.

[15] Gabizon, A. and D. Papahadjopoulos. 1988. "Liposome formulations with prolonged circulation time in blood and enhanced uptake by tumors". *Proc Natl Acad Sci U S A* 85(18): 6949-6953.

[16] Nie, Y., L. Ji, H. Ding, L. Xie, L. Li, B. He, Y. Wu, and Z. Gu. 2012. "Cholesterol derivatives based charged liposomes for doxorubicin delivery: preparation, in vitro and in vivo characterization". *Theranostics* 2(11): 1092-103.

[17] Vemuri, Sriram and C. T. Rhodes. 1995. "Preparation and characterization of liposomes as therapeutic delivery systems: a review". *Pharmaceutica Acta Helvetiae* 70(2): 95-111.

[18] Plessis, J., C. Ramachandran, N. Weiner, and D. G. Muller. 1996. "The influence of lipid composition and lamellarity of liposomes on the physical stability of liposomes upon storage". *International Journal of Pharmaceutics* 127: 273-278.

[19] Gao, W., C. M. Hu, R. H. Fang, and L. Zhang. 2013. "Liposome-like Nanostructures for Drug Delivery". *J Mater Chem B Mater Biol Med* 1(48).

[20] Gómez-Hens, A. and J. M. Fernández-Romero. 2005. "The role of liposomes in analytical processes". *TrAC Trends in Analytical Chemistry* 24(1): 9-19.

[21] Casals, Elisenda, Ana María Galán, Ginés Escolar, Montserrat Gallardo, and Joan Estelrich. 2003. "Physical stability of liposomes bearing hemostatic activity". *Chemistry and Physics of Lipids* 125(2): 139-146.

[22] Frohlich, M., V. Brecht, and R. Peschka-Suss. 2001. "Parameters influencing the determination of liposome lamellarity by P-NMR". *Chemistry and Physics of Lipids* 109: 103-112.

[23] Sharma, A. and U. Sharma. 1997. "Liposomes in drug delivery: progress and limitations". *International Journal of Pharmaceutics* 154: 123-140.

[24] Li, Jing, Xuling Wang, Ting Zhang, Chunling Wang, Zhenjun Huang, Xiang Luo, and Yihui Deng. 2015. "A review on phospholipids and their main applications in drug delivery systems". *Asian Journal of Pharmaceutical Sciences* 10(2): 81-98.

[25] Movahedi, F., R. G. Hu, D. L. Becker, and C. Xu. 2015. "Stimuli-responsive liposomes for the delivery of nucleic acid therapeutics". *Nanomedicine* 11(6): 1575-84.

[26] Andresen, Thomas L., Simon S. Jensen, and Kent Jørgensen. 2005. "Advanced strategies in liposomal cancer therapy: Problems and prospects of active and tumor specific drug release". *Progress in Lipid Research* 44(1): 68-97.

[27] Simões, Sérgio, João Nuno Moreira, Cristina Fonseca, Nejat Düzgüneş, and Maria C. Pedroso de Lima. 2004. "On the formulation of pH-sensitive liposomes with long circulation times". *Advanced Drug Delivery Reviews* 56(7): 947-965.

[28] Lopes, S. C. A., M. V. M. Novais, C. S. Teixeira, K. Honorato-Sampaio, M. T. Pereira, L. A. M. Ferreira, F. C. Braga, and M. C. Oliveira. 2013. "Preparation, Physicochemical Characterization, and Cell Viability Evaluation of Long-Circulating and pH-Sensitive Liposomes Containing Ursolic Acid". *Biomedical Research International* 2013: 7.

[29] Hamaguchi, Shigeaki, Iwai Tohnai, Akira Ito, Kenji Mitsudo, Toshio Shigetomi, Masafumi Ito, Hiroyuki Honda, Takeshi Kobayashi, and Minoru Ueda. 2003.

"Selective hyperthermia using magnetoliposomes to target cervical lymph node metastasis in a rabbit tongue tumor model". *Cancer Science* 94(9): 834-839.

[30] Geusens, Barbara, Tine Strobbe, Stefanie Bracke, Peter Dynoodt, Niek Sanders, Mireille Van Gele, and Jo Lambert. 2011. "Lipid-mediated gene delivery to the skin". *European Journal of Pharmaceutical Sciences* 43(4): 199-211.

[31] Vora, Bhavana, Ajay J. Khopade, and N. K. Jain. 1998. "Proniosome based transdermal delivery of levonorgestrel for effective contraception". *Journal of Controlled Release* 54(2): 149-165.

[32] Verma, Ashish Kumar and Mahesh Bindal. 2012. "A review on niosomes: an ultimate controlled and novel drug delivery carrier". *International journal of nanoparticles* 5(1): 73-87.

[33] Rahimpour, Yahya and Hamed Hamishehkar. 2012. *Niosomes as carrier in dermal drug delivery*. INTECH Open Access Publisher.

[34] Cevc, G. and F. Paltauf. 1995. *Phospholipids: characterization, metabolism, and novel biological applications : proceedings of the 6th International Colloquium*. AOCS Press.

[35] Gangwar, Mayank, Ragini Singh, R. K. Goel, and Gopal Nath. 2012. "Recent advances in various emerging vescicular systems: An overview". *Asian Pac J Trop Biomed* 2(2): S1176-S1188.

[36] Rajan, Reshmy, Shoma Jose, V Biju Mukund, and Deepa Vasudevan. 2011. "Transferosomes - A vesicular transdermal delivery system for enhanced drug permeation". *Journal of Advanced Pharmaceutical Technology & Research* 2(3): 138-143.

[37] Touitou, E., N. Dayan, L. Bergelson, B. Godin, and M. Eliaz. 2000. "Ethosomes — novel vesicular carriers for enhanced delivery: characterization and skin penetration properties". *Journal of Controlled Release* 65(3): 403-418.

[38] Verma, Poonam and K Pathak. 2010. "Therapeutic and cosmeceutical potential of ethosomes: An overview". *Journal of Advanced Pharmaceutical Technology & Research* 1(3): 274-282.

[39] Sudhakar, C. K., N. Upadhyay, S. Jain, and R. N. Charyulu. "Ethosomes as non-invasive loom for transdermal drug delivery system", in *Nanomedicine and drug delivery*, M. Sebastian, N. Ninan, and A.K. Haghi, Editors. 2013, Apple Academic Press: Canada.

[40] Oliveira, Lidiane Correia de, Eliseu José Fleury Taveira, Leonardo Gomes Souza, Ricardo Neves Marreto, Eliana Martins Lima, and Stephânia Fleury Taveira. 2012. "Aplicações das Nanopartículas Lipídicas no Tratamento de Tumores Sólidos: Revisão de Literatura". *Revista Brasileira de Cancerologia* 58(4): 695-701.

[41] Woodle, Martin C. and Danilo D. Lasic. 1992. "Sterically stabilized liposomes". *Biochimica et Biophysica Acta (BBA) - Reviews on Biomembranes* 1113(2): 171-199.

[42] Felgner, P. L., T. R. Gadek, M. Holm, R. Roman, H. W. Chan, M. Wenz, J. P. Northrop, G. M. Ringold, and M. Danielsen. 1987. "Lipofection: A highly efficient, lipid-mediated DNA-transfection procedure". *Proc Natl Acad Sci* 84: 7413-7417.

[43] Kumar, Dinesh, Deepak Sharma, Gurmeet Singh, Mankaran Singh, and Mahendra Singh Rathore. 2012. "Lipoidal Soft Hybrid Biocarriers of Supramolecular Construction for Drug Delivery". *ISRN Pharm* 2012: 474830.

[44] Karthivashan, G., M. J. Masarudin, A. U. Kura, F. Abas, and S. Fakurazi. 2016. "Optimization, formulation, and characterization of multiflavonoids-loaded flavanosome by bulk or sequential technique". *Int J Nanomedicine* 11: 3417-34.

[45] Zorzi, Giovanni Konat, Edison Luis Santana Carvalho, Gilsane Lino von Poser, and Helder Ferreira Teixeira. 2015. "On the use of nanotechnology-based strategies for association of complex matrices from plant extracts". *Revista Brasileira de Farmacognosia* 25(4): 426-436.

[46] Semalty, A., M. Semalty, M. S. Rawat, and F. Franceschi. 2010. "Supramolecular phospholipids-polyphenolics interactions: the PHYTOSOME strategy to improve the bioavailability of phytochemicals". *Fitoterapia* 81(5): 306-14.

[47] Bonifácio, Bruna Vidal, Patricia Bento da Silva, Matheus Aparecido dos Santos Ramos, Kamila Maria Silveira Negri, Taís Maria Bauab, and Marlus Chorilli. 2014. "Nanotechnology-based drug delivery systems and herbal medicines: a review". *Int J Nanomedicine* 9: 1-15.

[48] Yan-yu, X., S. Yun-mei, C. Zhi-peng, and P. Qi-neng. 2006. "Preparation of silymarin proliposome: a new way to increase oral bioavailability of silymarin in beagle dogs". *Int J Pharm* 319(1-2): 162-8.

[49] Zhang, J., Q. Tang, X. Xu, and N. Li. 2013. "Development and evaluation of a novel phytosome-loaded chitosan microsphere system for curcumin delivery". *Int J Pharm* 448(1): 168-74.

[50] Jin, Y., J. Wen, S. Garg, D. Liu, Y. Zhou, L. Teng, and W. Zhang. 2013. "Development of a novel niosomal system for oral delivery of Ginkgo biloba extract". *Int J Nanomedicine* 8: 421-30.

[51] Ajazuddin and S. Saraf. 2010. "Applications of novel drug delivery system for herbal formulations". *Fitoterapia* 81(7): 680-9.

[52] Ghanbarzadeh, Babak, Afshin Babazadeh, and Hamed Hamishehkar. 2016. "Nano-phytosome as a potential food-grade delivery system". *Food Bioscience* 15: 126-135.

[53] Shakeri, A. and A. Sahebkar. 2016. "Phytosome: a fatty solution for efficient formulation of phytopharmaceutical". *Recent Pat Drug Deliv Formul* 10(1): 7-10.

[54] Pradhan, S. C. and C. Girish. 2006. "Hepatoprotective herbal drug, silymarin from experimental pharmacology to clinical medicine. ". *Indian J Med Res* 124: 491-504.

[55] Javed, S., K. Kohli, and M. Ali. 2011. "Reassessing Bioavailability of Silymarin". *Altern. Med. Rev.* 16(3): 239-249.

[56] Chu, C., S. S. Tong, Y. Xu, L. Wang, M. Fu, Y. R. Ge, J. N. Yu, and X. M. Xu. 2011. "Proliposomes for oral delivery of dehydrosilymarin: preparation and evaluation in vitro and in vivo". *Acta Pharmacol Sin* 32(7): 973-80.

[57] Chang, L. W., M. L. Hou, and T. H. Tsai. 2014. "Silymarin in liposomes and ethosomes: pharmacokinetics and tissue distribution in free-moving rats by high-performance liquid chromatography-tandem mass spectrometry". *J Agric Food Chem* 62(48): 11657-65.

[58] Kumar, N., A. Rai, N. D. Reddy, P. V. Raj, P. Jain, P. Deshpande, G. Mathew, N. G. Kutty, N. Udupa, and C. M. Rao. 2014. "Silymarin liposomes improves oral bioavailability of silybin besides targeting hepatocytes, and immune cells". *Pharmacol Rep* 66(5): 788-98.

[59] Angelico, Ruggero, Andrea Ceglie, Pasquale Sacco, Giuseppe Colafemmina, Maria Ripoli, and Alessandra Mangia. 2014. "Phyto-liposomes as nanoshuttles for water-insoluble silybin–phospholipid complex". *Int J Pharm* 471(1–2): 173-181.

[60] Elmowafy, Mohammed, Tapani Viitala, Hany M. Ibrahim, Sherif K. Abu-Elyazid, Ahmed Samy, Alaa Kassem, and Marjo Yliperttula. 2013. "Silymarin loaded liposomes for hepatic targeting: In vitro evaluation and HepG2 drug uptake". *European Journal of Pharmaceutical Sciences* 50(2): 161-171.

[61] Hamid, A. A., Z. Md. Shah, R. Muse, and S. Mohamed. 2002. "Characterisation of antioxidative activities of various extracts of *Centella asiatica* (L) Urban". *Food Chemistry* 77: 465-469.

[62] Lu, L., K. Ying, S. Wei, Y. Fang, Y. Liu, H. Lin, L. Ma, and Y. Mao. 2004. "Asiaticoside induction for cell-cycle progression, proliferation and collagen synthesis in human dermal fibroblasts". *International Journal of Dermatology* 43: 801-807.

[63] Kartnig, T. 1988. "Clinical applications of *Centella asiatica* (L) Urb.". *Herbs, Spices, and Medicinal Plants* 3: 145-173.

[64] Brinkhaus, B., M. Lindner, D. Schuppan, and E. G. Hahn. 2000. "Chemical, pharmacological and clinical profile of the east asian medical plant *Centella asiatica*". *Phytomedicine* 7(5): 427-448.

[65] Cunha, A. P. M. A. 2010. *Farmacognosia e Fitoquímica*. 3 ed. Brasil.

[66] Wang, J., C. Ma, C. Guo, R. Yuan, and X. Zhan. 2016. "CTG-loaded liposomes as an approach for improving the intestinal absorption of asiaticoside in Centella Total Glucosides". *Int J Pharm* 509(1-2): 296-304.

[67] Ren, Y., X. D. He, B. C. Shang, X. K. Bao, Y. F. Wang, and J. S. Ma. 2013. "[Analysis on preparation and characterization of asiaticoside-loaded flexible nanoliposomes]". *Zhongguo Zhong Yao Za Zhi* 38(19): 3282-6.

[68] Tsai, Wen-Che, Wei-Chu Li, Hsin-Yi Yin, Ming-Chiang Yu, and Hsiao-Wei Wen. 2012. "Constructing liposomal nanovesicles of ginseng extract against hydrogen peroxide-induced oxidative damage to L929 cells". *Food Chem* 132(2): 744-751.

[69] Zhang, Jing, Xizhen Han, Xiang Li, Yun Luo, Haiping Zhao, Ming Yang, Bin Ni, and Zhenggen Liao. 2012. "Core-shell hybrid liposomal vesicles loaded with panax notoginsenoside: preparation, characterization and protective effects on global cerebral ischemia/reperfusion injury and acute myocardial ischemia in rats". *Int J Nanomedicine* 7: 4299-4310.

[70] Choi, Jae-Hwan, Sun-Hang Cho, Je-Jung Yun, Young-Beob Yu, and Cheong-Weon Cho. 2015. "Ethosomes and Transfersomes for Topical Delivery of Ginsenoside Rh1 from Red Ginseng: Characterization and <I>In Vitro</I> Evaluation". *J Nanosci Nanotechnol* 15(8): 5660-5662.

[71] Park, Sung-Il, Eun-Ok Lee, Hee-Man Yang, Chan Woo Park, and Jong-Duk Kim. 2013. "Polymer-hybridized liposomes of poly(amino acid) derivatives as transepidermal carriers". *Colloids and Surfaces B: Biointerfaces* 110: 333-338.

[72] Hao, Fei, Yanxi He, Yating Sun, Bin Zheng, Yan Liu, Xinmei Wang, Yongkai Zhang, Robert J. Lee, Lirong Teng, and Jing Xie. 2016. "Improvement of oral availability of ginseng fruit saponins by a proliposome delivery system containing sodium deoxycholate". *Saudi J Biol Sci* 23(1, Supplement): S113-S125.

[73] Siviero, Angelo, Eugenia Gallo, Valentina Maggini, Luigi Gori, Alessandro Mugelli, Fabio Firenzuoli, and Alfredo Vannacci. 2015. "Curcumin, a golden spice with a low bioavailability". *Journal of Herbal Medicine* 5(2): 57-70.

[74] Kidd, P. M. 2009. "Bioavailability and Activity of Phytosome Complexes from Botanical Polyphenols: The Silymarin, Curcumin, Green Tea, and Grape Seed Extracts". *Alternative Medicine Review* 14(3): 226-246.

[75] Aditya, N. P., Geetanjali Chimote, Karthigayan Gunalan, Rinti Banerjee, Swati Patankar, and Basavaraj Madhusudhan. 2012. "Curcuminoids-loaded liposomes in combination with arteether protects against Plasmodium berghei infection in mice". *Experimental Parasitology* 131(3): 292-299.

[76] Amaral, A. C., L. A. Gomes, J. R. Silva, J. L. Ferreira, S. Ramos Ade, S. Rosa Mdo, A. B. Vermelho, and I. A. Rodrigues. 2014. "Liposomal formulation of turmerone-rich hexane fractions from Curcuma longa enhances their antileishmanial activity". *Biomed Res Int* 2014: 694934.

[77] Saengkrit, Nattika, Somsak Saesoo, Wanwisa Srinuanchai, Sarunya Phunpee, and Uracha Rungsardthong Ruktanonchai. 2014. "Influence of curcumin-loaded cationic liposome on anticancer activity for cervical cancer therapy". *Colloids and Surfaces B: Biointerfaces* 114: 349-356.

[78] Barui, Sugata, Soumen Saha, Goutam Mondal, Shaik Haseena, and Arabinda Chaudhuri. 2014. "Simultaneous delivery of doxorubicin and curcumin encapsulated in liposomes of pegylated RGDK-lipopeptide to tumor vasculature". *Biomaterials* 35(5): 1643-1656.

[79] Catalan-Latorre, Ana, Maryam Ravaghi, Maria Letizia Manca, Carla Caddeo, Francesca Marongiu, Guido Ennas, Elvira Escribano-Ferrer, José Esteban Peris,

Octavio Diez-Sales, Anna Maria Fadda, and Maria Manconi. 2016. "Freeze-dried eudragit-hyaluronan multicompartment liposomes to improve the intestinal bioavailability of curcumin". *European Journal of Pharmaceutics and Biopharmaceutics* 107: 49-55.

[80] Liu, Yujia, Dandan Liu, Li Zhu, Qian Gan, and Xueyi Le. 2015. "Temperature-dependent structure stability and in vitro release of chitosan-coated curcumin liposome". *Food Research International* 74: 97-105.

[81] Zheng, Bin, Lirong Teng, Gaoyang Xing, Ye Bi, Shuang Yang, Fei Hao, Guodong Yan, Xinmei Wang, Robert J. Lee, Lesheng Teng, and Jing Xie. 2015. "Proliposomes containing a bile salt for oral delivery of Ginkgo biloba extract: Formulation optimization, characterization, oral bioavailability and tissue distribution in rats". *European Journal of Pharmaceutical Sciences* 77: 254-264.

[82] Ripoli, Maria, Ruggero Angelico, Pasquale Sacco, Andrea Ceglie, and Alessandra Mangia. 2016. "Phytoliposome-Based Silibinin Delivery System as a Promising Strategy to Prevent Hepatitis C Virus Infection". *Journal of Biomedical Nanotechnology* 12(4): 770-780.

[83] Faezizadeha, Z., A. Ghariba, and M. Godarzeeb. 2015. "In-vitro and In-vivo Evaluation of Silymarin Nanoliposomes against Isolated Methicillin-resistant Staphylococcus aureus". *Iranian Journal of Pharmaceutical Research* 14(2): 627-633.

[84] El-Samaligy, Mohamed S., Nagia N. Afifi, and Enas A. Mahmoud. 2006. "Evaluation of hybrid liposomes-encapsulated silymarin regarding physical stability and in vivo performance". *Int J Pharm* 319(1-2): 121-129.

[85] Xiao, Yan-yu, Yun-mei Song, Zhi-peng Chen, and Qi-neng Ping. 2005. "Preparation of silymarin proliposomes and its pharmacokinetics in rats". *Acta pharmaceutica Sinica* 40(8): 758-763.

[86] Hao, F., Y. He, Y. Sun, B. Zheng, Y. Liu, X. Wang, Y. Zhang, R. J. Lee, L. Teng, and J. Xie. 2016. "Improvement of oral availability of ginseng fruit saponins by a proliposome delivery system containing sodium deoxycholate". *Saudi J Biol Sci* 23(1): S113-25.

[87] Choi, Jae-Hwan, Sun-Hang Cho, Je-Jung Yun, Young-Beob Yu, and Cheong-Weon Cho. 2015. "Ethosomes and Transfersomes for Topical Delivery of Ginsenoside Rh1 from Red Ginseng: Characterization and <I>In Vitro</I> Evaluation". *Journal of Nanoscience and Nanotechnology* 15(8): 5660-5662.

[88] Tsai, Wen-Che, Wei-Chu Li, Hsin-Yi Yin, Ming-Chiang Yu, and Hsiao-Wei Wen. 2012. "Constructing liposomal nanovesicles of ginseng extract against hydrogen peroxide-induced oxidative damage to L929 cells". *Food Chemistry* 132(2): 744-751.

[89] Zhang, J., X. Han, X. Li, Y. Luo, H. Zhao, M. Yang, B. Ni, and Z. Liao. 2012. "Core-shell hybrid liposomal vesicles loaded with panax notoginsenoside:

preparation, characterization and protective effects on global cerebral ischemia/reperfusion injury and acute myocardial ischemia in rats". *Int J Nanomedicine* 7: 4299-310.

[90] Park, S. I., E. O. Lee, H. M. Yang, C. W. Park, and J. D. Kim. 2013. "Polymer-hybridized liposomes of poly(amino acid) derivatives as transepidermal carriers". *Colloids Surf B Biointerfaces* 110: 333-8.

[91] Wang, H., M. Liu, and S. Du. 2014. "Optimization of madecassoside liposomes using response surface methodology and evaluation of its stability". *Int J Pharm* 473(1-2): 280-5.

[92] Paolino, D., D. Cosco, F. Cilurzo, E. Trapasso, V. M. Morittu, C. Celia, and M. Fresta. 2012. "Improved in vitro and in vivo collagen biosynthesis by asiaticoside-loaded ultradeformable vesicles". *J Control Release* 162(1): 143-51.

[93] Saesoo, S., I. Sramala, A. Soottitantawat, T. Charinpanitkul, and U. R. Ruktanonchai. 2010. "Enhanced stability and in vitro bioactivity of surfactant-loaded liposomes containing Asiatic Pennywort extract". *J Microencapsul* 27(5): 436-46.

[94] Yeh, C. C., Y. H. Su, Y. J. Lin, P. J. Chen, C. S. Shi, C. N. Chen, and H. I. Chang. 2015. "Evaluation of the protective effects of curcuminoid (curcumin and bisdemethoxycurcumin)-loaded liposomes against bone turnover in a cell-based model of osteoarthritis". *Drug Des Devel Ther* 9: 2285-300.

[95] Hasan, M., N. Belhaj, H. Benachour, M. Barberi-Heyob, C. J. F. Kahn, E. Jabbari, M. Linder, and E. Arab-Tehrany. 2014. "Liposome encapsulation of curcumin: Physico-chemical characterizations and effects on MCF7 cancer cell proliferation". *Int J Pharm* 461(1–2): 519-528.

[96] Kaur, C. and S. Saraf. 2011. "Topical vesicular formulations of Curcuma longa extract on recuperating the ultraviolet radiation–damaged skin". *Journal of Cosmetic Dermatology* 10: 260-265.

[97] Lima, C.A., A.J. Oliveira, A.J.L.A. Pedreira, and S.A.C. Castiglioni, 2006, . . . *Study on economic viability on the implementation of an apiary for honey and propolis production*, in *XLIV Meeting of the Brazilian Society for Rural Sociology and Economy.* July 23rd-27th 2006: Fortaleza, Brazil. Link: http://www.sober.org.br/palestra/ 5/869.pdf, accessed in May 22nd, 2016.

[98] Patil, Y. P. and S. Jadhav. 2014. "Novel methods for liposome preparation". *Chem Phys Lipids* 177: 8-18.

[99] Huang, Zhenjun, Xuan Li, Ting Zhang, Yanzhi Song, Zhennan She, Jing Li, and Yihui Deng. 2014. "Progress involving new techniques for liposome preparation". *Asian Journal of Pharmaceutical Sciences* 9(4): 176-182.

[100] Dua, J. S., A. C. Rana, and A. K. Bhandari. 2012. "Liposome: Methods of preparation and applications". *International Journal of Pharmaceutical Studies and Research* 3(3): 14-20.

[101] Torchilin, V. P. and V. Weissig. 2003. *Liposomes: A pratical approach.* 2 ed. New York: Oxford University Press.

[102] Morton, Leslie A., Jonel P. Saludes, and Hang Yin. 2012. "Constant Pressure-controlled Extrusion Method for the Preparation of Nano-sized Lipid Vesicles". *J Vis Exp* (64): 4151.

[103] Patty, Philipus J. and Barbara J. Frisken. 2003. "The Pressure-Dependence of the Size of Extruded Vesicles". *Biophys J* 85(2): 996-1004.

[104] Liang, Ming T., Nigel M. Davies, and Istvan Toth. 2005. "Encapsulation of lipopeptides within liposomes: Effect of number of lipid chains, chain length and method of liposome preparation". *Int J Pharm* 301(1–2): 247-254.

[105] Varona, Salima, Ángel Martín, and María José Cocero. 2011. "Liposomal Incorporation of Lavandin Essential Oil by a Thin-Film Hydration Method and by Particles from Gas-Saturated Solutions". *Industrial & Engineering Chemistry Research* 50(4): 2088-2097.

[106] Szoka, F. and D. Papahadjopoulos. 1978. "Procedure for preparation of liposomes with large internal aqueous space and high capture by reverse-phase evaporation". *Proc Natl Acad Sci U S A* 75(9): 4194-4198.

[107] Batzri, Shmuel and Edward D. Korn. 1973. "Single bilayer liposomes prepared without sonication". *Biochimica et Biophysica Acta (BBA) - Biomembranes* 298(4): 1015-1019.

[108] Phetdee, M., A. Polnok, and J. Viyoch. 2008. "Development of chitosan-coated liposomes for sustained delivery of tamarind fruit pulp's extract to the skin". *International Journal of Cosmetic Science* 30(4): 285-295.

[109] Wagner, Andreas, Karola Vorauer-Uhl, and Hermann Katinger. 2002. "Liposomes produced in a pilot scale: production, purification and efficiency aspects". *European Journal of Pharmaceutics and Biopharmaceutics* 54(2): 213-219.

[110] Kremer, J. M. H., M. W. Van der Esker, C. Pathmamanoharan, and P. H. Wiersema. 1977. "Vesicles of variable diameter prepared by a modified injection method". *Biochemistry* 16(17): 3932-3935.

[111] Stano, Pasquale, Simone Bufali, Claudio Pisano, Federica Bucci, Marcella Barbarino, Mosè Santaniello, Paolo Carminati, and Pier Luigi Luisi. 2004. "Novel Camptothecin Analogue (Gimatecan)-Containing Liposomes Prepared by the Ethanol Injection Method". *Journal of Liposome Research* 14(1-2): 87-109.

[112] Lasch, J, VR Berdichevsky, VP Torchilin, Regine Koelsch, and K Kretschmer. 1983. "A method to measure critical detergent parameters. Preparation of liposomes". *Analytical biochemistry* 133(2): 486-491.

[113] Enoch, H. G. and P. Strittmatter. 1979. "Formation and properties of 1000-A-diameter, single-bilayer phospholipid vesicles". *Proc Natl Acad Sci U S A* 76(1): 145-149.

[114] Alpes, H, K Allmann, H Plattner, J Reichert, R Rick, and S Schulz. 1986. "Formation of large unilamellar vesicles using alkyl maltoside detergents". *Biochimica et Biophysica Acta (BBA)-Biomembranes* 862(2): 294-302.

[115] Danenberg, Haim D., Gershon Golomb, Adam Groothuis, Jianchuan Gao, Hila Epstein, Rajesh V. Swaminathan, Philip Seifert, and Elazer R. Edelman. 2003. "Liposomal Alendronate Inhibits Systemic Innate Immunity and Reduces In-Stent Neointimal Hyperplasia in Rabbits". *Circulation* 108(22): 2798-2804.

[116] Deamer, D and AD Bangham. 1976. "Large volume liposomes by an ether vaporization method". *Biochimica et Biophysica Acta (BBA)-Nucleic Acids and Protein Synthesis* 443(3): 629-634.

[117] Sun, Feng, Jian Li, Qiang Yu, and Eli Chan. 2012. "Loading 3-deazaneplanocin A into pegylated unilamellar liposomes by forming transient phenylboronic acid–drug complex and its pharmacokinetic features in Sprague–Dawley rats". *European Journal of Pharmaceutics and Biopharmaceutics* 80(2): 323-331.

[118] Frézard, F., M.S.M. Michalick, C.F. Soares, and C. Demicheli. 2000. "Novel methods for the encapsulation of meglumine antimoniate into liposomes". *Brazilian Journal of Medical and Biological Research* 33: 841-846.

[119] Chonn, Arcadio and Pieter R. Cullis. 1998. "Recent advances in liposome technologies and their applications for systemic gene delivery". *Advanced Drug Delivery Reviews* 30(1–3): 73-83.

[120] Cortesi, R. 1999. "Preparation of liposomes by reverse-phase evaporation using alternative organic solvents". *Journal of Microencapsulation* 16(2): 251-256.

[121] Mozafari, M Reza. 2005. "Liposomes: an overview of manufacturing techniques". *Cellular and Molecular Biology Letters* 10(4): 711.

[122] Otake, K., T. Imura, H. Sakai, and M. Abe. 2001. "Development of a new preparation method of lipossomes using supercritical carbon dioxide". *Langmuir* 17: 3898-3901.

[123] Campardelli, Roberta, Islane Espirito Santo, Elaine Cabral Albuquerque, Silvio Vieira de Melo, Giovanna Della Porta, and Ernesto Reverchon. 2016. "Efficient encapsulation of proteins in submicro liposomes using a supercritical fluid assisted continuous process". *The Journal of Supercritical Fluids* 107: 163-169.

[124] Massing, U., S. Cicko, and V. Ziroli. 2008. "Dual asymmetric centrifugation (DAC)--a new technique for liposome preparation". *J Control Release* 125(1): 16-24.

[125] Hirsch, M., V. Ziroli, M. Helm, and U. Massing. 2009. "Preparation of small amounts of sterile siRNA-liposomes with high entrapping efficiency by dual asymmetric centrifugation (DAC)". *J Control Release* 135(1): 80-8.

[126] Charcosset, C. 2006. "Membrane processes in biotechnology: an overview". *Biotechnol Adv* 24(5): 482-92.

[127] Jaafar-Maalej, Chiraz, Catherine Charcosset, and Hatem Fessi. 2011. "A new method for liposome preparation using a membrane contactor". *J Liposome Res* 21(3): 213-220.

[128] Laouini, A., C. Jaafar-Maalej, S. Sfar, C. Charcosset, and H. Fessi. 2011. "Liposome preparation using a hollow fiber membrane contactor--application to spironolactone encapsulation". *Int J Pharm* 415(1-2): 53-61.

[129] Pham, T. T., C. Jaafar-Maalej, C. Charcosset, and H. Fessi. 2012. "Liposome and niosome preparation using a membrane contactor for scale-up". *Colloids Surf B Biointerfaces* 94: 15-21.

[130] Chen, C., D. Han, C. Cai, and X. Tang. 2010. "An overview of liposome lyophilization and its future potential". *J Control Release* 142(3): 299-311.

[131] Ingvarsson, P. T., M. Yang, H. M. Nielsen, J. Rantanen, and C. Foged. 2011. "Stabilization of liposomes during drying". *Expert Opin Drug Deliv* 8(3): 375-88.

[132] Wang, T., Y. Deng, Y. Geng, Z. Gao, J. Zou, and Z. Wang. 2006. "Preparation of submicron unilamellar liposomes by freeze-drying double emulsions". *Biochim Biophys Acta* 1758(2): 222-31.

[133] Wang, T., N. Wang, T. Li, and Y. Deng. 2008. "Freeze drying of double emulsions to prepare topotecan-entrapping liposomes featuring controlled release". *Drug Dev Ind Pharm* 34(4): 427-33.

[134] Wang, T., N. Wang, X. Jin, K. Zhang, and T. Li. 2009. "A novel procedure for preparation of submicron liposomes-lyophilization of oil-in-water emulsions". *J Liposome Res* 19(3): 231-40.

[135] Patil-Gadhe, Arpana and Varsha Pokharkar. 2014. "Single step spray drying method to develop proliposomes for inhalation: A systematic study based on quality by design approach". *Pulmonary Pharmacology & Therapeutics* 27(2): 197-207.

[136] Wang, Lijuan, Xiongwei Hu, Baode Shen, Yunchang Xie, Chengying Shen, Yi Lu, Jianping Qi, Hailong Yuan, and Wei Wu. 2015. "Enhanced stability of liposomes against solidification stress during freeze-drying and spray-drying by coating with calcium alginate". *Journal of Drug Delivery Science and Technology* 30: 163-170.

[137] Sweeney, Lyle G., Zhaolin Wang, Raimar Loebenberg, Jonathan P. Wong, Carlos F. Lange, and Warren H. Finlay. 2005. "Spray-freeze-dried liposomal ciprofloxacin powder for inhaled aerosol drug delivery". *Int J Pharm* 305(1–2): 180-185.

[138] Brunner, G. 1994. *Gas extraction: An Introduction to Fundamentals of Supercritical Fluids and the application to separation processes*. 1 ed, ed. S. Verlag.

[139] Pasquali, Irene and Ruggero Bettini. 2008. "Are pharmaceutics really going supercritical?". *Int J Pharm* 364(2): 176-187.

[140] Zhao, Lisha and Feral Temelli. 2015. "Preparation of liposomes using supercritical carbon dioxide via depressurization of the supercritical phase". *Journal of Food Engineering* 158: 104-112.

[141] Frederiksen, Lene, Klaus Anton, Peter van Hoogevest, Hans Rudolf Keller, and Hans Leuenberger. 1997. "Preparation of Liposomes Encapsulating Water-Soluble Compounds Using Supercritical Carbon Dioxide". *Journal of Pharmaceutical Sciences* 86(8): 921-928.

[142] Campardelli, R., L. Baldino, and E. Reverchon. 2015. "Supercritical fluids applications in nanomedicine". *The Journal of Supercritical Fluids* 101: 193-214.

[143] Meure, L. A., N. R. Foster, and F. Dehghani. 2008. "Conventional and dense gas techniques for the production of liposomes: a review". *AAPS PharmSciTech* 9(3): 798-809.

[144] Santo, Islane Espirito, Roberta Campardelli, Elaine Cabral Albuquerque, Silvio Vieira de Melo, Giovanna Della Porta, and Ernesto Reverchon. 2014. "Liposomes preparation using a supercritical fluid assisted continuous process". *Chemical Engineering Journal* 249: 153-159.

[145] Whitesides, George M. 2006. "The origins and the future of microfluidics". *Nature* 442(7101): 368-373.

[146] Tsai, Wen-Chyan and Syed S. H. Rizvi. 2016. "Liposomal microencapsulation using the conventional methods and novel supercritical fluid processes". *Trends in Food Science & Technology* 55: 61-71.

[147] Yu, Bo, Robert J. Lee, and L. James Lee. 2009. "Microfluidic Methods for Production of Liposomes". 465: 129-141.

[148] van Swaay, Dirk and Andrew deMello. 2013. "Microfluidic methods for forming liposomes". *Lab on a Chip* 13(5): 752-767.

[149] Pautot, Sophie, Barbara J. Frisken, and D. A. Weitz. 2003. "Production of Unilamellar Vesicles Using an Inverted Emulsion". *Langmuir* 19(7): 2870-2879.

[150] Matosevic, S. and B. M. Paegel. 2011. "Stepwise synthesis of giant unilamellar vesicles on a microfluidic assembly line". *J Am Chem Soc* 133(9): 2798-800.

[151] van Swaay, D. and A. deMello. 2013. "Microfluidic methods for forming liposomes". *Lab Chip* 13(5): 752-67.

[152] Jahn, A., F. Lucas, R. A. Wepf, and P. S. Dittrich. 2013. "Freezing continuous-flow self-assembly in a microfluidic device: toward imaging of liposome formation". *Langmuir* 29(5): 1717-23.

[153] Balbino, Tiago A., Nayla T. Aoki, Antonio A. M. Gasperini, Cristiano L. P. Oliveira, Adriano R. Azzoni, Leide P. Cavalcanti, and Lucimara G. de la Torre. 2013. "Continuous flow production of cationic liposomes at high lipid concentration in microfluidic devices for gene delivery applications". *Chemical Engineering Journal* 226: 423-433.

[154] Tien Sing Young, R. V. and M. Tabrizian. 2015. "Rapid, one-step fabrication and loading of nanoscale 1,2-distearoyl-sn-glycero-3-phosphocholine liposomes in a simple, double flow-focusing microfluidic device". *Biomicrofluidics* 9(4): 046501.

[155] Mandal, S., M. Moudgil, and S. K. Mandal. 2009. "Rational drug design". *Eur J Pharmacol* 625(1-3): 90-100.

[156] Singh, Bhupinder, Rajiv Kumar, and Naveen Ahuja. "Optimizing Drug Delivery Systems Using Systematic "Design of Experiments." Part I: Fundamental Aspects", in *Critical Reviews in the Therapeutic Drug Carrier Systems*. 2005: New York. 27-105.

[157] Montgomery, Douglas C. 2012. *Design and Analysis of Experiments*, ed. I. John Wiley & Sons. Tempe, Arizona.

[158] Alund, Siv Jorunn, Gro Smistad, and Marianne Hiorth. 2013. "A multivariate analysis investigating different factors important for the interaction between liposomes and pectin". *Colloids and Surfaces A: Physicochemical and Engineering Aspects* 420: 1-9.

[159] Loukas, Yannis L. 1998. "A computer-based expert system designs and analyzes a 2(k-p) fractional factorial design for the formulation optimization of novel multicomponent liposomes". *Journal of Pharmaceutical and Biomedical Analysis* 17(1): 133-140.

[160] Raj, R., P. M. Raj, and A. Ram. 2016. "Lipid based noninvasive vesicular formulation of cytarabine: Nanodeformable liposomes". *Eur J Pharm Sci* 88: 83-90.

[161] Padamwar, M. N. and V. B. Pokharkar. 2006. "Development of vitamin loaded topical liposomal formulation using factorial design approach: drug deposition and stability". *Int J Pharm* 320(1-2): 37-44.

[162] Seth, A. Kumar, Ambikanandan Misra, and Dipak Umrigar. 2004. "Topical Liposomal Gel of Idoxuridine for the Treatment of Herpes Simplex: Pharmaceutical and Clinical Implications". *Pharmaceutical development and technology* 9(3): 277-289.

[163] Stensrud, Gry, Sverre A. Sande, Solveig Kristensen, and Gro Smistad. 2000. "Formulation and characterisation of primaquine loaded liposomes prepared by a pH gradient using experimental design". *Int J Pharm* 198(2): 213-228.

[164] Casals, Elisenda, Montserrat Gallardo, and Joan Estelrich. 1996. "Factors influencing the encapsulation of thioguanine in DRV liposomes". *Int J Pharm* 143(2): 171-177.

[165] Antony, Jiju. "2 - Fundamentals of Design of Experiments", in *Design of Experiments for Engineers and Scientists*. 2003, Butterworth-Heinemann: Oxford. 6-16.

In: Recent Developments in Phytomedicine Technology ISBN: 978-1-53611-977-0
Editors: L. A. Pedro de Freitas et al.

Chapter 9

STANDARDIZATION AND QUALITY CONTROL OF HERBAL MEDICINES

Luiz Alberto L. Soares and Magda R. A. Ferreira
Laboratory of Pharmacognosy, Federal University of Pernambuco

ABSTRACT

Standardization is an essential step in the development and production of herbal medicines in order to assure the reproducibility of quality, efficacy and safety. The quality of raw materials plays an important role on the successful manufacture of phytopharmaceuticals. However, the acquisition of herbal materials in quantity and quality remains a challenge, due to the influence of several factors such as: biological variability, source of starting herbal materials (cultivation/wildness) and drug processing (drying/grinding/storage). Additionally, the plant materials are susceptible to adulterations, contaminations and deterioration (physicochemical and chemical). Thus, the herbal drugs must comply with detailed specifications or monographs of identity, as well as purity and content; preferably established from clinical studies. The quantitative determination of markers plays a major role on the clinical properties of herbal drug, and it is closely linked to the standardization of herbal medicines. Nevertheless, the chemical homogeneity of herbal materials is also dependent on their intrinsic variability and becomes more critical due to the chemical complexity of such matrices. Thus, crude extracts manufactured directly from herbal materials show qualitative and quantitative data in accordance to the quality of the respective starting raw material. The lack of chemical uniformity observed from batch-to-batch undermines the efficacy and the safety. Subsequently, chemical standardization is a major step in the reproducibility of the efficacy and safety of Phytopharmaceuticals. Regarding the industrial manufacture and the quality control of herbal products, in spite of the complex mixture of phytochemicals, the analytical task has been simplified by modern instrumentation such as the hyphenated-techniques. Notwithstanding, the identification of markers and the availability of Pharmacopeial Reference Materials (standardized extracts/chemical reference substances) are currently a challenge.

Keywords: standardization, quality control, herbal medicine product

INTRODUCTION

The quality of active pharmaceutical ingredients (API), whether of animal, vegetable, mineral, or biotechnological synthesis origin; is based on the assurance of the reproducibility of its efficacy and safety. Once the efficacy and safety are established by clinical and toxicological tests at the early stages of product development, the maintenance of such properties is ensured through a rigorous and continuous evaluation of pre-established specifications for all the factors able to interfere in the reproducibility of the quality of raw materials, manufacturing processes and finished products. This approach is widely known as Quality Assurance and includes Quality Control and the Risk Management; which are key parts for the implementation of good manufacturing practices (GMP) [1, 2].

Taking into account the manufacturing of herbal medicinal products (HMP), the quality control is more critical due to its susceptibility to several sources of variability such as geographical origin, stage and development conditions (age, soil, and climate), and processing (harvesting, transport, drying and storage). In addition, the HMP can be adulterated by addition of ingredients [3], misidentified or even contaminated (heavy metals, pesticides, microorganisms, radioactivity or BSE) [4]. In this context, good agricultural practices and harvesting has an important role in minimizing authenticity problems and meeting minimum safety requirements [5].

The legal specifications for HMP are reported in the respective monographs of national or regional pharmacopeias [6-10]. The minimum legal requirements of quality must be addressed in order to classify the HMP as API. Thus, the quality of such materials is established by the evaluation of authenticity/identity (botanical/DNA), purity and chemical composition (fingerprints and/or quantitative analysis). Among the parameters of quality of HMPs, special attention is given to the chemical analysis. The chemical content (qualitative and quantitative) plays a key role in assuring the effectiveness of the herbal API and has special relevance to therapeutic practices that use crude vegetable drug *in natura* or dried (herbalism); or even simple preparations obtained directly from plant material (crude extracts) [11].

On the other hand, some HMPs are technically elaborated products and are manufactured by several operations and processes of transformation. In order to maintain the biological properties of the herbal materials, the use of high quality raw materials is mandatory. Anyway, inappropriate manufacture adjustment (temperature, time, solvents and others), can easily result in innocuous products or increase the toxic effects [12, 13].

Therefore, safety and efficacy studies have a crucial role in the development of new herbal medicines. Then, after proving the safety and efficacy of the HMP, the product quality is assured by the reproducibility of the manufacturing process. However, the complex nature of herbal materials can introduce important variability in the biological (activity) quality of the final product [14-16]. Additionally, the absence of simple, fast and low cost biological tests is a limitation for the identification and quantification of efficacy/safety deviations due to process failures (setups, traders, raw materials, etc.), making it difficult to use this approach as a decisive tool of corrective procedures to provide the immediate normalization of the manufacturing conditions. In this context, the employment of control methods based on chemical markers is the most widespread strategy for the process and quality control of herbal medicines [13, 17].

The markers are chemically defined compounds from the secondary metabolism of plants and their choice is based on their indispensability to the product's efficacy (clinical markers) in its pharmacological importance (active markers) or only for analytical purposes (analytical markers). Thus, the herbal extracts can be typified according to the knowledge of their chemical content as follows: "Standardized extracts" (the clinical compound(s) is(are) known - clinical marker), "Quantified extracts" (the therapeutically constituent(s) is(are) unknown and the efficacy is attributed to a concentration range of pharmacologically relevant substances) and "Other herbal extracts" (the efficacy is connected to the reproducibility of the manufacturing procedure, and analytical markers are used for in the control process). The full characterized herbal extracts (standardized/ quantified/other), also described as native extracts, are widely used as API in the development of pharmaceutical dosage forms [9, 11, 13, 18].

Regarding the quality control of dosage forms containing herbal extracts, the assays are performed by similar requirements observed for classical dosage forms. However, the chemical complexity and the high dosage of herbal products require more effort either for technological development or for validation of analytical tools [19].

Thus, in this chapter, the quality and standardization requirements and strategies of herbal drug and herbal medicine will be revised and discussed.

THE QUALITY AND STANDARDIZATION OF HERBAL DRUGS

The quality of raw materials plays an important role on the successful manufacture of phytopharmaceuticals. However, the obtainment of drug materials in quantity and quality remains a challenge, due to the influence of several factors such as: biological variability; herbal material source (cultivation/wildness), geographical origin and drug processing (drying/grinding/storage). [20-22]. In addition, the herbal drug is easily susceptible to adulterations, contaminations and deterioration (physicochemical and chemical). Therefore, the quality control of herbal drugs and herbal medicine products (HMP) requires the correct identification of the specie (botanical authentication), seasonality studies (appropriately developed) standardization of techniques of postharvest processing, storage conditions which would minimize the risks of adulteration or substitution [16].

Due to the complex chemical composition and the natural variability of HMP, it is not easy to establish the quality control parameters of such materials. However, the evolution of analytical techniques helped overcome many of these difficulties. Thus, in the quality control of herbal API, their intermediate and final products, it is a parameter of utmost importance and essential for their acceptance in the modern system of health. The WHO has emphasized the use of modern and standardized procedures for conducting quality analyses; in addition to conventional techniques commonly used and reported by various herbal monographs [23].

The quality parameters and respective minimum acceptable limits for API or finished products are reported in pharmacopoeia monographs or other recognized documents such as international guidelines [9, 11, 18, 24-26]. However, just the establishment and evaluation of specifications of the API are not sufficient to ensure the compliance of manufactured products resulting from several operations/processes of transformation. Regarding herbal drugs and HMP, the specifications of quality and the respective analytical procedures are described in detail in specific pharmacopeial monographs [6, 9, 13]. In addition to the pharmacopeias, there are some valid sources such as monographs and guidelines from several organizations such as WHO [27-30], ESCOPE [31, 32] and Commission E [33]. If there is not documentation for the species, the manufacturer must provide the necessary and validated data that addresses the requirements of identity, purity and content [25].

The procedures and methods of evaluation of API quality described in the Pharmacopoeias and equivalent codes are intended to prove the identity, purity and quantification of chemical compounds of interest present in the material. The quantification of substances of interest is the most difficult test because many of the compounds responsible for the effectiveness of API are still unknown. For this reason, often some compounds are elected as markers only with the purpose for quality control, even if there is no evidence of their participation or responsibility for the clinical response. Regardless of the purpose of the test performed (identity, purity or content), all analytical procedures adopted must be described in Pharmacopoeias, recognized or otherwise, which have been properly validated. Considering these aspects, the steps involved in the quality control and standardization of raw materials are described briefly below:

Identity

The first step to perform the standardization of drug materials is the identification. The analysis includes the verification of drug origin, collection area, climate conditions and confirmation of the part of the plant material. Then, the authenticity is performed by botanical micro and macroscopic evaluation of sensory, morphological and anatomical characteristics of the herbal material [23, 34].

So firstly the material is submitted to the analyzes. The research also allows for the search and identification of adulterations and substitutions. Material is whole or coarsely strike-through, and macroscopic analysis with the aid of botanical illustrations present in pharmacopoeia monographs and sensory information (color, form, texture and odor) allow for identification without great difficulty [6, 35].

Macroscopic Analysis

Macroscopic analysis of whole and fragmented coarsely cut herbal materials can be easily performed with the aid of botanical illustrations from specific monographs and sensory data (color, form, texture and odor). The analysis describes general macroscopic properties such as texture, color and consistency. The macroscopic examination can be carried out with the naked eye, but also with the aid of a magnifying glass. Therefore, it is also possible to recognize the presence of different species of analyzed material (adulterants or contaminants), or to identify other parts of the material that are not allowed or not originally integrate into API [6, 9, 35].

Microscopic Analysis

The analysis of the powdered material is complex and requires analysis of microscopic structure characteristics [6, 9, 35]. For microscopic analysis, the material needs to be prepared properly. The blades can be prepared from whole or fragment drug by making histological sections. Depending on the plant tissue or part, specific preparation might be necessary. Firstly, dried materials must be softened before fixed, then, the material can be transferred to the microscopic slides, solution is added to dissolve the starch grains and the cover slip is put on. Finally, the material is stained to distinguish the structures and tissues. In addition, some histochemical reactions may be carried out as a complement to characterize some chemical groups that help the identification of microscopic structures [36-38]. Moreover, with the histochemical data it is also possible to perform a qualitative evaluation of the chemical profile of the material which plays an important role in the identification of varieties and cultivars [39, 40].

DNA Fingerprints

Another alternative used to confirm the drug authenticity is the DNA fingerprints. This tool allows for the indisputable identification of drug materials, improving the ability of detection of substitutions and adulterations, especially in species that exhibit high chemical composition and morphological similarity. Therefore, the herbal drug authenticity can also be ensured through the use of different techniques for determining DNA fingerprints (Simples Sequence Repeats – SSR; Restriction Fragment Length

Polymorphism – RFLP; Amplified Fragment Length Polymorphism – AFLP; Random Amplified Polyphormic DNA – RAPD) [41, 42].

Purity

The purity analysis of herbal API and HMP aims to identify and quantify undesirable components (contaminants) from various sources. The main purity tests include researching foreign materials, moisture content, ash, extractives content and, in some specific cases, also the determination of swelling, bitterness and foam indices. However, additional tests not included in the specific monographs, are also recommended for the residue of heavy metals and pesticides, microbial contamination, mycotoxins, radioactivity and assay for BSE [6-9, 43].

Foreign Materials

Foreign material is defined as undesired additives to the herbal API, such as insects and parts of the same species that do not meet the specifications of the drug or fungi [35]. The pharmacopoeias recommend visual inspection with the naked eye or with the aid of a magnifying glass to search, identify and determine the percentage of foreign elements in the sample or to search by microscopy.

Water Content

The water content is an important parameter for maintaining the quality of the API, since excess water encourages microbial growth, the appearance of fungus contributes to the deterioration of the material followed by hydrolysis. Fresh material has relatively high water content, so the appropriate drying and stabilization of the API is essential so that residual moisture does not compromise its chemical and/or physicochemical properties.

Ash (Total, Sulfated and Insoluble in Acid)

The determination of total ash allows verification of non-volatile inorganic impurities in vegetable API of physiological origin, such as carbonates, phosphates, chlorides and oxides; and non-physiological such as sand, stone and earth, which may be present as contaminants in the API [44]. Thus, the material must be subjected to high temperatures in an oven until all organic matter is burned leaving only mineral waste in the form of gray ash. However, variations are sometimes observed in tests to determine ash due to the volatility of alkali metal and alkaline earth metal chlorides. In this case, the material should be subjected to combustion in the presence of sulfuric acid to obtain sulfated ash content. Finally, the residue of sulfated ash is treated with hydrochloric acid for the presence of ash that is not from a physiological source such as siliceous residues.

Total Content of Extractives Material

The extractives content is the amount of substances that can be extracted with a particular solvent (ethanol, water, or other specified solvent), employing particular methods (maceration, reflux or soxhlet) and pre-defined extraction conditions (hot or cold). The evaporation residue is the result of this parameter

Other Assays: Swelling Indices, Bittering and Foam

These assays are based on typical properties of APIs and act as indicators of quality of herbal drugs. The swelling index is a simple method to indicate the amount of polysaccharides present in API. The bitterness index is used to assess the quality of API rich in bitter principles. The foam index indicates the presence of saponins in plant drugs through foam persistence after vigorous agitation of the material in water.

Microbiological Parameters

Microbiological analysis includes the content of viable microorganisms, the total mold count and the total coliforms count. Thresholds can be used as a quantitative or semi-quantitative tool to determine and control the amount of impurities [23, 45]. Contamination can be derived from the soil, the natural microflora of the species or a contaminant introduced during handling. Therefore, appropriate management conditions are necessary for drying or storage, so as to avoid the development of viable microorganisms intensifying contamination and definitely compromising the API. Microbiological contamination is of toxicological concern, for hygienic reasons and because of the possibility of production of toxins by bacteria and fungi. The microbial load is determined by the number of colony forming units (CFU) using one of the following methods: membrane filtration, plate count or serial dilution [35].

Agrochemicals and Pesticides

Pesticides are used to prevent infestation of plant material in quantities of unwanted species from other species (herbicides), fungi (fungicides), insects (pesticides) or animal (rat poison), and may cause damage or interference during the steps of the productive chain. Plant species, mainly those that are cultivated, can be contaminated by DDT, toxaphene, and aldrin, these pesticides can cause serious side-effects in human [46]. The WHO and FAO (Food and Agricultural Organization of United Nations) set limits for pesticides, and limit tests are necessary to find the acceptable levels of pesticide contamination in herbal ingredients [47].

Heavy Metals

Heavy metals are common constituents of the earth's surface and can infect plant roots. The contamination of plant materials can also occur through industrial emissions. The most relevant heavy metals in order of exposure frequency are lead, cadmium and mercury. The control of heavy metals is important due to the cumulative effect and the existence of several sources of contamination. There are qualitative and quantitative tests recommended by Pharmacopoeias such as atomic spectrometry which permits the quantification of each dopant element in the sample, in addition to setting specific limits for each element according to its toxicity [6].

Radioactive Analysis

The API from nearby regions or regions with possible radioactive contamination should be tested for radioactivity or radiation. However, there is no general method of analysis due to the variability generated by radiation. Therefore, when there is evidence of contamination of the API, samples under study should be directed to competent laboratories. The radioactivity of the raw materials should be checked accordingly with the guidelines of the International Atomic Energy Agency [48] from Vienna and that of WHO [35].

The Analyses of Chemical Markers

The identification and quantification of chemical compounds (markers) is one of the most important tools for the actual quality control of raw materials and products of herbal origin. For this purpose, one or more compounds from the herbal drug can be used as an indicator of the HMP efficacy. Besides the active or analytical marker, there are some important compounds that must also be controlled due to allergenic or toxic properties such as nephotoxicity and hepatotoxicity [49, 50].

However, in addition to the major markers (clinical, active, analytical or negative), the dependency of safety and efficacy of HMP from the chemical complexity is well known. Thus, the multi-component analysis is much more representative and sensitive to detect variations in the chemical quality of HMP and therefore the chemical profiles play a crucial role in the identification and quality control of herbal drugs and products.

The chemical profiles (fingerprints) are widely studied by chromatographic methods such as thin layer chromatography (TLC), high performance liquid chromatography (HPLC) and gas chromatograhy (GC); and they are practically mandatory in herbal monographs. Due to its simplicity, low cost and easy interpretation (identification), the TLC is the most commonly used technique for figerprinting herbal materials. By using high performance TLC (HPTLC) the resolution and reproducibility of herbal fingerprints allows for precise sample application (automatized systems) and optimized separation conditions (controlled chambers). Additionally, the TLC-plates can be scanned and a quantitative analysis carried out by densitometry. Besides the TLC, the fingerprint by HPLC is also popular and its major advantage is the diversity of detectors (usually UV/DAD, MS or NMR). Thus, after chromatographic separation, the compounds can be indentified and quantified. The evaluation of volatile substances from essential oils by GC is mandatory. Similar to HPLC, the GC can be easily hyphened with a MS-detector improving the analyses with identification and quantifications of the substances [43, 51-54].

Regarding the quantitative analysis of chemical markers from HMP, the content requirements reflect the intrinsic variability of such biological matrices, which often have significant batch-to-batch fluctuations, either within the same or different harvests. Therefore, the use of validated analytical methods is required to ensure the performance and stability of the method during its use throughout the analytical routine. All the steps to evaluate the analytical methods are summarized in the guidelines on validation of the International Conference of Harmonization: "Validation of Analytical Procedures: Text and Metodology Q2 (R1)". The guideline summarizes the scientific state-of-art methods of validation [55].

Since the herbal API and HMP are natural products, some issues should be taken into account during analytical method development: sample preparation (clean-up, concentration, solvent system, and extraction procedure and time), sample stability and reaction conditions [56-59].

Chromatographic and Spectroscopic Analysis

The development of effective procedures to carry out the control of herbal materials can be hindered by the lack of information on the substance or group of substances that are responsible for the biological/pharmacological activity [12, 60, 61].

In the last decades, the marker-based quality control of HMP has become well known and is well accepted in the scientific community. However, the synergic effects reported in HMP, in which pharmacological or clinical mechanisms remain totally or partially unexplained, improved in recent years, due to a multi-target approach in the multi-compound mixture from herbal products (API and HMP). Therefore, the qualitative analysis of HMP by chemical fingerprint plays an important role in ensuring the reproducibility of therapeutic efficacy [13, 62].

Subsequently, herbal fingerprints are widely recommended to perform the quality control of HMP, emphasizing the use of a chromatographic or spectroscopic data of biologically active chemical compounds [24, 54, 63].

The identification and evaluation of HMP can be made accurately using several compounds, even if their diversity and concentration are not exactly the same [64]. However, the success of this approach relies on the chromatographic and/or spectroscopic data. Since the HMP presents a complex chemical composition, a chromatographic separation is essential to provide a satisfactory profile [65].

The WHO and Pharmacopoeias recommend the use of chromatographic analysis (TLC, HPTLC, HPLC, GC) and/or spectroscopic (UV, IR, FT-IR, LC-MS, GC-MS) methods to obtain qualitative profiles and for quantification of the main active constituents present in the raw materials and their derivatives. The quality control and standardization of raw materials and herbal medicines by chromatographic and spectrometric analysis help to provide batch to batch comparability and the chromatogram/spectra may be used as a fingerprint by demonstrating the profile of some common plant constituents.

The chemical composition of plant materials is variable because it depends on factors such as the biological variability, stage of development, soil and weather interference, seasonality, and pests, among others [66]. Therefore, the composition needs to be defaulted to ensure the therapeutic efficacy and efficiency. Thus, obtaining fingerprints has been used to detect active compounds that have a measurable concentration, and to obtain the profile of substances present in the material. Recently, new technologies have become available to obtain the profiles, such as infrared spectroscopy, metabolite profiling and determinations based on NMR [67].

Thin layer chromatography (TLC), High performance liquid chromatography (HPLC), High performance thin layer chromatography (HPTLC), and Gas chromatography (GC) can be employed in order to establish the constant composition of herbal preparations. Depending on whether the active principles of the preparation are known or unknown, different concepts such as "normalization versus standardization" have to be applied in order to establish relevant criteria for uniformity. The major challenge of the quality analysis of HMP is the quantitative analysis of phytocompounds, notably for those species in which the active components are unknown. Thus, chemical markers can be used. However, there are several species whose phytochemicals (either active or marker) weren't yet reported, the content of extractable matter using with water or alcohol as solvent, can be accept as a quality assay described by several pharmacopeias [34, 35]. Another special form of assay is the determination of essential oils by hydrodistillation or steam distillation [14]. Regarding HMP whose phytocompounds are known, the chemical analyses can be carried out by a lot of modern analytical tools such spectroscopy/spectrometry (UV/VIS, IR, NMR, MS), chromatographic (TLC, HPLC, HPTLC, GC), or hyphened techniques (GC-MS, LC-PDA, LC-MS, LC-MS/MS, LC-NMR, etc.) [68-70].

The quantitative determination of markers plays a major role on the clinical properties of herbal drug and it is closely linked to standardized herbal medicines. However, the chemical homogeneity of herbal materials is also dependent on their intrinsic variability and becomes more critical due to the chemical complexity of such matrices. Thus, crude extracts manufactured directly from herbal materials show qualitative and quantitative data in accordance to the quality of the respective starting raw material. The lack of chemical uniformity observed from batch-to-batch undermines the efficacy and the safety. Subsequently, chemical standardization is a major step in the reproducibility of the efficacy and safety of Phytopharmaceuticals [14, 71, 72].

Nevertheless, there are several plant species in which the active constituents are not yet known and the chemical standardization of such products is not possible. In these cases, the efficacy and safety are assured by the use of standardized industrial processes. The in-process control is performed by chromatographic profiles (qualitatively) and by an analytical marker(s) (quantitatively). The uses of high-quality herbal materials play a fundamental role in the successful production of such herbal medicines with lower content variation.

THE STANDARDIZATION AND QUALITY OF HERBAL MEDICINES

Standardization of Herbal Medicines

The practice of traditional medicine using herbal drugs (Herbalism) or simple preparations (such as teas and tinctures), imposes a great challenge to their standardization. The intrinsic variability of herbal materials provides significant inconsistency in the content of markers (clinical, analytical or assets), whose profiles are reproduced in the crude extracts. Thus, even if high quality raw materials are used, there will always be fluctuation in the chemical content of crude extracts. Therefore, the factors that can affect the quality of vegetable drugs (origin: cultivated/wild; harvesting and post-harvest procedures) must be optimized, controlled and the variation minimized, since the efficacy and safety of HMP are ensured by reproducibility of the amount of herbal drug in the crude extracts. Thus, after complying with the legal quality requirements (identity, purity and content), the standardization of HMP can be achieved by blending different batches of herbal materials (cultivated and/or wild).

Since the type and concentration of extracted compounds are guided by the physicochemical properties from the solvent systems, the reproducibility of the chemical profiles of crude extracts are directly linked to the quality of the extractive solvent. In addition, extractive parameters and adjustments should also be observed. Drug characteristics such as quantity and particle size, the extractive procedure (infusion, decoction, percolation, turboextraction, etc.) and/or the extractive conditions (temperature, time and velocity), can increase or decrease the extraction performance. Therefore, as reported for herbal drugs, the standardization of crude extract is carried out by setting the extractive conditions in order to comply with the minimum quality specifications. There are in the literature several studies reporting the evaluation and optimization of extractive procedures in order to achieve higher quality extracts with maximum levels of chemical markers (individual/groups) and/or extractive matters [48, 73-85].

The natural variability of herbal drugs plays an important role in the industrial manufacture of herbal medicines (phytopharmaceuticals), and the chemical spectrum should be taking into account the batch-to-batch homogeneity in order to provide medicines with the same quality (including efficacy and safety). Thus, some issues such as: chemo-varieties and cultivars; harvesting and post-harvesting procedures, are fundamental for the herbal drug quality, and can be addressed through cultivation under controlled conditions by applying good agricultural and manufacturing practices [5, 26, 62, 86].

After fulfilling the legal requirements for the minimum quality (identity, purity and physicochemical), the influence of biological variability on chemical content, should be addressed. This variability can be reduced but cannot be completely eliminated and should be tracked and balanced so that the material shows a uniform content. The adjustment can be initially achieved by the blending of batches of herbal materials and/or crude extracts to meet a specific or restricted range of chemical compounds. However, the final adjustment is performed by the extraction conditions (solvents, enrichment steps, methods and equipment) and at the manufacture of the dosage form [12, 13].

The extraction conditions and manufacturing processes should be defined to provide the adjustments in accordance with the knowledge of the pharmacological/therapeutic properties of the herbal drug and respective chemical content. Thus, the herbal extracts can be classified into three types: standardized, quantified or other extracts [25, 87]:

In standardized extracts the efficacy is attributed to a known substance or a group of substances (clinical markers). Thus, these extracts show a narrow range of markers and the standardization is achieved by adding excipients and/or by blending several batches of the herbal native extracts. Such adjustments (normalization) provide a final extract with a constant concentration of chemical markers and a variable content of excipients [13, 87].

A similar approach is applied to quantified extracts. The efficacy of such extracts is assured by the adjustment of the chemical content to a specific range of its pharmacologically relevant substance or group of substances. Then, the quantified extracts make sense only if the pharmacological and toxicological data from chemical markers (active markers) are available. Also, the clinical data of the extract play an important role in the establishment of marker concentration range. The addition of excipients is not allowed.

Regarding the other extracts, the quality is assured by the reproducibility of the manufacturing process (standardized manufacture). The use of chemical markers (analytical markers) plays a key role in the control process, as they match the chemical quality of raw materials. So, although the analytical markers are effective to evaluate the consistency of the production process, their concentrations in the final extract show the same variability observed for the herbal drug. For these extracts the content adjustments either by blend of herbal materials or by excipients are not allowed.

Besides the type of extracts described by pharmacopoeias [9], there is another possibility to classify extracts, known as special or purified extracts. Unlike the previous types of extracts, the manufacture of enriched or purified extract employs several processes that are able to improve the content of active substances (clinical or active markers); and/or, to reduce/eliminate toxic substances such as allergens or carcinogens, and are present in the herbal drug. In this way, several operational steps are widely used for the manufacturing of special extracts, *among which* we *can highlight:* selective extraction process; fractioning/partitions; precipitation followed by filtration; and chromatographic separations. Despite the challenge and effort necessary in the technological development and production of special/purified extracts, the advantage is the possibility of intellectual property protection of products and processes [87, 88].

Strategies for Herbal Medicines Standardization

The major challenges related to the standardization of herbal medicine products starts with the lack of scientific information about its clinical efficacy. Added to this, the complex chemical composition (many of them active, but not always directly responsible for the clinical activity), which requires a very complex standardization task. Accordingly, standardization based on a single marker is often inappropriate and in many cases other substances must also be controlled, because they may have an important role in the processes of bioavailability, metabolization or excretion of the active compounds [89, 90]. Finally, the already known variability of biological matrices such plant material must be taken into account, as well as all the factors that can affect their quality, as discussed above.

Some strategies have been reported in order to try to establish patterns that ensure the reproducibility of the activity and safety of HMP. The simplest approach which is widely reported in the literature deals with the standardization of the manufacturing process (drug: solvent ratio; solvent characteristics; extractive process and conditions), and after confirmation of the activity of HMP, the resultant chemical quality is adopted as the quantitative and qualitative specifications [80, 85, 91-95].

The qualitative chemical profile (TLC, HPLC, GC, etc.) and/or the content/contents compounds or chemical groups are used as a reference for reproducible biological quality of HMP. However, the variations in this analysis either qualitative (number and intensity of peaks/spots) or quantitative (content of compounds or chemical groups) indicate only a lack of compliance with the specifications and are not enough to infer about the safety and effectiveness of such products. Therefore, this kind of data is sufficient for assessing the quality of products typified as “Quantified” extracts and “Other” extracts (based on the standardization of manufacturing process). Thus, before the adoption of these requirements as references, the sources of variability for each process step should be studied to know and predict the quality deviation of the raw materials (batch of herbal drug) as well as the stability of the manufacturing procedure [13, 87].

Although these studies aren't enough to assure the therapeutic markers, they are important references to deepen knowledge of the relevant chemical compounds in species or HMP. Thus, they can be used in the development of new standardized and purified/special extracts. An interesting approach to illustrate this method is shown in Figure 1.

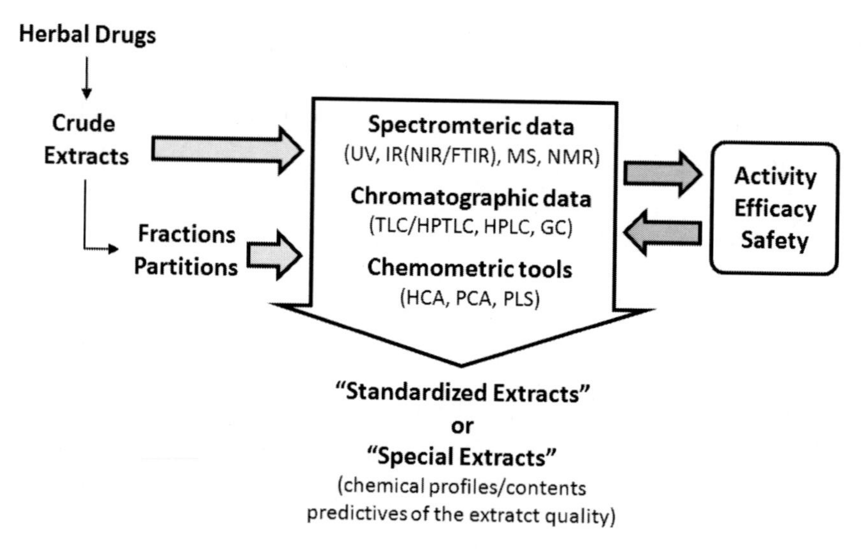

Figure 1. Strategy for herbal medicine standardization.

Accordingly, crude extracts from well known traditional herbal species are chemically characterized and then subjected to *in vivo* and *in vitro* models. After the confirmation of biological properties, the extracts can be enriched by liquid-liquid extraction [70, 85, 96-104]. The fraction is characterized and tested in biological models. The protocol can be repeated until the main compounds or groups of compounds responsible for the biological activity are identified. Thereafter, the fraction is finally characterized qualitatively (chemical profile) and quantitatively (marker content), which are predictive of safety and efficacy of the extract. Finally, the typical chromatographic profiles (fingerprints) and the ranges of marker concentrations can be established as a quality specification of extracts or fractions.

Several modern analytical tools (IR, MS, NMR, HPLC and GC) have been used to aid the elucidation of the qualitative and quantitative compositions from crude extracts and fractions. However, the nature of the analytical responses (spectroscopic and chromatographic), added to the chemical complexity inherent in herbal matrices, provide a high volume of chromatographic and/or spectroscopic data, imposing great difficulty in the interpretation of such data. Thus, chemometric tools play a crucial role in the data treatment and are mandatory before interpretation and correlations. The chemometric approach improves significantly the ability of comparative analysis and detects unexpected changes through mathematical simplification, but without losing any critical information from the original data [51, 53, 72, 86, 105, 106].

Among the chemometric techniques most used for pattern recognition in vegetable derived fingerprinting studies are the principal component analysis (PCA) and hierarchical cluster analysis (HCA). This approach allows for the classification of the sample into different groups according to their similarities. As well as the PCA and HCA there are other statistical methods used to identify or classify herbal samples such as linear discriminant anlaysis [107] [108]; partial least squares (PLS) and partial last square-discriminant analysis (PLS-DA) [109]; and orthogonal partial least squares (OPLS) and the respective discriminant analysis (OPLS-DA) [110, 111].

The Chemometric Techniques and the Analysis of Complex Mixtures

Since the quality control of HMP is based on traditional use or on the quantitative analysis of chemical markers, the identification and quantification of such substance markers are usually chosen from one or more pharmacologically important substances present in the sample [86, 112].

Therefore, the *fingerprint* technique is recognized and accepted by the World Health Organization (WHO) and regulatory agencies (*Brazilian Health Surveillance Agency-ANVISA, Food and Drug Administration-FDA* and *European Medicine-EMA*) as a strategy for the evaluation of natural products [24, 63, 113], emphasizing the use of qualitative and quantitative comparative analysis of spectroscopic and chromatographic *fingerprint* of herbal materials/extracts/products (herbal drugs, extracts or certified chemicals) to ensure the identity and quality [114].

The *fingerprint* of traditional products, such as spectrum or chromatogram obtained by a specific procedure, is unique and allows the researcher to typify the chemical profile of this type of material [53]. This profile must be characterized by identifying multicompounds used in traditional medicine and can be made according to the similarities or differences. However, the major challenge is to develop approaches capable of obtaining useful information, considering the abundance of raw data produced when analyzing data generated by chromatograms and spectra [115, 116].

The combination of fingerprint with chemometric methods increases the speed and reliability of processing of data, providing maximum relevant chemical information [106]. Among the most commonly used chemometric procedures are: optimization of experiments; pattern recognition (methods of exploratory analysis and classification); selection of samples and spectral variables; multivariate calibration [117].

Most studies in the scientific literature focus on *fingerprints* for correlation with biological activity; pattern recognition and quantification of markers by spectroscopic methods with multivariate calibration [118, 119].

Pattern Recognition

Principal Component Analysis (PCA) and Cluster Analysis (CA)

Even with the amount of information generated in herbal drugs analysis (spectra, chromatograms or chemical data), the ultimate goal is to find similarities and trends in the analyzed data. Considering these aspects, the chemometric *Principal Component Analysis* (PCA) and *Cluster Analysis* (CA) have been exploited for the assessment and classification of plant extracts based on discriminatory analysis for mainly similarity research [120].

PCA is the basis of pattern recognition methods, classification and multivariate calibration. It is usually applied to fingerprint analysis and other data in order to visualize the data structure, finding similarities between samples to detect outlier samples and reduce the dimensionality of the data set [112, 120]. The cluster analysis is based on quantitative characteristics to classify samples and to evaluate the quality of medicinal plants, the most used is the hierarchical clustering analysis (HCA), due to technical flexibility, in addition to using dendograms that allow better visualization of results [121]. Currently, the herbal drug analysis of extracts and products using the combination of PCA and HCA has been widespread. Santos et al. [122] studied the authenticity of *Phyllanthus* species by NMR and FT-IR techniques coupled with PCA and HCA analysis. Gad et al. [112] used PCA and HCA to verify the authenticity of *Thymus* species associated with spectrophotometry in the ultraviolet region.

Multivariate Calibration

A part of chemometrics used for quantitative analysis is a multivariate calibration, a process in which models are built that can provide characteristics or properties of interest of unknown samples [123, 124]. A variety of regression methods have been widespread in the construction of multivariate calibration models, among these which have been highlighted in the literature are: *Classical Least Square* (CLS), *Multiple Linear Regression* (MLR), *Principal Component Regression* (PCR) and *Partial Least Square* (PLS).

Recent works with natural products have been aimed at the determination and quantification of secondary metabolites in some species groups [125, 126]. Such is the case of this technique in the study of phenolic compounds in grapefruit; to identify the natural extracts containing polyphenols in its composition or in the identification/ differentiation of plants which may have the same common name, although they are characterized as different plant species [127, 128]. Wang et al. [129] achieved excellent results in the determination of isoflavone in *Pueraria lobata* by NIR. Viegas et al. [130] determined the quality of fruits of *Syzygium malaccense* by NIR.

STANDARDIZED EXTRACTS BY PHARMACOLOGICAL ACTIVITY

Although the herbal standardization approach related to traditional knowledge or adoption of markers is recommended by official codes to establish quality specifications for most medicinal plant, the design does not ensure the therapeutic quality of HMP since the biological activity is often related to the complex chemical composition of herbal materials. Hence, minor variations in the diversity and/or the concentration of the chemical constituents may affect the therapeutic and/or toxic properties due to the synergistic action (often unknown) of the multiple secondary metabolites present in herbal drugs [131].

Given the difficulties in standardizing and defining quality parameters for herbal drugs, the *metabolic profiling* technique has been widely used in recent years. This technique consists of using the *fingerprint* of the species to identify key markers and other compounds in order to correlate their synergistic contribution with the expected effectiveness [52, 53, 116].

Recent studies have been conducted to standardize extracts based on pharmacological activity, demonstrating the use of chromatographic profile to characterize the extract and/or the groups responsible for such activity. Araujo et al. [98] evaluated the antimicrobial, analgesic and anti-inflammatory activivity of aqueous and acetone-water extracts of *Libidibia ferrea*, *Parapiptadenia rigida* and *Psidium guajava*, and associated these activities with the presence of phenolic compounds evidenced in the *fingerprint* obtained by HPLC. Oliveira et al. [104] found that the low toxicity, non-genotoxicity and inhibitory effect of acute inflammation of the hydroalcoholic extract of *Morus alba* was probably due to the presence of chlorogenic acid and flavonoids in the composition, as evidenced in the *fingerprint* obtained by HPLC.

DEVELOPMENT, PRODUCTION AND QUALITY CONTROL OF HERBAL MEDICINES

Since herbal teas contain powdered or sliced materials for tea sachets, the pharmacognostical standardization of high quality drug materials plays an important role in order to assure the safety and the expected activity. The pharmacopeial definition of this herbal product is a herbal drug(s) for aqueous preparations obtained by infusion, decoction or maceration for use immediately after preparation [9]. Alongside the standardized preparation conditions (drug amount, water volume, temperature and/or time); the drug processing, such as drying (residual moisture) and milling (mean particle size), are also important [9, 12, 19, 87].

Some advantages can be attributed to the tea sachet, such as handling, reproducibility of dose (drug amount per bag) and possibility of fine milled material in order to reach maximum extraction. However, some disadvantages are also observed, these being the sachets are unable to retain volatile compounds and the material can undergo oxidative degradations due to the low particle size. In addition, contaminants cannot be observed after production. The quality control of such products is performed in accordance to the respective herbal monograph, including identification (macroscopic and microscopic analysis), chemical content (qualitative and quantitative), and contaminations (microbial, pesticide, radioactivity, and heavy metals) [9, 13, 132].

Regarding the production of herbal extracts, as discussed above, the extract manufacturing is guided by the type of chemical marker to produce Standardized, Quantified or Other extracts. The herbal extracts are mainly manufactured by percolation or maceration to produce Tinctures or Fluid Extracts. These primary extracts are known as "genuine/native extracts" [13, 87, 88].

The manufacture of Tinctures follows the traditional pharmacopeial procedure using drug:extract ratio (DER) of 1:5 or 1:10 (w:v), where the mixtures of ethanol are used as extractive solvent and the extraction occurs by percolation or maceration [6, 9, 13].

Moreover, Fluid Extracts are liquid preparations in which a part of volume or mass corresponds to a part of dry mass of herbal drug used in its manufacture. They are prepared at DEV of 1:1 (w/v) and, if necessary, these preparations can also be specified in relation to the solvent concentration, markers content or dry residue. Since the quality of the raw material plays an important role in the quality of genuine/native liquid extracts, the evaluation of such extracts includes the analysis of contaminants (microbial, heavy metals, mycotoxin, and pesticides). In addition, the content of marker (clinical, active or analytical) and the physicochemical analysis (density, dry residue, content of ethanol, methanol and 2-propanol) are required [6, 9, 13].

However, in most cases, the native extracts cannot be used directly in the manufacturing of final Phytopharmaceuticals. Thus, several native extracts are widely used as intermediary products in the preparation of soft or dry extracts [133]. If an organic solvent such as acetone or methanol is used as extractive medium, the solvent should be completely eliminated and the dry residue should be determined in relation to the initial native extract. Following this, the pre-concentrated extract is further concentrated until reaching a minimum extractive content of 50% (p.ex. using a falling fill evaporator). The concentrated extract can be used to produce instant granulated teas by agglomeration with a filler material such as sucrose or maltodextrin; or it can be completely dried by using spray dryers or vacuum belt dryers [88, 134-136].

The herbal dried extracts are widely produced as an important technological intermediary to produce solid dosage forms. The dried extracts have several advantages such as stability (physical and chemical), mean particle size, density (tapped and bulk), flowability and content uniformity. In addition, the use of excipients can improve the technological properties of the dried extracts, specifically the stability, density and compressibility [137-142]. However, only the spray dried extracts can be obtained as finished products. Other drying procedures for herbal extracts such as vacuum belt dryers required other processing steps such as milling.

Beside their rheological properties, the quality of dried extract is performed by identity (fingerprints: by TLC, HPLC, GC, etc.), purity (moisture, mycotoxin, heavy metals, pesticides and microbial), residual solvents (genuine extracts prepared by organic solvents) and chemical content (qualitative and quantitative analysis). The quantitative analysis of chemical marker is based on the extract types: Standardized, Quantified or Other extracts. In this context, the adjustments of chemical content are widely performed by different charges of dried extracts or by the addition of excipients. Regarding the Special or Purified Extracts, the content is adjusted during the extractive process by steps such as: selective solvents, partition/fraction (liquid-liquid extraction), adsorption and precipitation/ filtration [9, 13, 87].

The stability of dried extracts is carried out in order to evaluate organoleptic properties (odor or taste), physical (solubility, homogeneity, agglomeration and color), chemical (marker content, fingerprint and degradation products), and microbial contaminations. The stability tests are performed at short (6 months), intermediate (12 months) and long term (until 24 months) periods [25, 87].

The study of pre-formulation of herbal medicines or phytopharmaceuticals is a challenging and time-consuming task. The chemical complexity, physic-chemical properties and the high dosage of herbal derivate should be taken into account during the technological development and production of such medicines [142-144].

The liquid preparation (herbal extract) can be manufactured directly as a final product (Fluid Extracts and Tinctures) or, by direct incorporation/dilution, it can also be used in the production of other liquid products (solution, lotions, syrups, emulsions, etc.) and semi-solid dosage forms (creams, gels, ointments, etc.). In the same way, the herbal oils and volatile oils can be directly incorporated into semi-solid systems either in the lipophilic phase of disperse systems or direct dissolution in lipophilic excipients. The quality of such products is based on the specifications for herbal derivate (identity, purity and marker content) and the properties of the pharmaceutical dosage form (content uniformity, density, refraction index, pH, moisture, ethanol concentration, viscosity, dispersitivity, interface tension, stabilities, etc.) [9, 145-147].

On the other hand, herbal dried extracts have been used successfully to produce phytopharmaceuticals. In comparison to liquid preparations, dried extracts have shown some advantages such as stability, density and handling. Additionally, dried extracts can easily be used as intermediaries to produce several dosage forms, from instantaneous teas to tablets. The solid dosage forms are preferable due to their higher stability, accurate dosage, lower volume per dose, high throughput screening and relatively low cost to produce [141, 142, 144, 148].

Some difficulties are reported in the manufacture of solid dosage form containing dried herbal extracts as active pharmaceutical ingredient (API), these include:

- the lower uniformity of mass for standardized/quantified extracts;
- high amount of API per dosage; lower technological properties (hygroscopicity, lower density and flowability); and,
- dissolution/disintegration difficulties (lipophilic composition, especially for purified extracts).

To overcome such difficulties, several technological strategies were developed in the last two decade. First of all, the easiest way is the addition of excipients such as high disperse colloidal silicon, microcrystalline cellulose and maltodextrin, among others [142, 146, 149-156]. The excipients can be added by dispersion in the liquid extract before drying (spray-dryer) or by blending after drying (vacuum belt dryer). In any case, the purpose of the excipients is to improve the technological properties of the dried product. Moisture stability, flowability, packing density, particle size and compressibility are some examples of the particle bed improvements. However, in many cases the addition of excipients isn't enough to ensure the minimum requirements necessary to enable the production of solid forms such as capsules or tablets. Thus, as well as the direct compression of dried extracts blended with excipients, alternatives of agglomeration have been studied, such as wet granulation, dried granulation and extrusion [140, 142, 143, 148, 157-159]. Either as final medicine product or as an intermediary to produce another solid dosage form, the quality control of granules from dried extracts is performed by the determination of residual moisture, hygroscopicity (water sorption and desorption isotherms), density (apparent, real, bulk and tapped), porosity, flowability, particle size and granulometry, disintegration, dissolution, content uniformity, friability and hardness [6, 9, 160]. Regarding capsules containing granules from dried herbal extracts, the quality control also includes the analysis of the final dosage form by uniformity of mass, uniformity of content, disintegration and dissolution [6, 9, 146, 161].

Tablets containing herbal dried extracts require more attention during development and production. The physical properties of particle bed (powdered or granulated), plays an important role in the success of compaction and in the final properties of the tablet. Therefore, direct compression of dried herbal extracts is complex due to their quite often poor compressional properties (hygroscopicity, flowability, density and compressibility). Notwithstanding, several studies about the compressional performance of dried extracts have been reported [142, 143, 162], with the findings that pre-processing by dry granulation seems to be the more effective strategy to enable the compression of such materials [142, 143, 148, 159, 163, 164]. The quality control of tablets containing dried herbal extracts are described in the literature and include: dimensions (height, diameter and thickness), uniformity of mass and content, hardness, friability, disintegration and dissolution [144, 164-169].

Therefore, the quality control of pharmaceutical dosage forms containing herbal drugs or herbal drug derivates are performed exactly as classic dosage forms, and their specifications are summarized below in Table 1.

Table 1. Quality control assays for HMP dosage forms [6, 9, 13, 19, 145, 146]

	Dosage Form			
Assay	**Herbal teas**	**Extracts and other liquid preparations**	**Semi-solid**	**Solid**
Characteristics	Visual appearance (color and form), taste, smell, texture.	Color, appearance, smell	Color, appearance, form	Color, appearance, form
Pharmaceutical test	Mean particle size, granulometry, residual moisture	Relative density, refraction index, pH, uniformity of volume/masse, water and ethanol contents, viscosity, dry residue	Fats and fixed oils ratio (hydroxyl, iodine, acid and saponification values; unsaponificable matter), pH, water content, uniformity of volume/mass, reology (consistency, viscoelasticity), *in vitro* release (open diffusion cell systems).	Powder/granules: densities, porosity, flow, particle size, moisture, hygroscopicy, friability, hardness, solubility, content uniformity. Capsules/Tablets: dimensions (height, diameter and mass), uniformity of mass, content, moisture, friability, hardness, disintegration, *in vitro* dissolution,
Identity	Macroscopic and microscopic analysis, Chromatographic fingerprint	Chromatographic fingerprint	Chromatographic fingerprint	Chromatographic fingerprint
Purity	Foreign matter, ashes, extractable matter, microbial limits, heavy metals, mycotoxins, pesticides, fumigation agents, radioactivity, degradation products,	Methanol, 2-propanol, microbial limits, heavy metals, mycotoxins, pesticides, degradation products,	Microbial limits, heavy metals, mycotoxins, pesticides, degradation products,	Microbial limits, heavy metals, mycotoxins, pesticides, degradation products,
Content	• Standardized extracts: ± 5% of declared concentration of clinical marker declared; • Quantified extracts: ± 5% of declared value of active marker declared; • Other extracts: ± 5% until 10% of the analytical marker declared.			
Others	Volatile oils, swelling index, bitterness value, foaming index	Interfacial tension, conductivity, mean particle/droplets size, sedimentation velocity, zeta potential	Interfacial tension, melt point, mean particle/droplet size, sedimentation velocity, zeta potential	Film integrity (modified release), compressional behavior (API/mixture).

REFERENCES

[1] Haleem, Reham M., Maissa, Y. Salem., Faten, A. Fatahallah. & Laila, E. Abdelfattah. (2015). "Quality in the pharmaceutical industry – A literature review.". *Saudi Pharmaceutical Journal*, *23*, 463–469.

[2] WHO. (2007). Guideline on good manufacturing practices (GMP) for herbal medicines. World Health Organization: Geneve.

[3] Calahan, Dylan Howard., Ahmad, J. Almalki., Mahabir, P. Gupta. & Angela, I. Calderón. (2016). "Chemical Adulterants in Herbal Medicinal Products: A Review". *Planta Medica*, *82*, 505-515.

[4] WHO. (2007). Guidelines for assessing quality of herbal medicines with reference to contaminants and residues. World Health Organization: Geneve., p. 105.

[5] WHO. (2003). Guidelines on good agricultural and collection practices (GACP) for medicinal plants. World Health Organization: Geneva.

[6] FB5. Brazilian Pharmacopoeia. 2010, ANVISA: Brasília.

[7] China, The State Pharmacopoeia Commission of P. R. Pharmacopoeia of the People´s Republic of China. 2010, People's Medical Publishing House: Beijing.

[8] BP2016. British Pharmacopoeia. 2016, Stationery Office: United Kingdom.

[9] PhEur9. European Pharmacopoeia. 2015, Strassbourg: Council of Europe.

[10] WHO. (2015). The International Pharmacopoeia. World Health Organization

[11] EMA. Reflection paper on markers used for quantitative and qualitative analysis of herbal medicinal products and traditional herbal medicine products, C.o.H.M.P. (HMPC), Editor. 2008, European Medicines Agency: London.

[12] Bart, H. J. & Pilz, S. (2011). Industrial Scale Natural Product Extraction. Wheinheim: Wiley-VCH.

[13] Gaedcke, F. & Steinhoff, B. (2003). Herbal Medicinal Products: scientific and regulatory basis fr development, quality assurance and marketing authorisation. Stuttgart: Medpharm.

[14] Kunle, O. F., Egharevba, H. O. & Ahmadu, P. O. (2012). "Standardization of herbal medicines - A review". *International Journal of Biodiversity and Conservation*, *4*(3), 101-112.

[15] Pacifico, Severina, Simona Piccolella, Silvia Galasso, Antonio Fiorentino, Nadine Kretschmer, San-Po Pan, Rudolf Bauer, and Pietro Monaco. (2016). "Influence of harvest season on chemical composition and bioactivity of wild rue plant hydroalcoholic extracts". *Food and Chemical Toxicology*, *90*, 102-11.

[16] Dhami, Namraj. & Akkal, Dev Mishra. (2015). "Phytochemical variation: How to resolve the quality controversies of herbal medicinal products?". *Journal of Herbal Medicine*, *5*(2), 118-127.

[17] Beek, Teris A. Van. & Paola, Montoro. (2009). "Chemical analysis and quality control of Ginkgo biloba leaves, extracts, and phytopharmaceuticals". *Journal of Chromatography A*, *1216*(11), 2002-32.

[18] EMA. Guideline on declaration of herbal substances and herbal preparations in herbal medicinal products/traditional herbal medicinal produtcs. 2009, London. p. 21.

[19] List, Paul Heinz. & Peter, C. Schmidt. (1991). *Phytopharmaceutical Technology*. Wiley-Blackwell., *374*.

[20] Sidhu, O. P., Sanjay, Annarao., Sandipan, Chatterjee., Rakesh, Tuli., Raja, Roy. & Khetrapal, C. L. (2011). "Metabolic alterations of Withania somnifera (L.) dunal fruits at different developmental stages by NMR spectroscopy". *Phytochemical Analysis*, *22*(6), 492-502.

[21] Lubbe, Andrea., Henk, Gude., Robert, Verpoorte. & Young, Hae Choi. (2013). "Seasonal accumulation of major alkaloids in organs of pharmaceutical crop Narcissus Carlton". *Phytochemistry*, *88*, 43-53.

[22] Siriwardane, A. S., Dharmadasa, R. M. & Kosala, Samarasinghe. (2013). "Distribution of withaferin A, an anticancer potential agent, in different parts of two varieties of Withania somnifera (L.) Dunal. grown in Sri Lanka". *Pakistan Journal of Biological Sciences*, *16*(3), 141-4.

[23] Patel, C. J., Satyanand, T., Patel, K. J., Patel, T., Patel, H. K. & Patel, P. H. (2014). "Standardization of Herbal Medicine: A Concise Review". *Journal of Pharmaceutical and Biological Research*, *2*(1), 97-101.

[24] EMA. (2011). Guideline on quality of herbal medicinal products/traditional herbal medicinal products. European Medicines Agency: London. p. 13.

[25] EMA. Guideline on specifications: test procedures and acceptance criteria for herbal substances, herbal preparations and herbal medicinal products/traditional medicinal products. (2006). European Medicines Agency: London.

[26] He, Tian-Tian., Carolina, Oi Lam Ung., Hao, Hu. & Yi-Tao, Wang. (2015). "Good manufacturing practice (GMP) regulation of herbal medicine in comparative research: China GMP, cGMP, WHO-GMP, PIC/S and EU-GMP". *European Journal of Integrative Medicine*, *7*(1), 55-66.

[27] WHO. (1999). *WHO monographs on selected medicinal plants. Vol. 1*. Vol. 1, Malta: World Health Organization, 295.

[28] WHO. (2004). *WHO monographs on selected medicinal plants. Vol. 2*. Vol. 2, Geneve: World Health Organization, 358.

[29] WHO. (2007). *WHO monographs on selected medicinal plants. Vol. 3*. Vol. 3, Spain: World Health Organization, 390.

[30] WHO. (2009). *WHO monographs on selected medicinal plants. Vol. 4*. Vol. 4, Spain., 456.

[31] ESCOP. (2003). *ESCOP Monographs: The Scientific Foundation for Herbal Medicinal Products by ESCOP*. 2nd ed, ed. T.S.F.f.H.M. Products. Thieme., 568.

[32] ESCOP. (2009). *ESCOP Monographs. Second Edition Supplement 2009* 2nd 2009 ed, ed. T.S.F.f.H.M. Products. Thieme., 200.

[33] Blumenthal, Mark., Alicia, Goldberg. & Josef, Brinckmann. (2000). Herbal Medicine: Expanded Commission E Monographs. 1st ed. Austin: American Botanical Council., 519.

[34] Thakkar, K., Parmar, V., Patel, D. & Meshram, D. (2013). "Recent advances in herbal drug standardization – A Review". *International Journal of Advances in Pharmaceutical Research August*, *4*(8), 2130-2138.

[35] WHO. *Quality control methods for medicinal plant materials*. 2011, World Health Organization: Geneve., p. 173.

[36] Sá, Rafaela D., Asaph, S.c.o. Santana., Flávia, C. l. Silva., Luiz, Alberto L. Soares. & Karina, P. Randau. (2016). "Anatomical and histochemical analysis of Dysphania ambrosioides supported by light and electron microscopy". *Revista Brasileira de Farmacognosia*, *26*(5), 533-543.

[37] Silva, Márcia M.b. Da., Asaph, S.c.o. Santana., Rejane, M.m. Pimentel., Flávia, C. l. Silva., Karina, P. Randau. & Luiz, A. l. Soares. (2013). "Anatomy of leaf and stem of Erythrina velutina". *Revista Brasileira de Farmacognosia*, *23*(2), 200-206.

[38] Santos, Rafaela F., Bárbara, M. Nunes., Rafaela, D. Sá., Luiz, A. l. Soares. & Karina, P. Randau. (2016). "Morpho-anatomical study of Ageratum conyzoides". *Revista Brasileira de Farmacognosia*, *26*(6), 679-687.

[39] Seema, R. & Seshu, Lavania. (2015). "Histochemical localization of curcumin and its significance in chemotypic characterization of selected species of Curcuma L". *Industrial Crops and Products*, *65*, 175-179.

[40] Aladdin, Nor-Ashila., Jamia, Azdina Jamal., Noraini, Talip., Nur, Ain M. Hamsani., Mohd, Ruzi A. Rahman., Carla, W. Sabandar., Kartiniwati, Muhammad., Khairana, Husain. & Juriyati, Jalil. (2016). "Comparative study of three Marantodes pumilum varieties by microscopy, spectroscopy and chromatography". *Revista Brasileira de Farmacognosia*, *26*(1), 1-14.

[41] Garg, V., Dhar, V. J., Sharma, A. & Dutt, R. (2012). "Facts about standardization of herbal medicine: a review". *Zhong Xi Yi Jie He Xue Bao*, *10*(10), 1077-83.

[42] Jadhav, P. T., Jadhav, S. M., Salunkhe, M. N., Singh, S. R. & Pawar, H. A. (2014). "Modern approach to herbal drug standardisation". *International Journal of Chemical And Pharmaceutical Analysis*, *1*(2), 35-43.

[43] Kulkarni, K. M., Patil, L. S., Khanvilkar, V. V. & Kadam, V. J. (2014). "Fingerprinting techniques in herbal standardization". *Indo American Journal of Pharmaceutical Research*, *4*(2), 1049-1062.

[44] Brazil. *Dispõe sobre o registro de medicamentos fitoterápicos e o registro e a notificação de produtos tradicionais fitoterápicos. RDC nº 26, de 13 de maio de*

2014. DOU, 14 de maio de 2014, M.d. Saúde, Editor. 2014, Agência Nacional de Vigilância Sanitária: Brasília.

[45] Neeraj, C. & Bhupinder, S. S. (2011). "An overview of advances in the standardization of herbal drugs". *Journal of Pharmacetical Education and Research*, *2*(2), 55-70.

[46] Corrêa Junior, C. & Scheffer, M. C. (2013). Boas Práticas Agrícolas (BPA) de Plantas Medicinais, Aromáticas e Condimentares. Curitiba: Instituto Emater., *52*.

[47] FAO. *Manual on Development and Use of FAO and WHO Specifications for Pesticides*. 2016, WHO and FAO: Rome. p. 305.

[48] Klein-Júnior, Luiz C., Johan, Viaene., Juliana, Salton., Mariana, Koetz., André, L. Gasper., Amélia, T. Henriques. & Yvan, Vander Heyden. (2016). "The use of chemometrics to study multifunctional indole alkaloids from Psychotria nemorosa (Palicourea comb. nov.). Part I: Extraction and fractionation optimization based on metabolic profiling". *Journal of Chromatography A*, *1463*, 60-70.

[49] Pu, Xue-Yan., Jia-Ying, Shen., Zhong-Ping, Deng. & Ze-An, Zhang. (2016). "Oral exposure to aristolochic acid I induces gastric histological lesions with non-specific renal injury in rat". *Experimental and Toxicologic Pathology*, *68*(6), 315-320.

[50] Li, Songlin., Quanbin, Han., Chunfeng, Qiao., Jingzheng, Song., Chuen Lung, Cheng. & Hongxi, Xu. (2008). "Chemical markers for the quality control of herbal medicines: an overview". *Chinese Medicine*, *3*(7), 1-33.

[51] Liu, S., Liang, Y. Z. & Liu, H. T. (2016). "Chemometrics applied to quality control and metabolomics for traditional Chinese medicines". *Journal of Chromatography B: Biomedical and Life Sciences*, 1015-1016, 82-91.

[52] Wolfender, Jean-Luc., Guillaume, Marti., Aurélien, Thomas. & Samuel, Bertrand. (2015). "Current approaches and challenges for the metabolite profiling of complex natural extracts". *Journal of Chromatography A*, *1382*, 136-164.

[53] Gad, Haidy A., Sherweit, H. El-Ahmady., Mohamed, I. Abou-Shoer. & Mohamed, M. Al-Azizi. (2013). "Application of chemometrics in authentication of herbal medicines: a review". *Phytochemical Analysis*, *24*(1), 1-24.

[54] Giri, Lalit., Harish, C. Andola., Vijay, Kant Purohit., Rawat, M. s. m., Rawal, R. s. & Bhatt, I. d. (2010). "Chromatographic and Spectral Fingerprinting Standardization of Traditional Medicines: An Overview as Modern Tools". *Research Journal of Phytochemistry*, *4*(4), 234-241.

[55] ICH. *International Conference on Harmonization of Technical Requiriments for Registration on Pharmaceuticals for Human Use Q2A. Text on Validation of Analytical Procedures*., 2005, Genebra.

[56] Waksmundzka-Hajnos, M., Oniszczuk, A., Szewczyk, K. & Wianowska, D. (2007). "Effect of sample-preparation methodos on the hplc quantification of some phenolics acids in plants materials". *Acta Chromatographica*, *19*, 10.

[57] Chauthe, S. K., Sharma, R. J., Aqil, F., Gupta, R. C. & Singh, I. P. (2012). "Quantitative NMR: an applicable method for quantitative analysis of medicinal plant extracts and herbal products". *Phytochemical Analysis*, *23*(6), 689-96.

[58] Kustrin, Snezana A. (2014). "Quantitative High Performance Thin Layer Chromatography for the Analysis of Herbal Medicines: Problems and Advantages". *Modern Chemistry & Applications*, *02*(01).

[59] Yang, Xihui., Yichen, Hu., Weijun, Kong., Xianfeng, Chu., Meihua, Yang., Ming, Zhao. & Zhen, Ouyang. (2014). "Ultra-fast liquid chromatography with tandem mass spectrometry determination of ochratoxin A in traditional Chinese medicines based on vortex-assisted solid-liquid microextraction and aptamer-affinity column clean-up". *Journal of Separation Science*, *37*(21), 3052-9.

[60] Both, Simon., Iraj, Koudous., Urban, Jenelten. & Jochen, Strube. (2014). "Model-based equipment-design for plant-based extraction process – considering botanic and thermodynamic aspects". *Comptes Rendus Chimie*, *17*, 187-196.

[61] Pferschy-Wenzig, Eva-Maria. & Rudolf, Bauer. (2015). "The relevance of pharmacognosy in pharmacological research on herbal medicinal products". *Epilepsy & Behavior*, *52*(Part B), 344-362.

[62] Mok, Daniel K. w. & Foo-Tim, Chau. (2006). "Chemical information of Chinese medicines: A challenge to chemist". *Chemometrics and Intelligent Laboratory Systems*, *82*(1–2), 210-217.

[63] FDA. *Guidance for Industry Botanical Drug Products*, F.a.D.A. U.S. Department of Health and Human Services, Center for Drug Evaluat ion and Research (CDER) Editor. 2004, US Food and Drug Administration (FDA): Rockville.

[64] Liang, Y. Z., Xie, P. & Chan, K. (2004). "Quality control of herbal medicines". *Journal of Chromatography B: Biomedical Sciences and Applications*, *812*(1–2), 53-70.

[65] Ardila, Jorge Armando., Cristiano, Soleo Funari., André, Marques Andrade., Alberto, José Cavalheiro. & Renato, Lajarim Carneiro. (2015). "Cluster Analysis of Commercial Samples of Bauhinia spp. Using HPLC-UV/PDA and MCR-ALS/PCA Without Peak Alignment Procedure". *Phytochemical Analysis*, *26*(5), 367-373.

[66] Gobbo-Neto, L. & Lopes, N. P. (2007). "Plantas medicinais: fatores de influência no conteúdo de metabólitos secundários". *Química Nova*, *30*(2), 374-381.

[67] Efferth, Thomas. & Greten, H. J. (2012). "Quality Control for Medicinal Plants". *Medicinal & Aromatic Plants*, *1*(7), e131.

[68] Kumari, R. & Kotesha, M. (2016). "A review on the Standardization of herbal medicines". *International Journal of Pharma Sciences and Research*, *7*(2), 97-106.

[69] Bandaranayake, Wickramasinghe M. (2006). "Quality Control, Screening, Toxicity and Regulation of Herbal Drugs ", in *Modern Phytomedicine: Turning Medicinal Plants into Drugs*, I. Ahmad, F. Aqil, and M. Owais, Editors. Wiley-VCH: Germany., 404.

[70] Fernandes, Júlia M., Juliana, Félix-Silva., Lorena, M. Cunha., Jacyra, A. S., Gomes, Emerson M. S., Siqueira, Luisa P. Gimenes., Norberto, P. Lopes., Luiz, A. L. Soares., Matheus, F. Fernandes-Pedrosa. & Silvana, M. Zucolotto. (2016). "Inhibitory Effects of Hydroethanolic Leaf Extracts of Kalanchoe brasiliensis and Kalanchoe pinnata (Crassulaceae) against Local Effects Induced by Bothrops jararaca Snake Venom". *PLoS One*, *11*(12), e0168658.

[71] Arun, R., Sravya, R. B. & Roja, C. (2012). "A review on standardisation of herbal formulation". *International Journal of Phytotherapy*, *2*(2), 74-88.

[72] Bansal, A., Chhabra, V., Rawal, R. K. & Sharma, S. (2014). "Chemometrics: A new scenario in herbal drug standardization". *Journal of Pharmaceutical Analysis*, *4*(4), 223-233.

[73] Martins, Frederico. S., Henrique, Pascoa., Josérealino, R. Paula. & Edemilson, C. Conceicao. (2015). "Technical aspects on production of fluid extract from Brosimum gaudichaudii Trecul roots". *Pharmacognosy Magazine*, *11*(41), 226-31.

[74] Pavlić, Branimir., Senka, Vidović., Jelena, Vladić., Robert, Radosavljević., Marina, Cindrić. & Zoran, Zeković. (2016). "Subcritical water extraction of sage (Salvia officinalis L.) by-products—Process optimization by response surface methodology". *The Journal of Supercritical Fluids*, *116*, 36-45.

[75] Qu, Yan., Chunxue, Li., Chen, Zhang., Rui, Zeng. & Chaomei, Fu. (2016). "Optimization of infrared-assisted extraction of Bletilla striata polysaccharides based on response surface methodology and their antioxidant activities". *Carbohydrate Polymers*, *148*, 345-53.

[76] Tacon, Luciana. A. & Luis, A. P. Freitas. (2013). "Box-Behnken design to study the bergenin content and antioxidant activity of Endopleura uchi bark extracts obtained by dynamic maceration". *Revista Brasileira de Farmacognosia*, *23*, 65-71.

[77] Xia, Yong-Gang., Bing-You, Yang., Jun Liang, Di Wang., Qi, Yang. & Hai-Xue, Kuang. (2014). "Optimization of simultaneous ultrasonic-assisted extraction of water-soluble and fat-soluble characteristic constituents from Forsythiae Fructus Using response surface methodology and high-performance liquid chromatography". *Pharmacognosy Magazine*, *10*(39), 292-303.

[78] Xu, Wen-Jing., Jia-Wen, Zhai., Qi, Cui., Ju-Zhao, Liu., Meng, Luo., Yu-Jie, Fu. & Yuan-Gang, Zu. (2016). "Ultra-turrax based ultrasound-assisted extraction of five organic acids from honeysuckle (Lonicera japonica Thunb.) and optimization of extraction process". *Separation and Purification Technology*, *166*, 73-82.

[79] Belwal, Tarun., Praveen, Dhyani., Indra, D. Bhatt., Ranbeer, Singh Rawal. & Veena, Pande. (2016). "Optimization extraction conditions for improving phenolic content and antioxidant activity in Berberis asiatica fruits using response surface methodology (RSM)". *Food Chemistry*, *207*, 115-24.

[80] Coelho, Angélica G., José, S. Lima Neto., Arkellau, K. s. Moura., Taciana, Oliveira De Sousa., Ilmara, C.p.s. Morais., Gabriela, D. Carvalho., Francisco, Valmor M.

Cunha., Maria, Das Graças F. Medeiros., Eilika, A.f. Vasconcelos., Aldeídia, P. Oliveira., Daniel, D.r. Arcanjo., Lívio, C.c. Nunes. & Antônia, M.g.l. Citó. (2015). "Optimization and standardization of extraction method from Lippia origanoides H.B.K.: Focus on potential anti-hypertensive applications". *Industrial Crops and Products*, *78*, 124-130.

[81] Dranca, Florina. & Mircea, Oroian. (2016). "Optimization of ultrasound-assisted extraction of total monomeric anthocyanin (TMA) and total phenolic content (TPC) from eggplant (Solanum melongena L.) peel". *Ultrasonics Sonochemistry*, *31*, 637-646.

[82] Martins, Frederico. S., Edemilson, C. Conceicao., Elane, S. Bandeira., José, O. Silva-Jr. & Rose, M. Costa. (2014). "The effects of extraction method on recovery rutin from Calendula officinalis L. (Asteraceae)". *Pharmacognosy Magazine*, *10*(Suppl 3), S569-73.

[83] Paulucci, Viviane. P., Rene, O. Couto., Cristiane, C. C. Teixeira. & Luis, A. P. Freitas. (2013). "Optimization of the extraction of curcumin from Curcuma longa rhizomes". *Revista Brasileira de Farmacognosia*, *23*(1), 94-100.

[84] Wakte, P. S., Sachin, B. S., Patil, A. A., Mohato, D. M., Band, T. H. & Shinde, D. B. (2011). "Optimization of microwave, ultra-sonic and supercritical carbon dioxide assisted extraction techniques for curcumin from Curcuma longa". *Separation and Purification Technology*, *79*(1), 50-55.

[85] Lima, Bruno S., Cledison, S. Ramos., João, P.a. Santos., Thallita, K. Rabelo., Mairim, R. Serafini., Carlos, A.s. Souza., Luiz, A. l. Soares., Lucindo, J. Quintans Júnior., José, C.f. Moreira., Daniel, P. Gelain., Adriano, A.s. Araújo. & Francilene, A. Silva. (2015). "Development of standardized extractive solution from Lippia sidoides by factorial design and their redox active profile". *Revista Brasileira de Farmacognosia*, *25*(3), 301-306.

[86] Govindaraghavan, Suresh. & Nikolaus, J. Sucher. (2015). "Quality assessment of medicinal herbs and their extracts: Criteria and prerequisites for consistent safety and efficacy of herbal medicines". *Epilepsy & Behavior*, *52*(Pt B), 363-71.

[87] Sticher, O., Heilmann, J. & Zündorf, I. (2015). *Pharmakognosie Phytopharmazie*. Stuttgart.

[88] Blaschek, Wolfgang. (2016). *Wichtl-Teedrogen und Phytopharmaka: Ein Handbuch für die Praxis: Ein Handbuch für die Praxis*. 6 Auf ed. Stuttgart: WVG.

[89] Brand, Walter., Maaike, E. Schutte., Gary, Williamson., Jelmer, J. Van Zanden., Nicole, H. p. Cnubben., John, P. Groten., Peter, J. Van Bladeren. & Ivonne, M.c.m. Rietjens. (2006). "Flavonoid-mediated inhibition of intestinal ABC transporters may affect the oral bioavailability of drugs, food-borne toxic compounds and bioactive ingredients". *Biomedicine & Pharmacotherapy*, *60*(9), 508-519.

[90] Srinivas, Nuggehally. R. (2015). "Recent trends in preclinical drug-drug interaction studies of flavonoids-Review of case studies, issues and perspectives". *Phytotherapy Research*, *29*(11), 1679-91.

[91] Couto, Angélica G., Marli, L. Kunzler., Bárbara, Spaniol., Pedro, M. Magalhães., George, G. Ortega. & Pedro, R. Petrovick. (2013). "Chemical and technological evaluation of the Phyllanthus niruri aerial parts as a function of cultivation and harvesting conditions". *Revista Brasileira de Farmacognosia*, *23*, 36-43.

[92] Lima-Landman, M. T., Borges, A. C., Cysneiros, R. M., De Lima, T. C., Souccar, C. & Lapa, A. J. (2007). "Antihypertensive effect of a standardized aqueous extract of Cecropia glaziovii Sneth in rats: an *in vivo* approach to the hypotensive mechanism". *Phytomedicine*, *14*(5), 314-20.

[93] Jambaninj, D., Sulaiman, S. A., Gillani, S. W., Davaasuren, T. S., Erdenetsetseg, G. & Dungerdorj, D. (2012). "Technological study of preparing gel from semi-solid extract of Cacalia hastata L". *Journal of Advanced Pharmaceutical Technology & Research*, *3*(1), 25-9.

[94] Ladva, Bhaktij., Vijaym, Mahida., Rinah, Gokani. & Urmid, Kantaria. (2014). "Marker based standardization of polyherbal formulation (SJT-DI-02) by high performance thin layer chromatography method". *Journal of Pharmacy & Bioallied Sciences*, *6*(3), 213-9.

[95] Tsai, Chin-Hsien., Sheue-Fen, Tzeng., Shih-Chuan, Hsieh., Chih-Yu, Lin., Chia-Jui, Tsai., Yet-Ran, Chen., Yu-Chih, Yang., Ya-Wen, Chou., Ming-Ting, Lee. & Pei-Wen, Hsiao. (2015). "Development of a standardized and effect-optimized herbal extract of Wedelia chinensis for prostate cancer". *Phytomedicine*, *22*(3), 406-14.

[96] Araujo Junior, R. F., Souza, T. P., Pires, J. G., Soares, L. A. L., de Araujo, A. A., Petrovick, P. R., Macedo, H. D., Oliveira, A. L. S. L. & Guerra, G. C. (2012). "A dry extract of Phyllanthus niruri protects normal cells and induces apoptosis in human liver carcinoma cells". *Experimental Biology and Medicine*, *237*(11), 1281-8.

[97] Vieira, Daniela., Cristina, Padoani., Janaína, Dos S. Soares., Jerusa, Adriano., Valdir, Cechinel Filho., Márcia, M. De Souza., Tania, M. b. Bresolin. & Angélica, G. Couto. (2013). "Development of hydroethanolic extract of Ipomoea pes-caprae using factorial design followed by antinociceptive and anti-inflammatory evaluation". *Revista Brasileira de Farmacognosia*, *23*, 72-78.

[98] Araújo, Aurigena A., Luiz, Alberto L. Soares., Magda, R. A. Ferreira., Manoel, André S. Neto., Giselle, R. Silva., Raimundo, F. Araújo., Gerlane, C. B. Guerra. & Maria, C. N. Melo. (2014). "Quantification of polyphenols and evaluation of antimicrobial, analgesic and anti-inflammatory activities of aqueous and acetone-water extracts of Libidibia ferrea, Parapiptadenia rigida and Psidium guajava". *Journal of Ethnopharmacology*, *156*, 88-96.

[99] Vasconcelos, C. F., Maranhao, H. M., Batista, T. M., Carneiro, E. M., Ferreira, F., Costa, J., Soares, L. A. L., Sa, M. D., Souza, T. P. & Wanderley, A. G. (2011). "Hypoglycaemic activity and molecular mechanisms of Caesalpinia ferrea Martius bark extract on streptozotocin-induced diabetes in Wistar rats". *Journal of Ethnopharmacology*, *137*(3), 1533-41.

[100] Lima, C. R., Vasconcelos, C. F., Costa-Silva, J. H., Maranhao, C. A., Costa, J., Batista, T. M., Carneiro, E. M., Soares, L. A., Ferreira, F. & Wanderley, A. G. (2012). "Anti-diabetic activity of extract from Persea americana Mill. leaf via the activation of protein kinase B (PKB/Akt) in streptozotocin-induced diabetic rats". *Journal of Ethnopharmacology*, *141*(1), 517-25.

[101] Dimech, Gustavo S., Luiz, Alberto L. Soares., Magda, A. Ferreira., Anne, G. V. Oliveira., Maria, C. Carvalho. & Eulália, A. Ximenes. (2013). "Phytochemical and antibacterial investigations of the extracts and fractions from the stem bark of Hymenaea stigonocarpa Mart. ex Hayne and effect on ultrastructure of Staphylococcus aureus induced by hydroalcoholic extract". *The Scientific World Journal*, 2013, 862763.

[102] Silva-Rocha, Walicyranison. P., Vitor, L. B. Lemos., Magda, R. Ferreira., Luis, Albeto Soares., Terezinha, I. Svidzisnki., Eveline, P. Milan. & Guilherme, M. Chaves. (2015). "Effect of the crude extract of Eugenia uniflora in morphogenesis and secretion of hydrolytic enzymes in Candida albicans from the oral cavity of kidney transplant recipients". *BMC Complementary and Alternative Medicine*, *15*, 6.

[103] Biasi-Garbin, Renata P., Fernanda, O. Demitto., Renata, C. R. Amaral., Magda, R. Ferreira., Luiz, Alberto Lira Soares., Terezinha, I. E., Svidzinski, Lilian C. Baeza. & Sueli, F. Yamada-Ogatta. (2016). "Antifungal Potential of Plant Species from Brazilian Caatinga against Dermatophytes". *Revista do Instituto de Medicina Tropical de Sao Paulo*, *58*, 18.

[104] Oliveira, Alisson M., Matheus, F. Nascimento., Magda, R. A. Ferreira., Danielle, F. Moura., Talita, G. S. Souza., Gabriela, C. Silva., Eduardo, H. S. Ramos., Patricia, M. G. Paiva., Paloma, L. Medeiros., Tersinha, G. Silva., Luis, Alberto L. Soares., Cristiano, A. Chagas., Ivone, A. Souza. & Thiago, H. Napoleão. (2016). "Evaluation of acute toxicity, genotoxicity and inhibitory effect on acute inflammation of an ethanol extract of Morus alba L. (Moraceae) in mice". *Journal of Ethnopharmacology*, *194*, 162-168.

[105] Huang, Y., Wu, Z., Su, R., Ruan, G., Du, F. & Li, G. (2016). "Current application of chemometrics in traditional Chinese herbal medicine research". *Journal of Chromatography B: Biomedical and Life Sciences*, *1026*, 27-35.

[106] Razmovski-Naumovski, Valentina., Wannit, Tongkao-On., Benjamin, Kimble., Vincent, L. Qiao., Lin, Beilun., Kong, M. Li., Basil, Roufogalis., Yang, Depo., Yao, Meicun. & George, Q. Li. (2010). "Multiple Chromatographic and

Chemometric Methods for Quality Standardisation of Chinese Herbal Medicines". *World Science and Technology*, *12*(1), 99-106.

[107] Geldart, D., Abdullah, E. C., Hassanpour, A., Nwoke, L. C. & Wouters, I. (2006). "Characterization of powder flowability using measurement of angle of repose". *China Particuology*, *4*, 104-107.

[108] Shawky, Eman. (2016). "Multivariate analyses of NP-TLC chromatographic retention data for grouping of structurally-related plant secondary metabolites". *Journal of Chromatography B: Biomedical and Life Sciences*, 1029-1030, 10-5.

[109] Zhao, Yan., Ya, N. Sun., Min, J. Lee., Young, Ho Kim., Wonjae, Lee., Kyeong, H. Kim., Kyung, T. Kim. & Jong, S. Kang. (2016). "Identification and discrimination of three common Aloe species by high performance liquid chromatography–tandem mass spectrometry coupled with multivariate analysis". *Journal of Chromatography B*, 1031, 163-171.

[110] Boccard, Julien. & Douglas, N. Rutledge. (2013). "A consensus orthogonal partial least squares discriminant analysis (OPLS-DA) strategy for multiblock Omics data fusion". *Analytica Chimica Acta*, *769*, 30-9.

[111] Chagas-Paula, Daniela., Tiago, Oliveira., Tong, Zhang., Ruangelie, Edrada-Ebel. & Fernando, Da Costa. (2015). "Prediction of Anti-inflammatory Plants and Discovery of Their Biomarkers by Machine Learning Algorithms and Metabolomic Studies". *Planta Medica*, *81*(6), 450-8.

[112] Gad, Haidy A., Sherweit, H. El-Ahmady., Mohamed, I. Abou-Shoer. & Mohamed, M. Al-Azizi. (2013). "A modern approach to the authentication and quality assessment of thyme using UV spectroscopy and chemometric analysis". *Phytochemical Analysis*, *24*(6), 520-6.

[113] WHO. General Guidelines for Methodologies on Research and Evaluation of Traditional Medicine. (2000). World Health Organization: Geneve.

[114] Zhang, J., Wider, B., Shang, H., Li, X. & Ernst, E. (2012). "Quality of herbal medicines: challenges and solutions". *Complementary Therapies in Medicine*, *20*(1-2), 100-6.

[115] Choi, Young H. & Robert, Verpoorte. (2014). "Metabolomics: what you see is what you extract". *Phytochemical Analysis*, *25*(4), 289-90.

[116] Wolfender, Jean-Luc., Serge, Rudaz., Young, H. Choi. & Hye, K. Kim. (2013). "Plant metabolomics: from holistic data to relevant biomarkers". *Current Medicinal Chemistry*, *20*(8), 1056-90.

[117] Neto, Benício De Barros., Ieda, S. Scarminio. & Roy, E. Bruns. (2006). "25 anos de quimiometria no Brasil". *Química Nova*, *29*(6), 1401-1406.

[118] Sârbu, Costel., Rodica, D. Naşcu-Briciu., Agata, Kot-Wasik., Shela, Gorinstein., Andrzej, Wasik. & Jacek, Namieśnik. (2012). "Classification and fingerprinting of kiwi and pomelo fruits by multivariate analysis of chromatographic and spectroscopic data". *Food Chemistry*, *130*(4), 994-1002.

[119] Soares, Patricia K., Roy, E. Bruns. & Ieda, S. Scarminio. (2012). "Principal component and Tucker3 analyses of high performance liquid chromatography with diode-array detection fingerprints of crude extracts of Erythrina speciosa Andrews leaves". *Analytica Chimica Acta*, *736*, 36-44.

[120] Souza, A. M. & Poppi, R. J. (2012). "Teaching experiment of chemometrics for exploratory analysis of edible vegetable oils by mid infrared spectroscopy and principal component analysis: a tutorial, part I". *Química Nova*, *35*(1), 223-229.

[121] Jing, D., Deguang, W., Linfang, H., Shilin, C. & Minjian, Q. (2011). "Application of chemometrics in quality evaluation of medicinal plants ". *Journal of Medicinal Plants Research*, *5*(17), 4001-4008.

[122] Santos, Maiara S., Edenir, R. Pereira-Filho., Antonio, G. Ferreira., Elisangela, F. Boffo. & Glyn, M. Figueira. (2012). "Authenticity study of Phyllanthus species by NMR and FT-IR techniques coupled with chemometric methods". *Química Nova*, *35*(11), 2210-2217.

[123] Beebe, Kenneth R., Randy, J. Pell. & Mary, Beth Seasholtz. (1998). Chemometrics: A practical guide. New York: Wiley Interscience.

[124] Geladi, Paul. (2003). "Review Chemometrics in spectroscopy. Part 1. Classical chemometrics". *Spectrochimica Acta Part B: Atomic Spectroscopy*, *58*, 767–782.

[125] Navarro Escamilla, M., Rodenas Sanz, F., Li, H., Schonbichler, S. A., Yang, B., Bonn, G. K. & Huck, C. W. (2013). "Rapid determination of baicalin and total baicalein content in Scutellariae radix by ATR-IR and NIR spectroscopy". *Talanta*, *114*, 304-10.

[126] Schonbichler, S. A., Bittner, L. K., Pallua, J. D., Popp, M., Abel, G., Bonn, G. K. & Huck, C. W. (2013). "Simultaneous quantification of verbenalin and verbascoside in Verbena officinalis by ATR-IR and NIR spectroscopy". *Journal of Pharmaceutical and Biomedical Analysis*, *84*, 97-102.

[127] Choong, Yew K., Jin, Lan., Han, L. Lee., Xiang-Dong, Chen., Xiao-Guang, Wang. & Yu-Ping, Yang. (2016). "Differential identification of mushrooms sclerotia by IR macro-fingerprint method". *Spectrochimica Acta Part A: Molecular and Biomolecular Spectroscopy*, *152*, 34-42.

[128] Fragoso, Sandra., Laura, Aceña., Josep, Guasch., Olga, Busto. & Montserrat, Mestres. (2011). "Application of FT-MIR spectroscopy for fast control of red grape phenolic ripening". *Journal of Agricultural and Food Chemistry*, *59*(6), 2175-83.

[129] Wang, Pei. & Zhiguo, Yu. (2015). "Species authentication and geographical origin discrimination of herbal medicines by near infrared spectroscopy: A review". *Journal of Pharmaceutical Analysis*, *5*(5), 277-284.

[130] Viegas, Thayna R., Ana, L. M. L., Mata, Márcia M. Duarte. & Kássio, M. G. Lima. (2016). "Determination of quality attributes in wax jambu fruit using NIRS and PLS". *Food Chemistry*, *190*, 1-4.

[131] Govindaraghavan, Suresh., James, R. Hennell. & Nikolaus, J. Sucher. (2012). “From classical taxonomy to genome and metabolome: towards comprehensive quality standards for medicinal herb raw materials and extracts”. *Fitoterapia*, *83*(6), 979-88.

[132] Carvalho, A. C. B., Perfeito, J. P. S., Silva, L. V. C., Ramalho, L. S., Marques, R. F. O. & Silveira, D. (2011). “Regulation of herbal medicines in Brazil: advances and perspectives”. *Brazilian Journal of Pharmaceutical Sciences*, *47*, 467-473.

[133] De Paula, I. C., Ortega, G. G., Bassani, V. L. & Petrovick, P. R. (1998). “Development of ointment formulations prepared with Achyrocline satureioides spray-dried extracts”. *Drug Development and Industrial Pharmacy*, *24*(3), 235-41.

[134] Liu, X. S., Qiu, Z. F., Wang, L. H., Ji, Y., Cheng, Y. Y. & Qu, H. B. (2008). “Optimization for vacuum belt drying process of Panax notoginseng extract”. *Zhongguo Zhong Yao Za Zhi*, *33*(4), 4.

[135] Liu, Xuesong., Zhifang, Qiu., Longhu, Wang., Yiyu, Cheng., Haibin, Qu. & Yong, Chen. (2009). “Mathematical modeling for thin layer vacuum belt drying of Panax notoginseng extract”. *Energy Conversion and Management*, *50*(4), 928-932.

[136] Liu, Xuesong., Zhifang, Qiu., Longhu, Wang. & Yong, Chen. (2011). “Quality evaluation of Panax notoginseng extract dried by different drying methods”. *Food and Bioproducts Processing*, *89*(1), 10-14.

[137] Cortés-Rojas, Diego Francisco., Cláudia Regina, Fernandes Souza. & Wanderley, Pereira Oliveira. (2015). “Optimization of spray drying conditions for production of Bidens pilosa L. dried extract”. *Chemical Engineering Research and Design*, *93*, 366-376.

[138] Peixoto, Maria Paula G. & Luis, A. P. Freitas. (2013). “Spray-dried extracts from Syzygium cumini seeds: physicochemical and biological evaluation”. *Revista Brasileira de Farmacognosia*, *23*, 145-152.

[139] Souza, Claudia R. f., Danielle, N. Ramos., Diego, F. Cortes-Rojas. & Wanderley, P. Oliveira. (2013). “Stability testing and shelf live prediction of a spouted bed dried phytopharmaceutical preparation from Maytenus ilicifolia”. *The Canadian Journal of Chemical Engineering*, *91*(11), 1847-1855.

[140] Yatsu, Francini K. J., Greice, S. Borghetti., Fagner, Magalhães., Humberto, G. Ferraz., Eloir, Paulo Schenkel. & Valquiria, L. Bassani. (2016). “Ilex paraguariensis Pellets from a Spray-Dried Extract: Development, Characterization, and Stability”. *AAPS PharmSciTech*, *17*(2), 358-67.

[141] Souza, T. P., Gomez-Amoza, J. L., Martinez-Pacheco, R. & Pedro, R. Petrovick. (2006). “Compression behavior of formulations from Phyllanthus niruri spray dried extract”. *Pharmazie*, *61*(3), 213-7.

[142] Soares, Luis Alberto L., George, Gonzalez Ortega., Pedro, R. Petrovick. & Peter, C. Schmidt. (2005). “Dry granulation and compression of spray-dried plant extracts”. *AAPS PharmSciTech*, *6*(3), E359-66.

[143] Spaniol, Bárbara., Vinicius, C. Bica., Lisias, R. Ruppenthal., Maria, R. Volpato. & Pedro, R. Petrovick. (2009). "Compressional behavior of a mixture of granules containing high load of Phyllanthus niruri spray-dried extract and granules of adjuvants: comparison between eccentric and rotary tablet machines". *AAPS PharmSciTech*, *10*(3), 1013-23.

[144] Linden, R., Ortega, G. G., Pedro, R. Petrovick. & Bassani, V. L. (2000). "Response surface analysis applied to the preparation of tablets containing a high concentration of vegetable spray-dried extract". *Drug Development and Industrial Pharmacy*, *26*(4), 441-6.

[145] Fahr, A. (2015). *Voigt - Pharmzeutische Technologie*, *12* Auf. ed. Stuttgart: WVG. 688.

[146] Bauer, Kurt H., Karl-Heinz, Frömming. & Claus, Führer. (2012). *Pharmazeutische Technologie - Mit Einführung in die Biopharmazie.*, *9* Auf. ed. Stuttgart: WVG. 784.

[147] Jain, Nimisha., Kusums, Valli. & Vkusum, Devi. (2010). "Importance of novel drug delivery systems in herbal medicines". *Pharmacognosy Reviews*, *4*(7), 27-31.

[148] Qusaj, Ylber., Andreas, Leng., Firas, Alshihabi., Blerim, Krasniqi. & Thierry, Vandamme. (2012). "Development strategies for herbal products reducing the influence of natural variance in dry mass on tableting properties and tablet characteristics". *Pharmaceutics*, *4*(4), 501-16.

[149] Fernandes, Luciana P., Regina, C. Candido. & Wanderley, P. Oliveira. (2012). "Spray drying microencapsulation of Lippia sidoides extracts in carbohydrate blends". *Food and Bioproducts Processing*, *90*(3), 425-432.

[150] Frascareli, E. C., Silva, V. M., Tonon, R. V. & Hubinger, M. D. (2012). "Effect of process conditions on the microencapsulation of coffee oil by spray drying". *Food and Bioproducts Processing*, *90*(3), 413-424.

[151] Chatterjee, Dipan, Paramita Bhattacharjee, Gour Gopal Satpati, and Ruma Pal. 2014. "Spray Dried Extract of Phormidium valderianum as a Promising Source of Natural Antioxidant". *International Journal of Food Science* 2014: 897497.

[152] Guajardo-Flores, Daniel., Curtis, Rempel., Janet, Gutiérrez-Uribe. & Sergio, Serna-Saldívar. (2015). "Influence of Excipients and Spray Drying on the Physical and Chemical Properties of Nutraceutical Capsules Containing Phytochemicals from Black Bean Extract". *Molecules*, *20*(12), 21626-35.

[153] Vidović, Senka S., Jelena, Z. Vladić., Žužana, G. Vaštag., Zoran, P. Zeković. & Ljiljana, M. Popović. (2014). "Maltodextrin as a carrier of health benefit compounds in Satureja montana dry powder extract obtained by spray drying technique". *Powder Technology*, *258*, 209-215.

[154] Krishnaiah, Duduku., Awang, Bono., Rosalam, Sarbatly., Rajesh, Nithyanandam. & Anisuzzaman, S. M. (2015). "Optimisation of spray drying operating conditions of

Morinda citrifolia L. fruit extract using response surface methodology". *Journal of King Saud University - Engineering Sciences*, *27*(1), 26-36.

[155] Andersson, J. M., Lindahl, S., Turner, C. & Rodriguez-Meizoso, I. (2012). "Pressurised hot water extraction with on-line particle formation by supercritical fluid technology". *Food Chemistry*, *134*(4), 1724-31.

[156] De Souza, K. C., Pedro, R. Petrovick., Bassani, V. L. & Ortega, G. G. (2000). "The adjuvants aerosil 200 and Gelita-Sol-P influence on the technological characteristics of spray-dried powders from Passiflora edulis var. flavicarpa". *Drug Development and Industrial Pharmacy*, *26*(3), 331-6.

[157] Souza, Tatiane P., Rámon, Martinez-Pacheco., José, L. Gomez-Amoza. & Pedro, R. Petrovick. (2007). "Eudragit E as excipient for production of granules and tablets from Phyllanthus niruri L spray-dried extract". *AAPS PharmSciTech*, *8*(2), Article 34.

[158] Amin, Purnima. & Ketkee, Deshmukh. (2013). "Meltlets((R)) of soy isoflavones: process optimization and the effect of extrusion spheronization process parameters on antioxidant activity". *Indian Journal of Pharmaceutical Sciences*, *75*(4), 450-6.

[159] Eggelkraut-Gottanka, Stephan G. Von., Salah, Abu Abed., Wolfgang, Müller. & Peter, C. Schmidt. (2002). "Roller compaction and tabletting of St. John's wort plant dry extract using a gap width and force controlled roller compactor. II. Study of roller compaction variables on granule and tablet properties by a 3(3) factorial design". *Pharmaceutical Development and Technology*, *7*(4), 447-55.

[160] Bauer-Brandl, A. & Ritschl, W. A. (2012). Die Tablette. Handbuch der Entwicklung, Herstellung und Qualitäntssicherung. 3. Auf. ed. Aulendorf: ECV., 736.

[161] Carvalho, Helison De O., Benedito, J. Medeiros., Beatriz, M. De Sá., Jennifer, T. C De Araújo., Monique, Y. m. Kawakami., Hugo, A. S. Favacho. & José Carlos, T. Carvalho. (2013). "Study of dissolution profiles and desintegration of capsules containing the dried hydroethanolic extract of Calophyllum brasiliense". *Revista Brasileira de Farmacognosia*, *23*(1), 194-199.

[162] Emeje, Martins., Amaka, Izuka., Christiana, Isimi., Sabinus, Ofoefule. & Olobayo, Kunle. (2011). "Preparation and standardization of a herbal agent for the therapeutic management of asthma". *Pharmaceutical Development and Technology*, *16*(2), 170-8.

[163] Marczyinski, Z. (2009). "Tableting technology of a dry extract from Solidago virgaurea L. with the use of silicified microcrystalline cellulose (Prosolv) and other selected auxiliary substances". *Polimery w Medycynie*, *39*(4), 51-60.

[164] Kulkarni, Alpanap., Shreerams, Savarikar., Maneesham, Barbhind. & Umakantk, Halde. (2011). "Pharmaceutical and analytical evaluation of triphalaguggulkalpa tablets". *Journal of Ayurveda and Integrative Medicine*, *2*(1), 21-5.

[165] Shaikh, Hamiduddin., Waris, Ali., Ansari, Abdullah. & Salma, Khanam. (2016). "Standardization of Unani Antidiabetic Tablet - Qurse Tabasheer". *Pharmacognosy Research*, *8*(2), 147-52.

[166] Klein, Traudi., Renata, Longhini., Marcos, Luciano Bruschi. & João, Carlos Palazzo De Mello. (2013). "Development of tablets containing semipurii ed extract of guaraná (Paullinia cupana)". *Revista Brasileira de Farmacognosia, 23*(1), 186-193.

[167] Chaves, Juliana S., Fernando, B. Costa. & Luis, A. P. Freitas. (2009). "Development of enteric coated tablets from spray dried extract of feverfew (Tanacetum parthenium L:)". *Brazilian Journal of Pharmaceutical Sciences, 45*, 573-584.

[168] Soares, Luis Alberto L., George, Gonzalez Ortega., Pedro, R. Petrovick. & Peter, C. Schmidt. (2005). "Optimization of tablets containing a high dose of spray-dried plant extract: a technical note". *AAPS PharmSciTech*, *6*(3), E367-71.

[169] Souza, Tatiane P., Bassani, V. L., George Gonzalez Ortega, T. C., Dalla, Costa. & Pedro, R. Petrovick. (2001). "Influence of adjuvants on the dissolution profile of tablets containing high doses of spray-dried extract of Maytenus ilicifolia". *Pharmazie*, *56*(9), 730-3.

EDITORS CONTACT INFORMATION

Dr. Luis Alexandre Pedro de Freitas, PhD
Faculdade de Ciências Farmacêuticas de Ribeirão Preto da
Universidade de São Paulo
Núcleo de Pesquisas em Produtos Naturais e Sintéticos
Ribeirão Preto, São Paulo, Brazil
Email: lapdfrei@fcfrp.usp.br

Dr. Cristiane Cardoso Correia Teixeira, PhD
Faculdade de Ciências Farmacêuticas de Ribeirão Preto da
Universidade de São Paulo
Núcleo de Pesquisas em Produtos Naturais e Sintéticos
Ribeirão Preto, São Paulo, Brazil
Email: cricorreia@yahoo.com.br

Dr. Cristina Mara Zamarioli, PhD
University of São Paulo at Ribeirão Preto College of Nursing,
Núcleo de Pesquisas em Produtos Naturais e Sintéticos,
Ribeirão Preto, São Paulo, Brazil
Email: cristinazamarioli@usp.br

INDEX

F

G

H

I

L

M

N

O

P

Q

R

S

T

U

V

W

X